T0134337

Wissen über Waren –
Historische Studien zu Nahrungs- und Genussmitteln

herausgegeben von

Prof. Dr. Frank Jacob
Dr. Swen Steinberg

Band 2

Jonathan Lewy

Drugs in Germany and the United States, 1819–1945

The Birth of Two Addictions

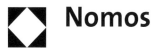 **Nomos**

© Coverpicture:
Title: The new morality play exit demon rum—enter drug habit / / W.A. Rogers.
Creator(s): Rogers, W. A. (William Allen), 1854-1931, artist Date Created/Published: 1919.
Published in: New York Herald, Jan. 23, 1919. p. 15.
Cabinet of American Illustration.
Library of Congress, Prints & Photographs Division, [LC-USZ62-100528].

The Deutsche Nationalbibliothek lists this publication in the
Deutsche Nationalbibliografie; detailed bibliographic data
are available on the Internet at http://dnb.d-nb.de

a.t.: Jerusalem, Hebrew University, PhD 2011

Original title: Drug Policy as an Ideological Challenge: Germany and the United States
from the Birth of Addiction to the Second World War

ISBN   978-3-8487-3284-5 (Print)
         978-3-8452-7638-0 (ePDF)

British Library Cataloguing-in-Publication Data
A catalogue record for this book is available from the British Library.

ISBN   978-3-8487-3284-5 (Print)
         978-3-8452-7638-0 (ePDF)

Library of Congress Cataloging-in-Publication Data
Lewy, Jonathan
Drugs in Germany and the United States, 1819–1945
The Birth of Two Addictions
Jonathan Lewy
338 p.
Includes bibliographic references and index.

ISBN   978-3-8487-3284-5 (Print)
         978-3-8452-7638-0 (ePDF)

1. Edition 2017
© Nomos Verlagsgesellschaft, Baden-Baden, Germany 2017. Printed and bound in Germany.

Preface

"Was Hitler a drug addict?" Usually that is the first question I am asked when strangers hear that I have researched drugs in Germany. The claim that Adolf Hitler, the Führer of the thousand years Reich, was an addict is older than I am. Leonard and Renate Heston published this thesis in 1978 and since then every two or three years an enterprising journalist publishes a sensationalist article or a book about this "new" and "tantalizing" fact. However it is neither new nor tantalizing. Hitler was hardly the only world leader to have taken uppers.

Yes, Hitler's personal physician, Theodore Morell, injected him with drugs that are now considered illegal. However, Morell was not a particularly meticulous doctor and as such, he neglected to record the dosage or the exact drugs that he injected. Sometimes he mentioned pervitin – known to most readers as crystal meth – and sometimes he did not. Hitler was given numerous pills for his abdominal pains, and other drugs for real or imagined diseases he may have had. It is clear that at a certain point, sometime after the invasion of the Soviet Union, Hitler received a cornucopia of drugs from his doctor; but, none of his biographers attribute much to this fact. They insist that the basic traits of his personality never changed throughout the war. His temper was violent long before the war; he was certainly an anti-Semite when he wrote *Mein Kampf* in prison more than a decade before he met Morrel; and the claim that he reacted too slowly to Stalingrad because of a drug induced reverie simply ignores the fact that the German army was outnumbered and outmaneuvered in a terrible winter war that was probably impossible to win to begin with. So, was he an addict?

I normally answer the question with a query of my own: "What do you think addiction is?" And this is the question I would like you, dear reader, to ask yourself when you read the following pages. I hope that I shall be able to convince you that the understanding of addiction has changed over time, and also that it was different from one place to another. Whereas German doctors may have thought it to be X, American doctors insisted it was Y. That is why the subtitle of this book is "The Birth of Two Addictions. This concept can draw two different lineages: One as moral failing;

the other, as a disease like any other. At one point, the two ideas converged into a weird hybrid of a moral disease.

Most people think that the definition of addiction is simple. Like justice Potter Stewart who knew what pornography is when he saw it, they, too, think they could identify addiction when they see it. Nothing is further from the truth, or else the definition of the disease would not have changed on a regular basis. Addiction is not easy to define as might appear at first glance, and perhaps Thomas Szasz, the late professor of psychiatry from New York, was right; addiction only exists in our imagination and it simply describes the human condition, our cravings, desires, and habits.

The book does not only focus on Germany, but deals with the United States as well. For better or worse, America has set the standard for understanding drugs in the modern age. Ever since the acquisition of the Philippines and the inheritance of the Spanish Opium monopoly, the United States has been trying to convince the world that the drug problem was a foreign problem. By this view, Americans do not crave drugs more than others; they are simply seduced by foreigners, including Chinese, Mexicans, Canadians, Colombians or even Corsicans. The problem is always with the supply, and rarely with native demand. This notion influences American policy. Internally the United States uses a big stick and shows almost no compassion, a policy often known as "Zero Tolerance;" externally it puts pressure on foreign nations to adhere to an international control regime. The policy was, and still is, very strict to the point that President Nixon declared war on an inanimate material with no desires of its own. Recent legal changes in respect to medical marijuana, as well as the legalization of the drug in two states, may signify that a change in policy is coming. But it is too early to say whether a true policy shift will take place. One thing is certain; a change in policy will be caused by a change in the understanding of the concept of addiction.

I would like to thank the numerous people who had talked with me about this topic, and challenged my ideas; but drugs were so much on my mind, and I held so many conversations on the topic that I am unable to mention all of those who took the time to listen to me by name. This volume is the outcome of these challenges, resulting in a book that reads like two in one: Drugs in America and drugs in Germany. The comparisons between the two, as well as the conclusions, are left, for the most part, to the reader to make or draw on his own.

Finally, I would like to thank the editors of the series, Frank Jacob and Swen Steinberg, my doctoral advisor, Moshe Zimmermann, Oren Rawls,

Shai Dothan, Erika Hughes and Carolin Möbis, all of whom read numerous versions of the manuscript. I would also like to thank the Mosse Program and the Hebrew University for believing in my project. Above all, I want to thank my parents, whose support never failed me."

Rehovot, 2016

Table of Contents

Introduction

A specter is haunting the United States – the specter of drug use, misuse and addiction. An impressive array of bureaus, offices and administrations has entered into a holy alliance to exorcise this specter, with billions spent in vain on enforcement and treatment. For a century and a half, Americans have learned to prosecute, fear and loathe drugs, at the same time as they have come to love and consume them.

According to a 2014 estimate, nearly 1 in 10 Americans used drugs on a regular basis.[1] That number increases if one includes those who had tried drugs at least once in their lifetime. Drug use has become so widespread that the last three presidents in office each admitted to have consumed them. Yet American drug policy has hardly changed in the past century. Drug violators are punished and sent to overpopulated prisons, and drug dealers continue to supply demand.

The question of whether drug use is a vice or a disease plagued Americans for as long as drug use was first recorded in the New World, and it strikes right at the heart of the drug debate today, just as it did in the past. If addiction was a disease, doctors were charged with treating it. If it was a vice, drug users had to be punished. In the instances when addiction was seen as both a vice and a disease, doctors punished their patients. The tensions between vice and disease is most visible today in the ongoing debate over "medical marijuana." Exactly a hundred years after the first Federal Law against drugs was passed, no less than one-third of the country – 18 states and the District of Columbia – allow medically sanctioned marijuana; two states, Colorado and Washington, even legalized the drug. But the war on drugs is not over, and probably will not be over in the near future. Thanks to a Supreme Court decision (Gonzales v. Raich) federal prosecutors are within their rights to, if they so choose, indict users and suppliers even if they do not break any state laws. In fact, United States attorneys can also prosecute any financial institution, whether a

---

1 HHS, CBHSQ, SAMHSA and RTI, *National Survey on Drug Use and Health* (September, 2015) at: www.samhsa.gov/data/sites/default/files/NSDUHmrbSample Experience2014.pdf (Last access, 11.11.2015)

bank or a credit card company, that services a legal drugs retailer.[2] *Caveat Venditor!*

This book traces the origins of the ban on drugs in the United States, since it was and still remains the leading power supporting an uncompromising policy toward drugs. However, while the American example may be the most well known, it is hardly the only one, and certainly not the most successful. Germany's experience with drugs offers a compelling counterpoint to the American paradigm, and it is through this comparative lens that this book explores the history of drugs, focusing on the years between the birth of addiction in the 19th century and the end of World War II in 1945.

The comparison between Germany and the United States is not arbitrary. The former was not a democracy, save for a brief seven-year period of a stable government between 1924 and 1930. The latter is the epitome of a liberal democracy, where the self-evident truth of life, liberty and the pursuit of happiness were the inalienable rights for which the 13 colonies went to war against their king. At its most basic level, this book compares the drug policies pursued by two very different forms of government, one that controlled its own citizens and the other that promised absolute freedom. Yet, which country allowed more freedom to consume drugs?

Germany and the United States were also the two most important players in the international drug trade throughout the 19th and 20th centuries. Until World War I, German companies were the largest drug manufacturers in the world, responsible for the isolation or manufacture of many drugs, including cocaine, heroin and morphine. Parts of the United States, on the other hand, were the first in the West to ban drugs. Conflicts between the two powers over the production and consumption of drugs

---

2 *Gonzales v. Raich* 545 U.S. 1 (2005); "Banks say No to Marijuana Money; Legal or Not," *New York Times* (11 January 2014); "Legal Marijuana Businesses should have Access to Banks, Holder says," *New York Times* (23 January 2014). The Justice Department's promise to correct the situation would most likely never satisfy banks because otherwise Colorado and Washington would turn into money laundering states. The Federal government is expected to reserve its rights to prosecute anyone who deals with drugs regardless of state laws. Instead the Attorney General is expected to instruct federal prosecutors to "prioritize cases involving legal marijuana businesses that use banks." If this were to be implemented, federal prosecutors would always have a hanging sword over the necks of banks that accept drug money; a situation very few banks would be willing to live with. Only time will tell how the conflict between state and federal law will play out.

were inevitable. With the end of World War I, the United States pressured Germany to comply with the basic tenets of the American drug policy; these efforts were only successful in name, but rarely in practice.[3] Even after Germany had lost its monopoly, it remained reluctant to adhere to American or international pressures, and so economic interest could not account for Germany's policy. Instead, a different element dictated it. This book seeks the medical ideology of each country for the answer.

Without the concept of addiction, there would not have been a drug policy. The medical discourse was so prevalent that by the beginning of the 20th century not a single politician in either country questioned the fact that alcoholism or drug addiction troubled humanity. A mere century earlier, most politicians would have stared blankly and unknowingly if they were asked for their thoughts about drugs or addiction.

Any history of drugs must first begin with a basic definition of the term. Settling on a single definition, however, is surprisingly complicated. Drugs may mean different things to different people, from the tools of Satan in the eyes of many moralists to "God's Own Medicine," in the words of Sir William Osler (1849-1919), the first professor of medicine at Johns Hopkins University. To elucidate this gamut, one must first understand change and stasis in history. Historical phenomena and concepts hardly ever have a single definition, despite their false sense of a universal truth. Although freedom, democracy and equality might appear universal, they do not have a single meaning. Rather, they encapsulate myriad of definitions that were understood and misunderstood by multitudes of people over time. In a sense, the history of these concepts becomes their definition.

The same is true with drugs. Although a specific drug like cocaine is an inanimate object that is easily defined, the collective basket of 'drugs' lacks a single definition because the idea that drugs exist as a single concept is historical. Only in recent years, cocaine, opium, heroin, amphetamines and alcohol were lumped together into a single category of drugs. This was a historical event rather than an indefinite truth that is so common to inanimate objects like chairs and tables, or geometric shapes like squares and triangles.

---

3 For a similar claim after the Second World War, see H. Richard Friman, *NarcoDiplomacy: Exporting the U.S. War on Drugs* (Ithaca: Cornell University Press, 1996).

In English, the distinction between drugs and medicine, to the extent it exists, is barely noticeable. Since there has never been a clear neutral definition of drugs, this book deals with psychoactive substances that various governments deemed important enough to impose controlling measures, whether alcohol, opium or cocaine. This solution does not only circumvent the impossible task of finding a universal definition for drugs, but also provides a key according to which the biases were highlighted implicitly within each country.

To most modern readers when drugs or alcohol are consumed uncontrollably, a disease develops called addiction or alcoholism. This, however, was not the case throughout most of history. Alcoholism and drug addiction were not always understood as a disease. They share a similar, but not an identical history; therefore, this book deals with both though often times separately.

This book tells two stories in one, and should be read accordingly. The following subchapter opens the book with a prelude to the history of alcohol and drugs. It sets the stage by providing a brief history of drugs, alcohol and the mutating concept of addiction from ancient Greece to the modern era. It also deals with religion, medical opinion, morality and the mixing of the three in Europe and then crosses the Atlantic into pre-Revolutionary America, where an antagonistic attitude against alcohol prevailed among the elite; despite, or perhaps because of the love of the drink by the common people.

Part I of the book is devoted to Germany. Thus, the first chapter traces the birth of the alcohol disease in the early 19th century, and the second chapter turns to the birth of drug addiction six decades later. The chapter that follows explores the legal status and criminal responsibility of the diseased, which serves as a stepping stone for the fourth chapter on drug usage in Germany in the 1920s and 30s. The last two chapters deal with the German drug laws after the Treaty of Versailles and the Nazi policy towards drugs.

Part II is devoted to the United States and concentrates on drugs, racism and medicine, the three elements that created drugs as an enemy and the moral panic that followed. This is not to say that the book abandons the religious movements or alcohol prohibition altogether, but instead it refers to them when necessary to understand why Americans love to hate drugs. Consequently, chapter seven deals with opium and the anti-Chinese laws in America followed by chapter eight and a description of the drug panic. Chapter nine returns to the medical understanding of addiction in

America, which logically turns to chapter ten and the great experiment: Prohibition. The last two chapters deal with the legal measures taken against the drug trade both foreign and domestic and end with the American solution to the drug user problem.

Drugs and Alcohol in Short

Before the identification of addiction and alcoholism as a disease, Christians considered excessive drinking a sin. The lover of the drink, or the "perpetual drunkard" was often regarded a sinner, and excessive drinking considered Gluttony.[4] This notion was as old as the wandering clerics of the Middle Ages, who traveled from one university to the next, spending more time in taverns than with books.[5] As priests, they often drank wine as part of the Eucharist while engaged in the work of god; by drinking excessively outside their churches they committed a mortal sin, when the love of the drink superseded the love of god.[6] Negative attitudes towards excessive drinking survived the Reformation and crept into Protestant traditions, as indicated in a Calvinist text from the 18th century, which expressed suspicion of the drink because it robbed away the freedom of the will of the drinker.[7]

By the 17th and 18th centuries, two different traditions developed within the Protestant world: Puritans and Calvinists believed that the drink itself was the cause for loss of will, and as a result the drink, not the person was the danger. It stood to reason that the authorities should ban the drink itself to save man from temptation and degradation, an idea that many colonists carried with them to the New World.

---

4 On the connection between drunkenness and gluttony in the Middle Ages and the Reformation, see Beverly Ann Tlusty, *Bacchus and Civic Order: The Culture of Drink in Early Modern Germany* (Charlottesville: University of Virginia Press, 2001), 70-76, 82-84.

5 George F. Whicher (tr.), *The Goliard Poets: Medieval Latin Songs and Satires* (Norfolk CN: New Directions, 1949), 2-4; James H. Hanford, "The Progenitors of Golias" in *Speculum* 1:1 (1926), 38-58; Helen Waddell, *The Wandering Scholars* (Garden City NJ: Doubleday, 1955 [1926]), 181-182.

6 Beverly A. Tlusty, "Defining 'Drunk' in Early Modern Germany" *Contemporary Drug Problems* 2:2, (1994), 435-436.

7 Mariana Valverde, *Diseases of the Will: Alcohol and the Dilemmas of Freedom* (Cambridge: Cambridge University Press, 1998), 14-15.

Unlike Puritans and Calvinists, Lutherans believed that habitual drinkers suffered from a problem in the soul; thus, the drinking problem remained in the realm of healers. At first, they were priests, but over time, the care for the souls of humanity became secularized and was handed over to physicians, psychiatrists and psychologists who cured all matters relating to uncontrollable drinking and addiction.[8] Here one finds the most basic contrast between Germany and the United States: Lutherans sought treatment of the individual whereas Puritans and Calvinists implemented structural bans on society.

Men of medicine and men of the cloth often condemned drunkenness in early modern Europe. Laws against public drunkenness appeared in various German cities and principalities in the 16th and 17th centuries whether Catholic or Protestant, but without lasting results with the simple folk.. The *Saufteufel*, or boozing devil, spread its temptation throughout Germany with great success. Yet, addiction did not trouble the Germans as they continued to drink to their hearts' content well until the end of the long 19th century and the First World War. Only an economic depression caused Germans to drink less as many manufacturers were prevented from producing beer, and German workers from affording it.[9]

Heinrich Stromer of Auerbach (1476-1542), a reputable German physician of his time, identified *Rausch*, or intoxication, as an illness in 1531. Consequently, some doctors recommended their patients to drink moderately. Nevertheless, this did not prevent other physicians from using spirits liberally in their practice, calling the drink *aqua vitae*, or water of life.[10] Most doctors agreed that the joy caused by drinking was healthy, and some even recommended an occasional "medicinal intoxication" or drunkenness to the point of vomiting to purge the system from an excess of

---

8 Karl Wassenberg, "Die kulturelle Genese der Sucht" in *Suchtwirtschaft,* ed. Aldo Legnaro and Arnold Schmieder (Münster: LIT, 1999), 11-26; Valverde, *Diseases of the Will*, 47.

9 Mikuláš Teich, "The Industrialization of Brewing in Germany (1800-1914)" in *Production, Marketing and Consumption of Alcoholic Beverages since the Late Middle Ages*, ed. Erik Aerts et al. (Leuven: Leuven University Press, 1990), 102-113.

10 Hasso Spode, *Die Macht der Trunkenheit: Kultur- und Sozialgeschichte des Alkohols in Deutschland* (Opladen: Leske & Budrich, 1993), 117-118; Jean-Charles Sournia, *A History of Alcoholism* (Oxford: Oxford University Press, 1990), 17.

phlegm.[11] Medical men knew, however, that these spirits were not devoid of dangers; the water of life could become just as easily the water of death.

Stromer argued that drunkenness resulted from "superfluous use of wine," and that it was a "disease of the head, the brain and the veins growing out of the brain."[12] The physiological damage caused by drinking blocked these veins. The blockage resulted in the loss of their natural dryness, which was considered essential for the functioning of the body. The physical aberration of the drinker manifested itself in a variety of symptoms, from hangover to an early death. Moderate consumption of wine, however, was highly recommended in the treatment of illnesses and for the soul.[13]

Stromer sometimes called drunkenness or intoxication "diseases," but these ailments owed their origins to a vice or in other words, a moral failure of the patient. Disease and vice were often fused into one meaning. More importantly, he was still confined by the medical understanding of his time. He was not concerned with a causal link between an agent and the disease, but instead concentrated on the general environment of his patient in what historians dub "an unspecific cause of disease."[14]

Medical practices of early modern Europe drew their science from the ancient world of Greece and Rome; human behavior, objects and diseases were governed by the four humors of Hippocratic and Galenic medicine: sanguine, choleric, phlegmatic and melancholic, which corresponded to body fluids: blood, yellow bile, phlegm and black bile; and a combination of basic qualities: hot, cold, wet or dry.[15] Beverages, like people, bore traits and temperaments corresponding to their nature: cool, warm, light, heavy and so on. Spirits, for example, since they were produced with fire, were considered to be hot and dry. The qualities of spirits interacted with

---

11 Tlusty, "Defining 'Drunk' in Early Modern Germany," 433.
12 Hasso Spode, "The First Step Toward Sobriety: The 'Boozing Devil' in 16th Century Germany" *Contemporary Drug Problems*, vol. 2/2 (1994), 453-483, esp. 460; Heinrich Stromer, *Ein getrewe, vleissige und ehrliche Verwarnung widder des hesliche Laster der Trunkenheit* (Wittenberg, 1532 [1531]).
13 Ibid.
14 Claudia Wiesemann, *Die heimliche Krankheit: Eine Geschichte des Suchtbegriffs* (Stuttgart: Frommann-Holzboog, 2000), 69-74.
15 Noga Arikha, *Passions and Tempers: A History of Humours* (New York: Ecco, 2007); Andreas-Holger Maehle, *Drugs on Trial: Experimental Pharmacology and Therapeutic Innovation in the Eighteenth Century* (Amsterdam: Rodopi, 1999), 3.

the qualities of the drinker; for the drink to be beneficial or malefic, compatibility between the two was paramount.[16]

The interaction between the drinker's humors and the qualities of the drink was used to explain why some people reacted to alcohol lethargically and others violently. The balance of humors could have been affected by external causes such as illnesses and astrological conditions as well as food, drink, sex and age. For example, doctors cautioned against children drinking wine, claiming it was like adding fire to an existing fire. Warnings against drinks of a cool nature such as beer, fruit juice, or water were raised for women in labor or women trying to conceive; thus, infertility was sometimes blamed on the immoderate beer drinking of German women.[17]

For the ancient Greeks, the world was filled with various temptations, whether sexual, culinary or alcoholic. There were no specific drugs that caused addiction, but any object or activity could become addictive if gone unchecked. Anyone could be enticed by the lure of temptation. It was the goal of a civilized man, as opposed to a barbarian, to deny these temptations and limit them to specific social functions. For example, the symposium was a controlled environment in which alcohol was drunk, with a *symposiumarch* setting the rules on the number of glasses each participant was allowed to drink for the sake of keeping public order and morals.[18] Temptation was universal, a notion that Christianity, whether Catholic, Lutheran or Calvinist adopted in the form of the devil, essentially replacing the barbarian with Satan.

Immanuel Kant (1724-1804), when describing the duties of virtues to oneself in 1797, condemned the "dream euphoria" caused by drugs. Following the Greek example, he wrote that intoxication debased man, turning him into an animal. Moderate consumption of wine was useful to loosen men's tongues in conversation or symposia, but intoxication and opium (*Mohnsaft*) caused an immoral loss of reasoning, imagination and mental faculties. "They are seductive because, under their influence, people dream for a while that they are happy and free from care, and even

---

16 Tlusty, "Defining 'Drunk' in Early Modern Germany," 429.
17 Ibid., 431.
18 James Davidson, *Courtesans and Fishcakes: The Consuming Passions of Classical Athens* (New York: St. Martin's Press, 1998), 139-144. See also Michael A. Rinella, "Plato, Ecstasy and Identity," (Ph.D. Dissertation, State University New York-Albany, 1997), 294-395.

imagine that they are strong; but dejection and weakness follow and, worst of all, they create a need to use the narcotics [*Betäubungsmittel*] again and even to increase the amount."[19]

Therefore, Kant concluded that opium and other drugs should only be used in medicine. The urge to take drugs to satisfy an insatiable hunger with increasing dosage, a hallmark of addiction as it is understood today, was not viewed by Kant as a disease; that would come in a few decades. Instead, for him the insatiable hunger was a sign of loss of control, and this loss of control spelled out loss of free will and reason. Curiously, this breed of drug-moralism never took root in his native Germany.

* * *

When the American Republic was founded, many of the founding fathers, such as George Washington (1732-1799), John Adams (1735-1826) and Thomas Jefferson (1743-1826), considered alcohol drinking a vice, even though they consumed liquor themselves. They feared a bleak future in which the United States would turn into a nation of drunkards, not men.[20] Americans had a taste for the drink, but consumption did not mean approval. There were always those who were ready to condemn their brethren for their behavior. Many municipal ordinances and state laws were enacted against alcohol long before the final act of national Prohibition materialized in the 20th century in the form of the 18th amendment and the subsequent Volstead Act.

The prohibition of drugs and alcohol has been an undercurrent in American politics for over two centuries, always present in one way or form.[21] Many have tried to explain the shift from rampant drinking binges in the early days of America to the strict controls on drugs and alcohol in the 20th century. Since the Declaration of Independence theoretically sanctioned one's right to pursue happiness in the bottle, the discussion of why

---

19 Immanuel Kant, *The Metaphysics of Morals* (Cambridge: Cambridge University Press, 1996 [1797]), 180-181. See the original text in German at: http://www.korp ora.org/Kant/aa06/203.html (Last access, 19.12.2015), 427.

20 William J. Rorabaugh, *The Alcoholic Republic: An American Tradition* (New York: Oxford University Press, 1979), 5-6.

21 On the recurring waves of the prohibition of alcohol, see James A. Morone, *Hellfire Nation: The Politics of Sin in American History* (New Haven: Yale University Press, 2003), 281-317.

Americans chose to prohibit these substances resulted in discussions on the nature of the American character.

One scholar identified four fears that encompass American culture: "The fear of *being owned* (including fears of dependence and of being controlled and shaped by others); the fear of *falling apart* (a fear of anarchy and isolation); the fear of *winding down* (losing energy, dynamism, forward motion); and the fear of *falling away* from a past virtue and promise." These fears were the engine that propelled the United States in its greatest and disastrous endeavors.[22] While these four American fears might be a convincing basis that could explain the shift towards alcohol and drug prohibition, a look beyond the United States shows different responses to the same fears. After all, not only Americans fear for their liberty, fear anarchy, and fear a decline from a golden past. All these fears are as old as ancient Rome itself. The third fear – forward motion and dynamism – might not be as old; but it, too, was not a unique feature of the United States and was prevalent in Europe since the Renaissance; yet, the modern drug laws banning drug use for recreational purposes began in the United States at a specific time in history and nowhere else.

Perhaps the ban on drugs was the outcome of a struggle between the upper world and the underworld in America: a conflict between the respectable versus the unrespectable, of two cultures struggling against each other, one being the negative image of the other; one fitting the poor, the other the wealthy. The poor were not inherently part of the underworld by nature, but by physical proximity. Those who populated the underworld engaged in unrespectable activities and fell into bad habits.[23] Yet, one could argue against this thesis because Americans of all stripes used drugs, and not just the poor.

The questions whether addiction was a cause or effect of criminality, and whether the drug laws caused addicts to become criminal by definition or not were asked by numerous historians and sociologists over the years. Their answers usually reflected their own biases towards drugs; those who thought drugs were evil deemed them as the cause of crime. Those who

---

22 Rupert Wilkinson, *The Pursuit of American Character* (New York: Harper & Row, 1988), 2, 114-115.
23 John C. Burnham, *Bad Habits: Drinking, Smoking, Taking Drugs, Gambling, Sexual Misbehavior, and Swearing in American History* (New York: New York University Press, 1993), 1-22.

believed drugs to be benign asserted that criminality was simply a side effect of bad laws.

As one theory posits, the poor and criminals were the only ones left using drugs, after physicians who learned of the addictive nature of drugs in the first two decades of the 20th century cleaned respectable members of society from drug use.[24] Yet, perhaps the respectability of drug use was already on the decline with the drug panics of the mid to late 19th century before physicians learned of their errors.[25] Or as will be shown in the following chapters, a different mechanism propelled the United States to ban drugs altogether.

Throughout the 19th century, many Americans believed that "approximately all doctors were parasites of society' and that at least two-thirds of them were going to hell, individual practitioners, regardless of whether they were thought to be any good."[26] Benjamin Franklin (1706-1790), also a founding father of the first hospital and medical school in America, was known to say, "God heals and the doctor takes the fee." No wonder, then, that Americans remained suspicious of their doctors. Physicians and their remedies were seen more as a menace than a cure.

Oliver Wendell Holmes Sr.'s (1809-1894) speech before the Massachusetts Medical Society in 1860 should be read in light of this dread:

> Throw out opium, which the Creator himself seems to prescribe, for we often see the scarlet poppy growing in the cornfields, as if it were foreseen that wherever there is hunger to be fed there must also be pain to be soothed; throw out a few specifics which our art did not discover, and is hardly needed to apply; throw out wine, which is a food, and the vapours which produce the miracle of anaesthesia, and I firmly believe that if the whole materia medica, *as now used*, could be sunk to the bottom of the sea, it would be all the better for mankind – and all the worse for the fishes.[27]

---

24 See David T. Courtwright, *Dark Paradise: A History of Opium Addiction in America* (Cambridge MA: Harvard University Press, 2001).

25 See Joseph F. Spillane, *Cocaine: From Medical Marvel to Modern Menace in the United States, 1884-1920* (Baltimore: Johns Hopkins University Press, 2000).

26 Janice Rae McTavish, *Pain and Profits: The History of the Headache and its Remedies in America* (New Brunswick, NJ: Rutgers University Press, 2004), 43.

27 Oliver Wendell Holmes, "Currents and Counter-currents in Medical Science," (Annual Address before the Massachusetts Medical Society, 1860) in *The American Journal of the Medical Science* 40:80 (1860), 462-474.

Holmes was wary of his colleagues, urging them to seek professionalism, as was the case in Europe. But, more curiously, was his attitude towards ether, opium and wine. Opium was indeed a panacea. Ether was useful and wine was not only a cure, but also a foodstuff. These three drugs were the only medicines in the entire American *materia medica* worth saving. The suspicion of the medical profession continued in America, but the high esteem of opium and wine did not.

Once the American economic interests in the Asian opium trade subsided in the 1860s, and the trading firms of Boston, Philadelphia and New York abandoned it in favor of introducing American products to China; the path was cleared to damn the drug.[28] The moral bells rang out against the drug since the Opium War (1839-1842), but the federal government only took action after the opium trade was no longer lucrative.

Religious fervor against alcohol and drugs remained an undertone throughout the 19th and 20th centuries. Whereas the Puritans of centuries past, who sought shelter in the New World to escape the persecutions of the Old one, did not forget to bring with them their bottles of whiskey and rum,[29] the Puritan ethic turned into an ideal of living a life free of enslavement from tyranny. This changed over time to include a life free of the enslavement to alcohol and drugs. Freedom of the will, free from alcohol and drugs, became an essential component of the image of the City on the Hill, and those who failed to be free were either delinquents or diseased.[30]

Religion and morality played a marked role in American ethics, shaping common beliefs and attitudes. Damnations of alcohol and opium were

---

28 See Charles C. Stelle, "American Trade in Opium to China, Prior to 1820" *The Pacific Historical Review* 9:4 (1940), 425-444; Yen-P'ing Hao, "Chinese Teas to America-a Synopsis," in *America's China Trade in Historical Perspective*, ed. Ernst R. May & John K. Fairbank (Cambridge, MA: Harvard University Press, 1986), 12-31; Jacques M. Downs, "The Commercial Origins of American Attitudes Toward China, 1784-1944," in *America Views China: American Images of China then and now*, ed. Jonathan Goldstein, Jerry Israel & Hilary Conroy (Bethlehem PA: Leigh University Press, 1991), 56-66; Elizabeth Kelly Gray, "American Attitudes Toward British Imperialism, 1815-1860" (Ph.D. Dissertation, College of William and Mary, 2002); Sibing He "Russell and Company, 1818-1891: America's Trade and Diplomacy in Nineteenth-Century China" (Ph.D. Dissertation, University of Miami, 1997).

29 Rorabaugh, *The Alcoholic Republic,* 6-11.

30 Valverde, *Diseases of the Will.*

heard early in American history,[31] and in some cases, even before the Republic was declared. Reformed religious figures, be they Puritan, Quaker or Methodist, preached against the drink. They claimed that freedom was not only a political concept, but also a personal one. "A republic of free men," the Quaker Anthony Benezet (1713-1784) contended in the third quarter of the 18th century, "had no place for the bondage of men to either other men or to distilled spirits." Liberty transformed from a man's freedom to act as he pleased into a concept of self-sufficiency, self-dependence, self-control and moderation.[32] It took about a century and a half for Benezet's message to sink into American consciousness, motivating political action in the form of national prohibition, discounting the occasional local fervor against the drink. In fact, so much time elapsed as to suggest that religion and morality were not enough to forbid alcohol and drugs. Perhaps religion had nothing to do with the panic at all.

The shift against drugs coincided with racism, the Civil War, and the development of a rational, medical profession that sought legitimacy by controlling harmful and addictive substances. The pattern was a familiar one in American history: moralists discovered a problem in society, usually a sinful behavior, and rallied against it. That alone, however, was not enough to ban the sin or punish the sinners. Allies were needed to push bills through the "checks and balances of American politics," and the two crucial steps to attract allies were: "the right enemies and a good panic."[33]

* * *

Alcohol drinking, opium smoking and opium eating were not considered to be the same. Neither the morbid craving for cocaine, nor morphine nor heroin seemed to share common attributes. Different methods of consumption produced different results in different people. Physicians

---

31 Regarding opium, see Gray, "American Attitude Toward British Imperialism, 1815-1860."

32 Anthony Benezet, *The Mighty Destroyer Displaced and Some Account of the Dreadful Havoc Made by the Mistaken Use, As Well As the Abuse, of Distilled Spirituous Liquors* (1774) quoted in Rorabaugh, *The Alcoholic Republic*, 46.

33 Morone, *Hellfire Nation,* 476-477.

accepted opium eating and morphine in their practices for better or worse, whereas opium smoking was deemed utterly wicked and unnecessary.[34]

Throughout the 19th century, medical doctors turned their art into science first in Europe and much later across the Atlantic. Rigorous, secular studies were demanded from medical students; and they, in turn, demanded authority over their subject. The newfound authority was not only respected in the courtroom, but was present in day-to-day life. Individuals no longer sought out their local healer, barber, surgeon or priest for their physical or mental problems, but they went to the clinic, where the physician proudly nailed his Medical Doctor degree on the wall for all to see. Seen in hindsight, the physicians' domain spread into the realms formerly reserved for priests and law enforcers, as many sins turned into diseases: lust into nymphomania, gluttony into obesity, and drunkenness into addiction.[35]

Since the medical understanding of addiction in each country in the 19th century dictated future policy, the United States' extreme drug policy can be viewed as a preventative measure caused by the attitudes of physicians towards addiction, which in turn was influenced by the free market in drugs, as well as racial, economic and social biases in the 19th century. Germany followed a different pattern, which remained constant even during the most tumultuous political upheavals and revolutions that plagued the Kaiserreich, the Weimar Republic and the Third Reich.

But what is addiction? And if addiction is a modern concept,[36] when was it discovered? Alcohol and opium are two of the oldest medicines known to man, it should not come as a surprise that several physicians, botanists and chemists, or their contemporary equivalents, noticed their effects as early as the 16th century if not earlier. Opium and alcohol were known for their toxicity, habitual use, and euphoric effect, appearing in medical treatises for centuries. Even drug tolerance, not to be confused with addiction, was recorded as early as the 17th century.[37] If that is indeed the case, perhaps alcoholism and addiction are not modern concepts at all,

---

34 Courtwright, *Dark Paradise,* 61-62.
35 Sarah W. Tracy, *Alcoholism in America: From Reconstruction to Prohibition* (Baltimore: Johns Hopkins University Press, 2005), x, 226-228, 269-272, 292, note 2.
36 Sebastian Scheerer, *Sucht,* (Hamburg: Rowohlt, 1995) 9-15.
37 Maehle, *Drugs on Trial*; Mark David Merlin, *On the Trail of the Ancient Opium Poppy* (London: Associated University Press, 1984).

because physicians and society recognized intoxications throughout European history.[38]

The answer to when addiction was discovered cannot be satisfied with the citation of a specific treatise of one doctor or another. No medical Columbus or Magellan found addiction in a distant land, but instead a slow realization that addiction existed spread among physicians as they began to seek out single cause and effect for diseases. Addiction as a disease only appeared once physicians were concerned with it. Although doctors knew of the malefic effects of drugs and alcohol for centuries, not until the 19th century were they seriously concerned with direct causes and effects of diseases; addiction was a byproduct of this realization.[39]

Addiction, unlike other diseases, was hidden. As long as an addict kept a regular drug regimen, his general health remained intact. Addiction had no side effects to speak of, save for withdrawal symptoms. By dubbing addiction a disease, physicians assumed that this semblance of health was nothing more than a mirage. Instead of accepting the habitual use of drugs as a natural effect of drugs, a sinister problem emerged from within the patient.[40] Physicians first encountered addiction, in its broadest sense, while studying alcoholics and alcohol, rather than drug addicts and drugs. Once the alcoholic, the chronically inebriate, or the dipsomaniac was identified it was only a matter of time for the drug addict to join the diseased.

Not all physicians understood alcoholism and drug addiction in similar terms, though they often described one affliction by borrowing symptoms of the other. The two births of addiction could not have taken place without the conception of alcoholism as disease. After doctors acknowl-

---

38 Harry G. Levine, "The Discovery of Addiction: Changing Conceptions of Habitual Drunkenness in America," *Journal of Studies on Alcohol*, 39:1 (1978), 143-174; Roy Porter, "The Drinking Man's Disease: The 'Pre-History' of Alcoholism in Georgian Britain," *British Journal of Addiction*, 80:4 (1985), 385-396; Jessica Warner, "Before there was 'Alcoholism': Lessons from the Medieval Experience with Alcohol," *Contemporary Drug Problems*, 19:3 (1992), 409-428; Peter Ferentzy, "From Sin to Disease: Differences and Similarities between Past and Current Conceptions of Chronic Drunkenness," *Contemporary Drug problems*, 28:3 (2001), 363-390.

39 Wiesemann, *Die heimliche Krankheit,* 127-174. See also Virginia Berridge, *Opium and the People: Opiate Use in Nineteenth-Century England* (London: Free Association Books, 1999), 153; Gerald N. Grob, *The Deadly Truth: A History of Disease in America* (Cambridge MA: Harvard University Press, 2002), 2-3.

40 Wiesemann, *Die heimliche Krankheit*, 52-57.

edged alcoholism and drug addiction as diseases, the causes had to be identified. The three possible origins were: a moral weakness, making an individual prone to become an alcoholic; a biological deficiency, rendering the patient helpless in his condition; and finally, a universal threat, which would render anyone in contact with an excessive amount of alcohol or drugs sick. Somewhat related to the origins of the disease was its nature, either physical or mental, allowing for any number of combinations of these five components to devise a definition for the disease; for example, it could be caused by a biological deficiency with symptoms of mental inferiority, or perhaps caused by a moral weakness with signs of physical depravity. The adoption of each cause depended on religion, politics and the temperance movements in each country. The struggle against a moral weakness was the flag raised by temperance activists of a religious bent, the biological paradigm was held dear by secular physicians, and the universal model was adopted by physicians who were least affected by politics and sought a scientific solution to the addiction problem.

Historians crave to find the ever-elusive paradigm shift or the change in the assumptions that lead to a scientific revolution.[41] Similar to many other revolutions, a closer look reveals that the events that brought about the change were not revolutionary, but evolutionary. Old ideas were not immediately dropped when new ones were developed, and if the old was not retained it influenced the new. In this respect, the medicalization of addiction was no different.

Neither the alcohol disease nor drug addiction ever had a single definition; instead, competing concepts evolved almost simultaneously in the beginning of the 19th century. One of the first concepts of drinking disease that evolved in the German-speaking world stressed a physical cause for the disease. The second, popularized by the French physician Jean-Étienne Dominique Esquirol (1772-1840) in 1819, claimed that habitual drunkenness was a monomania, or a single mental disease, confined within the framework of society and civilization, without which the mentally ill

---

41 As described in Thomas S. Kuhn, *The Structure of Scientific Revolutions* (Chicago: University of Chicago Press, 1962). For some of the pitfalls of this theory regarding 18th and 19th century medicine, see Joseph F. Musser, "The Perils of Relying on Thomas Kuhn," *Eighteenth-Century Studies*, 18:2 (1985), 215-226.

could maintain a normal life.[42] Heredity played an important role in monomania.[43] This disease witnessed a short life and was replaced by a different concept developed by Esquirol's student, Jean-Pierre Falret (1794-1870) and his own student Bénédict-Augustin Morel (1809-1873), after the mid 19th century.[44] Yet, heredity retained a strong presence in the discussion of mental disorders, and resurfaced time and again throughout the 19th and 20th centuries.

Between the German and the French concepts of the disease, a third school emerged, claiming that habitual drunkenness had either mental or physical components and sometimes both, but was by definition a moral failure.[45] Adopted in the United States, the latter was reminiscent of ideas shared in previous centuries, often connected to moral and religious condemnations of spirits and habitual drunkards.

The word "addiction" existed for over two millennia, but it did not always have the same meaning. The Latin word *addictionis* meant the debt owed by a debtor, or the assigning of a debtor to the care of the creditor.[46] From its language of origin, addiction contained a sense of enslavement. In fact, an *addictus* was a man enslaved for his debts.[47] Over time, the meaning of the word mutated to denote dedication or devotion to a person, a thing or a belief,[48] until it had turned into an inclination to a person or a

---

42 On monomania in the 19th century, see B. Ball, "The History of Mental Medicine" *The Lancet*, 115:2941 (1880): 48-50. For a brief explanation of monomania in a historical context, see William F. Bynum, "Monomania" *The Lancet*, 362:9393 (2003), 1425. For the use of monomania to explain the alcohol disease, see Jan Ellen Goldstein, *Console and Classify: The French Psychiatric Profession in the Nineteenth Century* (Chicago: University of Chicago Press, 2001), 179.

43 William F. Bynum, "Alcoholism and Degeneration in 19th century European Medicine and Psychiatry," *British Journal of Addiction* 79 (1984), 61.

44 Goldstein, *Console and Classify*, 189-196.

45 Roy Porter's introduction in the facsimile of Thomas Trotter, *An Essay: Medical, Philosophical, and Chemical-On Drunkenness and its Effects on the Human Body* (London, 1988 [1804]), xii-xiii. The third concept that Porter mentioned, Magnus Huss' theory on alcoholism, as modern as it might have been, was an expansion of the German physical disease of the 1820s without the hereditary elements.

46 *Oxford Latin Dictionary* (Oxford: Oxford University Press, 1968), 36b-c;

47 Charlton T. Lewis and Charles Short, *A Latin Dictionary* (Oxford: Oxford University Press, 1969), 30c.

48 Ibid., 31a.

party,[49] or the assignment of property.[50] From Latin, the word found its way into the various vernacular tongues and was also anglicized. For example, on 13 March 1789, Thomas Jefferson wrote to Francis Hopkinson (1737-1791) of New Jersey:

> I am not a federalist, because I never submitted the whole system of my opinions to the creed of any party of men whatever, in religion, in philosophy, in politics or in anything else, where I was capable of thinking for myself. Such an addiction is the last degradation of a free and moral agent. If I could not go to heaven but with a party, I would not go there at all.[51]

The future third President of the United States preferred hell rather than addiction. Jefferson's fear of addiction; however, was not a metaphor and had little to do with drugs or alcohol. Instead, he spoke of his unwillingness to subscribe fully to a political party, or thought.

Addiction retained its negative connotation seventy years after Jefferson's letter, appearing in John Stuart Mill's (1806-1873) *On Liberty*:

> A man who causes grief to his family by addiction to bad habits…deserves reproach for his unkindness or ingratitude; but so he may for cultivating habits not in themselves vicious, if they are painful to those with whom he passes his life, or who from personal ties are dependent on him for their comfort.[52]

No bad deed should go unpunished if it kept a man from performing his duties for others. The meaning of addiction, however, was in reference to bad habits, rather than alcohol or drugs. These habits, according to Mill, varied from drunkenness, gambling and debt, to abandoning one's family.[53] Judging from the mutation of the word, it is clear that addiction was not understood in the 19th century as it is today. It was not necessarily a medical term relating to drug use. Instead, various uses were found for the word, from enslavement to addiction to bad habits, and from addiction to political ideas to an inclination to a neutral habit or pursuit.[54]

---

49 *Oxford English Dictionary* (Oxford: Oxford University Press, 1989); *Oxford Latin Dictionary*, 36b-c.
50 J. F. Niermeyer and C. van de Kieft, *Mediae Latinitatis Lexicon Minus*, vol. 1(Leiden: Brill, 2002), 22b.
51 "Thomas Jefferson to Francis Hopkins, (13 March 1789)," in Thomas Jefferson, *Letters, 1743-1826* (New York, 1984), 940-941.
52 John Stuart Mill, *On Liberty* (London, 1985 [1859]), 148-149.
53 Ibid.
54 *Oxford English Dictionary*

"Habit" was the word some physicians used to describe addiction in the 19th century, and addicts were known as habitués.[55] French rather than Latin described the condition. Physicians, who treated the habitués by the end of the 19th century, required a classical word to describe the disease, in the same manner that jaundice (French) of the 14th century turned into hepatitis (Greek) four centuries later. The transition from habit to addiction was gradual as old and new traditions and teachings lived side by side. Thus, aware of the many names of addiction, the *Journal of the American Medical Association* declared in 1906: "It matters little whether one speaks of the opium habit, the opium disease of the opium addiction."[56] By then, all three referred to one medical phenomenon.

In German a parallel process occurred, though it lacked the influence of a classic language. While today *Sucht* means addiction, it was not understood as such throughout most of the 19th century. *Sucht* or *Suht* were ancient Germanic words that meant "disease" since the 8th century.[57] Thus, they served as the root for words such as: *Seuche* or plague, *Fallsucht* or epilepsy, and *Gelbsucht* or jaundice.[58] Not until the mid 19th century did the association of addiction with *Sucht* become strong, but not yet exclusive. It served to describe a condition caused by a drug or alcohol as in the composite word *Morphiumsucht*, or the morphine disease, and *Alkoholsucht* or the alcohol disease. Only in the 20th century did the word attain

---

55 Timothy Alton Hickman, *The Secret Leprosy of Modern Days: Narcotic Addiction and Cultural Crisis in the United States, 1870-1920* (Amherst: University of Massachusetts Press, 2007), 8, 16-17.

56 Smith Ely Jelliffe, "Drug Addictions: Preliminary Report of the Committee in Section on Nervous and Mental Diseases," *Journal of the American Medical Association*, 46:9 (1906), 643-644.

57 See Jacob and Wilhelm Grimm, *Deutches Wörterbuch*, 20 (Leipzig, 1854-1960), 858-910.

58 *Fallsucht*, originally *Fallendsucht* literally meaning falling disease, is the German term for epilepsy. *Gelbsucht* literally means the yellow disease, and therefore corresponds well with jaundice. Since the 14th century, *Krankheit* served as a competing word for *Sucht* to mean disease. By the 19th century, as *Sucht* increasingly became associated with addiction, *Krankheit* remained as the word used to describe disease. In English, the word disease itself experienced an evolution from dis-ease, or discomfort, to illness. For additional information, see Grimm's *Deutsches Wörterbuch*, the *Oxford English Dictionary* and Porter's introduction to Trotter's *On Drunkenness*.

an autonomous state to mean solely addiction, losing its original meaning of disease.[59]

The birth of addiction, defined as a compulsion to take drugs, coincided with the medicalization of sins.[60] As stated above, addiction could have appeared in numerous contexts in the early 19th century, from an addiction to tobacco,[61] to a political party or to bad habits such as masturbation. By the end of the 19th century, the word was condensed into one meaning: the compulsive consumption of drugs. The dust has not settled and the meaning of addiction continues on changing to this day.

The evolution of the term best resembles an hourglass: until the mid 19th century, addiction had innumerable meanings that narrowed into a waist of a single meaning, only to expand in recent years to include numerous social ailments from gambling and eating food to viewing pornography. This expansion, however, has resulted in a decline in popularity of the term 'addiction' among physicians in favor of 'substance related disorder.'[62]

* * *

Many historians and drug enthusiasts maintained that only with the emergence of the modern state, drugs became illegal. The abstract bureaucratic machine desired to control and quantify every movement of its citizens, and drugs created unreliable citizens. To support this claim, historians attempted to draw distinctions between a ban on substances and a ban on users, claiming that restrictions were indeed imposed in the past, but only against certain drugs, and never against those who used them. However, drunkenness and intoxication always scared the public. Rules, laws or public norms were imposed on wine, beer, liquor, drugs and their consumers the moment use became widespread.

Throughout history, governments have had three possible distinct policies toward drugs: ban, control, and toleration. Of the three, drug

---

59 Wiesemann, *Die heimliche Krankheit*, 41-42. *Die Abhängigkeit*, the word used to describe addiction in modern German, struck root in the language only after 1964. See Ibid., 45-46.

60 Peter Conrad and Joseph W. Schneider, *Deviance and Medicalization: From Badness to Sickness* (Philadelphia: Temple University Press, 1992).

61 Samuel Johnson, *The Lives of the English Poets* (London, 1825 [1779-1781]), 87.

62 Valverde, *Diseases of the Will*, 26-28, 44; See also Gordon Coonfield, "Mapping Addiction" (Ph.D. dissertation, Michigan Technological University, 2003), 13-15.

control remains the most flexible, and therefore it has the most manifestations. Control has most often been a matter of taxation, place of use, or method of delivery, as in the case of the English Gin Laws of the 18th century, or current liquor laws in the United States. Another mode of control was the limitation of the drug trade to professionals such as chemists and pharmacists, or granting a prescription monopoly to physicians. Control could also appear in the form of a legal drinking age, or as a part of measures taken for professionalism or public safety as in forbidding policemen or truck drivers to drink while on duty. The number of measures to control drugs is endless, and yet, each country developed its own tradition of how to deal with mind-altering substances.

Popular historians and sensationalists found a fertile breeding ground in conspiracy theories regarding drugs, the most famous of which was the tale of how the paper industry banned marijuana in the United States. Popular among hippies and stoners in the 1970s who wished to protect their ganja from 'the man,' the following story even appeared in print. Andrew W. Mellon (1855-1937), the secretary of the Treasury, appointed Harry J. Anslinger (1892-1975) to the Federal Bureau of Narcotics in 1930. Anslinger was married to Mellon's niece and therefore owed his position to family ties. Mellon was also a banker of the DuPont Corporation, which patented a new method of making paper out of wood pulp in the 1930s.

Shortly afterwards, a different method of producing paper using cannabis was introduced to the market, threatening DuPont's new patent. William Randolph Hearst (1863-1951), who was DuPont's client and an owner of forests scheduled to be turned into pulp, ordered his newspapers to demonize marijuana, while Mellon told Anslinger to testify before Congress about the dangers of marijuana. This campaign led to the ban on the drug, which also saved the paper industry from bankruptcy.[63]

Conspiracies are difficult to disprove, as they tend to elude historians' eyes. It is true that Hearst's press empire printed sensationalist stories of murders induced by drugs, and Anslinger was indeed married to Mellon's niece, virtually no other fact supports the existence of a conspiracy, as can be discerned from the process of how cannabis was banned in 1937.

---

63 Peter McWilliams, *Ain't Nobody's Business if you do: The Absurdity of Consensual Crimes in a Free Society* (Los Angeles: Books on Demand, 1993), 536-541.

Biases do not only influence historical work, but also has influenced the sources. In 1913, John D. Rockefeller (1839-1937) established the Bureau of Social Hygiene, Inc. in New York with a special emphasis on criminology. In the following decade, the *Committee on Drug Addiction* was formed, which sponsored several studies on the drug problem and addiction, the most famous of which was Charles E. Terry (1878-1945) and Mildred Pellans' *The Opium Problem* first published in 1928.[64] The book was criticized shortly after publication for its leniency and liberal views towards addicts and addiction, advocating treatment instead of the incarceration of addicts. It was perhaps for this reason that the book was a commercial failure.[65] Although forgotten shortly after being published, historians later resurrected the study and hailed it as one of the most important compendia on the history of drug addiction.[66]

The dismissal and subsequent resurrection of the *Opium Problem* is a fitting metaphor for the trajectory of the history of drugs. As German psychiatrist Max Seige found in 1912, physicians often have a cyclical appreciation of new drugs: the discovery of a drug produces excitement, which results in the expansion of the use of the drug alongside high expectations for a panacea. Disappointment follows when the new drug fails to meet expectations, finally leading to limitations on the use of the drug.[67]

For much of the last century and half, this cycle has repeated itself.[68] The following chapters trace the rise and fall of opium, cocaine, morphine and other drugs, each once considered to be god's own medicine, only to be condemned as the scourge of mankind.

---

64 Nathan B. Eddy, *The National Research Council Involvement in the Opiate Problem, 1928-1971* (Washington DC: National Academy of Sciences, 1973), 5-8.

65 David T. Courtwright, "Charles Terry, the Opium Problem, and American Narcotic Policy," *Journal of Drug Issues* 16:3 (1986), 421-434.

66 H. Wayne Morgan, *Drugs in America: A Social History, 1800-1980* (Syracuse: Syracuse University Press, 1981), 224.

67 Stephen Snelders, Charles Kaplan, and Toine Pieters, "On Cannabis, Chloral Hydrate, and Career Cycles of Psychotropic Drugs in Medicine," *Bulletin of the History of Medicine* 80:1 (2006), 95-114. Max Seige, "Klinische Erfahrungen mit Neoronal," *Deutsche medizinische Wochenschrift* 38 (1912), 1828-1830. Seige made this off hand remark regarding drug cycles while seeking treatment for epilepsy with a drug called 'neuronal' after determining that the opium-bromide cure was mostly ineffective, see also Max Seige, "Erfolge der Flechsig'schen Brom-Opium-Kur," *Monatsschrift für Psychiatrie und Neurologie* 22:1 (1907), 84-92.

68 David F. Musto, *The American Disease* (Oxford: Oxford University Press, 1999).

Part I

1. The Drinking Disease

As early as the 9th century, if not earlier, efforts were made to sober the German nation. But it was not until the 19th century, when physicians began to speak of specific causes for diseases, that debate on the "drinking disease" found a base in medicine rather than morality. The leaders of this intellectual endeavor were German physicians, and the German language itself came to dominate the debate on the drinking disease. Indeed, all four words used to describe it shared a common German origin: *Trunksucht*, *Dipsomanie*, *Methysmus* and *Alcoholismus*.[69]

German dominance did not imply exclusive German development of the understanding of the drinking disease. Notable discoveries were also made elsewhere, the most important of which was Thomas Sutton's (1767-1835) identification of *delirium tremens* in England in 1813.[70] This discovery reinforced the notion that the drinking disease was an illness directly caused by one agent. Nevertheless, German dominance in the field was unquestioned, and the professionalism of German medicine had far-reaching implications, as the state relied on and allied itself with doctors. Public welfare, which first began in Prussia in the 1840s, and after the wars of unification spread to the rest of the Reich, funneled public money to medicine.[71]

The introduction of public medical insurance in 1883 and the general prosperity (despite a few hiccoughs) in the country in the following decades strengthened the role of physicians in Germany, as their numbers

---

69 William F. Bynum, "Chronic Alcoholism in the First Half of the 19th Century" *Bulletin of the History of Medicine* 42:2 (1968), 161. Other names for the disease, such as *Saufsucht* first appearing in 1823 never became popular.

70 Thomas Sutton, *Tracts on Delirium Tremens, on Peritonitis, and on some other internal inflammatory affections, and on Gout* (London, 1813), 1-77. English and French ideas were also known in Germany, such as Esquirol's theory on monomania or Thomas Trotter's disease concept. See Thomas Trotter, *An Essay: Medical, Philosophical, and Chemical-On Drunkenness and its Effects on the Human Body* (London, 1988 [1804]).

71 A similar process occurred in other German principalities, for the example in Baden see Arleen M. Tuchman, *Science, Medicine and the State in Germany: The Case of Baden, 1815-1871* (Oxford: Oxford University Press, 1993).

swelled and their influence over society and politics increased. They formed medical associations that both protected physicians and ensured professionalism. National health insurance assured that the urban poor and the upper classes were no longer the only patients being treated. Both peasants and workers, most of whom were insured by 1914, were able to afford professional medical care.[72]

In the pursuit of professionalism, early 19th-century physicians sought medical reform in a science devoid of god's presence. One theory that held the promise of propelling German medicine into a field of science was Brunonianism.[73] The theory, named after its founder John Brown (1735-1788), was based on the principle of excitability as the basic quality inherent in every living organism.[74] Brown first put forth his theory in *Elementa medicanae*, which was published in Edinburgh in 1781 under the name of one of his followers.[75]

Brown believed in mathematic certainty in medicine, and divided excitability into 80 degrees, with 40 indicating a healthy state.[76] Life could not exist without excitability, and if it were lacking, stimulants had to be administered to the organism to revive it.[77] Brown, himself an avid user of laudanum to ease his gout pains, divided diseases into two: sthenic, or the excessive amount of stimulation, and asthenic, or the lack of excitement.

---

72 Henry E. Sigerist, "From Bismarck to Beveridge: Developments and Trends in Social Security Legislation," *Journal of Public Health Policy* 20:4 (1999 [1943]), 484-489, 493-496. See also Ute Frevert, "Professional Medicine and the Working Classes in Imperial Germany," *Journal of Contemporary History* 20:4 (1985), 637-658; Claudia Huerkamp, "The Making of the Modern Medical profession, 1800-1914: Prussian Doctors in the Nineteenth Century," in *German Professions, 1800-1950*, ed. Geoffrey Cocks and Konrad H. Jarausch (New York: Oxford University Press, 1990), 66-84.

73 Nelly Tsouyopoulos, "The Influence of John Brown's Ideas in Germany," *Medical History* 8 (1988), 70.

74 Guenter B. Risse, "The History of John Brown's Medical System in Germany during the Years 1790-1806," (Doctoral dissertation, University of Chicago, 1971), 107.

75 Judith A. Overmier, "John Brown's *Elemena Medicinae*: An Introductory Bibliographical Essay," *Bulletin Medical Library Association* 70:3 (1982): 310-317.

76 Guenter B. Risse, "Medicine in the Age of Enlightenment," in *Medicine in Society: Historical Essays*, ed. Andrew Wear (Cambridge: Cambridge University Press, 1998), 165.

77 Risse, "The History of John Brown's Medical System in Germany," 110.

Since most ailments were the result of a lack of stimulation, according to Brown, administering stimulants such as opium and alcohol could restore health.[78] Following the publication of *Elementa medicanae*, the administration of opium and alcohol surged among physicians and those practicing quasi-medicine. It also rose among those without medical training, who were drawn to the simplicity of Brown's theory. Friedrich Schlegel (1772-1829), a philosopher with absolutely no medical background, felt comfortable enough with Brown's guidance to treat his wife Caroline with large doses of opium.[79]

Brunonianism attracted more followers in Germany than in England, but it nevertheless drew the wrath of many critics. In the beginning of the 19th century it was discredited as physicians turned to other scientific methods based on clinical observation. However, Brunonianism, like Mesmerism and homeopathy, left an indelible mark on German medicine; elements of excitability – the bond, according to Brown, that tied together all living organisms – were absorbed into clinical medicine, in the same manner that hypnosis entered psychiatry and herbal remedies turned into digestible pills.

The ideological struggle between Brunonianism and traditional medicine effected the inception of the birth of addiction in Germany.[80] Christoph Wilhelm Hufeland (1762-1836), arguably the most famous Prussian physician of his time, vocally opposed Brown and insisted that medicine should remain in the hands of professionals. Alarmed by the excesses of Brunonianists and amateurs like Schlegel, he wrote in his book on the art of living a long life published in 1796: "The first thing which, in regard to diet, can act as a shortener of life is immoderation," Hufeland warned. Eating and drinking too much was harmful for a healthy life, as was digesting "too refined cookery."[81] Immoderate consumption of anything, be it food or drink, was detrimental to one's health, Hufeland argued, in an unmistakable echo of ascetic Christian values. He was particularly critical of spirits:

---

78   Ibid., 88, 96-97, 112.
79   Marcus Boon, *The Road of Excess: A History of Writers on Drugs* (Cambridge: Harvard University Press, 2002), 26-27.
80   Claudia Wiesemann, *Die heimliche Krankheit: Eine Geschichte des Suchtbegriffs* (Stuttgart: Frommann-Holzboog, 2000).
81   Christoph Wilhelm Hufeland, *Art of Prolonging Life* (London, 1859), 150. [C. W. Hufeland, *Die Kunst, das menschliche Leben zu verlängern*, (1796)].

> Lastly, we may place in this class of things, that tend in a particular manner to shorten life, all preparations of spirituous liquors, which, under whatever name known, are, in that respect, highly prejudicial. When people drink these, they drink liquid fire. They accelerate vital consumption in a dreadful manner; and make life, in the properest sense, a process of burning.[82]

Liquid fire, or *Feuerwasser*, is a term often used in German to this day to describe spirits – a vestige of Hippocratic medicine in modern times. Burnt wine, or brandy wine (*Branntwein* in German) was produced by fire, and so retained the qualities of fire in the liquid. Thus, to Hufeland, when one consumed brandy the burning process continued inside the stomach. Continuing his attack against alcohol, he treated spirits as if they were *aqua mortis*, or water of death, poisoning the drinker's will, morality and self-control. Only in rare medicinal uses, he cautioned, should a physician prescribe alcohol, the true "enemy of mankind."

Alcohol was a dangerous stimulant that did not cause a mere disease, but a plague that poisoned many drinkers. Hufeland claimed there were two types of poisoning: quick and slow, depending on dosage and duration of consumption. Of the two, the slow and hidden poisoning was more dangerous, since the victim was unaware of his dangerous condition that could result in death or in other complications such as dropsy (edema).[83] This understanding should not be underestimated. For the first time, a modern physician acknowledged the possibility that alcohol could cause a hidden disease.

A like-minded physician in Berlin, Johann Ludwig Formey (1766-1823), wrote in 1796 that the "stupefying drink" caused an uncontrollable lethargy, which the drinker sought to satisfy by consuming more of the malefic beverage. Continuous consumption of spirits turned into an uncontrollable urge, but this uncontrollable urge was not a real disease, but rather a sin detrimental to one's health.[84] He was certain, however, that the disease was caused by a weakness in the human organism caused by over-stimulation of the senses, a notion borrowed from Brown, and shared by Hufeland.[85]

---

82 Ibid., 153.
83 Christoph Wilhelm Hufeland, *Ueber die Vergiftung durch Branntwein* (Berlin, 1802).
84 Johann Ludwig Formey, *Versuch einer medicinischen Topographie von Berlin* (Berlin, 1796), 79-80.
85 Ibid.; Hufeland, *Ueber die Vergiftung durch Branntwein*; Wiesemann, *Die heimliche Krankheit*, 146.

"Unfortunately I must confess that physicians themselves, deluded by the appearance of a false system, have shut their eyes to the detrimental effects of ardent spirits, and have recommended them freely to both the sick and the healthy,"[86] Hufeland wrote in 1802. His strident attacks against spirits must be seen as part and parcel of his animosity toward Brunonianism. Since Brown's theory called for excessive use of opium and alcohol, his opponents were concerned with the medical misuse of these drugs.[87] As a representative of traditional medicine – an eclectic doctor, as historians now call such physicians – Hufeland felt the need to protect the German public from Brown, whose theories had become popular among German Romantics and Romantic doctors.[88]

Nearly two decades later, Hufeland's writings again helped to reshape understanding of the drinking disease. In 1819, Russian-German physician C. von Brühl-Cramer published his seminal work on the drinking disease, "*Die Trunksucht und eine rationelle Heilmethode derselben.*"[89] In the preface to the German edition of the book, Hufeland praised Brühl-Cramer for demonstrating "how the bad habit brings out a disease, the *Trunksucht*, which has much analogy to nymphomania and therefore could be designated *dipsomania* nosologically."[90]

Hufeland, displaying a knack for coining new medical terms, kept the tradition of using a classical language for the systematic classification of diseases, which resulted in the adoption of dipsomania rather than *Trunk-*

---

86 Hufeland, *Ueber die Vergiftung durch Branntwein*, translated in Bynum, "Chronic Alcoholism in the First Half of the 19th Century," 162.

87 William F. Bynum, "Chronic Alcoholism in the First Half of the 19th Century," 161.

88 Andreas-Holger Maehle, *Drugs on Trial: Experimental Pharmacology and Therapeutic Innovation in the Eighteenth Century* (Amsterdam: Rodopi, 1999), 169.

89 C. von Brühl-Cramer, *Ueber die Trunksucht und eine rationelle Heilmethode derselben* (Berlin, 1819). Brühl-Cramer, though a descendant of a noble German family, remains a mystery. In fact, his first name has not yet been ascertained, sometimes appearing as Carl in Hasso Spode, *Die Macht der Trunkenheit: Kultur- und Sozialgeschichte des Alkohols in Deutschland* (Opladen: Leske & Budrich, 1993), 127; or Constantin in Maehle, *Drugs on Trial*, 185, and Wiesemann, *Die heimliche Krankheit*, 30. It is known that he practiced medicine in Russia first in Siberia and later in Moscow, dying there in 1821. See Friedrich-Wilhelm Kielhorn, "The History of Alcoholism: Brühl-Cramer's Concepts and Observations" *Addiction*, vol. 91/1 (1996), 121-128.

90 Brühl-Cramer, *Ueber die Trunksucht*, iii-iv.

sucht in other languages.[91] However, the translation of *Trunksucht* into dipsomania is misleading if the word is broken down into its parts – as Brühl-Cramer himself suggested in his own introduction.[92] Hufeland translated *Trunk* to *dipsa* in Greek, or thirst in English. *Sucht* was translated into *mania* in Greek and postclassical Latin, or madness in English. But Hufeland was imprecise. *Trunk* did not mean thirst, but rather meant "a drink, the act of drinking of any liquid though more likely of spirits, or drunkenness."[93] Nor was *Sucht* madness, but a disease. Thus, instead of dipsomania or the thirst madness, *Trunksucht* should have been translated as the drinking disease, or *morbus potus* in Latin.[94]

The drinking disease was a result of the immoderate consumption or enjoyment of intoxicating beverages.[95] According to Brühl-Cramer, it was "an evil influencing the population of many states, the morality of men, the domestic contentment of many families in a most detrimental way." Because the disease could hit anyone, Brühl-Cramer stressed that "it should be an object of intense attention of every man who as an upright citizen wants to contribute to the improvement and happiness of mankind. It is obvious that one can regard this topic from different standpoints: I, however, will try to investigate if the drinking disease is an object of pathology and if this illness can be consequently treated."[96] The disease, Brühl-Cramer argued, should remain in the realm of medicine, not morality, since the promise of a cure rested with doctors.[97]

Countering the common perception of both physicians and the general public, Brühl-Cramer argued:

> In general opinion, the excessive consumption of intoxicating beverages is not based on somatic, but on moral causes, and from this point of view it has

---

91 *Trunksucht* the noun should be separated from *trunksüchtig* the adjective, which is found in German as early as the 17th century and meant "devotion or degeneration [*verfallen*] to the drink." See Jacob and Wilhelm Grimm, *Deutsches Wörterbuch*, vol. 22 (Leipzig, 1854-1960), 1406. Dipsomania was used in English as early as 1843. See Bynum, "Chronic Alcoholism in the First Half of the 19th Century," 165.

92 Brühl-Cramer, *Ueber die Trunksucht*, viii.

93 Grimm, *Deutsches Wörterbuch*, 1375-1378, 1384.

94 Not until the 1870s, the word *Sucht* would attain a new meaning, that of addiction.

95 Brühl-Cramer, *Ueber die Trunksucht*, viii.

96 Ibid., 3. Translated with some modification in Kielhorn, "The History of Alcoholism," 121-128.

97 Spode, *Die Macht der Trunkenheit*, 127.

been supposed that the proper and only methods to remedy this malady might be those which produce aversion to spirituous liquors. For this reason certain cures were recommended or administered which provoke disgust or vomiting immediately after the consumption of inebriating beverages either by somatic means or by the contribution of imagination. Other measures based on prejudice are not to be mentioned.

The result of such a procedure most frequently had to be unsatisfactory; in other cases, however, it caused a breakdown of the remaining health. And so there is the popular, frequently not unfounded, opinion among the Russian people that a man would die soon after the cure of the drinking disease, but this opinion must not be applied to a rational method of treatment.[98]

The false appreciation of the disease as a moral failing resulted in poor treatment, causing fear and death among patients. Not only was the moral value attached to habitual drunkenness wrong, it was dangerous. Therefore, in order to find a rational treatment, a rational understanding of the disease was required. Morality had no place in the identification of the disease, nor did it have any place in its treatment. Nor, for that matter, was there a need to morally condemn the drinker, other than to note that the disease could cause moral weaknesses.[99]

"One could argue that the occasional cause of this illness may be immoral at least," Brühl-Cramer wrote. "The most frequent occasional cause is the consumption of spirits by itself. As long as the consumption of brandy is not considered immoral at all, it is difficult to decide in what degree morality can be invoked."[100] If a patient could not foresee that his drinking would result in a disease, he could not be morally condemned. Since, according to Brühl-Cramer, it was impossible to discern healthy drinkers from ill drinkers before they commenced drinking, morality could not serve as a measuring stick for identifying the sick from the healthy. In fact, as long as drinking alcohol remained a staple of society, the sick could not be blamed for their affliction. Observation led Brühl-Cramer to define seven characteristics of the disease:

1. Most patients felt that their illness was detrimental to their health and family. They tried to abstain from drinking, but their willpower betrayed them and an uncontrollable impulse forced them to drink, or otherwise suffer torturously.
2. The disease had a periodic cycle of remissions and intermissions.

---

98 Brühl-Cramer, *Ueber die Trunksucht*, 4-5, translated in Kielhorn, "The History of Alcoholism," 122.
99 Brühl-Cramer, *Ueber die Trunksucht*, 16-17.
100 Ibid., 8, translated in Kielhorn, "The History of Alcoholism," 123.

3. Early signs preceded attacks of the disease.
4. The length of each attack was within certain parameters.
5. Each attack ended with symptoms similar to other diseases.
6. Madness or even death might result if alcohol was withheld from a sick person at the beginning or during an outbreak of the disease.
7. The most important point: the disease could be cured.

Thus, Brühl-Cramer concluded, "the drinking disease is an involuntary evil, consequently a disease, and is not a reason for breach of morality, as is so often believed."[101] There were four types of the disease with varying degrees of severity from episodic to continuous. The episodic variety could be triggered by anger, shame or insults.[102] It functioned similar to gout attacks.[103] The continuous form of the disease was deemed the most serious, and described as an incessant desire for the drink, which resulted in daily vomiting.[104]

Brühl-Cramer's drinking disease had a significant insight which had hitherto been unheard of: the decision to drink was conscious and voluntary, but once the drinker fell ill, the continual desire to drink had turned into an involuntary urge. Alcohol dependence was not mere degeneration or an inability to control one's appetite, nor was it a moral failing. Rather, the disease manifested itself in a form of consciousness bound to an uncontrollable desire.[105] Naturally, this concept was only possible to articulate once humans were understood as independent and rational beings, and every person could realistically retain independence when living rationally.[106] The sick man's urge to drink consequently made his behavior irrational.

Perhaps the most revolutionary aspect of Brühl-Cramer's concept of the drinking disease was the fact that the disease was a physical disease, with physical manifestations such as abnormalities of the liver, swellings, hardening and inflammations.[107] The disease had other affects on the stomach,

---

101 Brühl-Cramer, *Ueber die Trunksucht*, 6-7.
102 Jann Schlimme, "Towards a Psychiatric Anthropology of Addiction" in *Philosophy and Psychiatry*, ed. Thomas Schramme and Johannes Thome (Berlin: De Gruyter, 2004), 275.
103 Bynum, "Chronic Alcoholism in the First Half of the 19th Century," 171.
104 Brühl-Cramer, *Ueber die Trunksucht*, 24-25.
105 Ibid., 10.
106 Schlimme, "Towards a Psychiatric Anthropology of Addiction," 275.
107 Brühl-Cramer, *Ueber die Trunksucht*, 60.

as well as neurological symptoms including trembling, and dullness and numbness of the senses.

Heredity was cited as one cause for the drinking disease, although Brühl-Cramer also noted external causes:[108]

> Violent annoyance, but mainly depressing feelings such as grief and sorrow produce – after an acquired disposition – an involuntary, more or less instinctive desire for the consumption of brandy which is drunk as a calming and amusing remedy, as a refreshing drink, and so this illness develops.

Disasters could also trigger the disease, he proposed, as in the case of the number of drinkers caused by Napoleon's capture of Moscow and the disaster that followed in 1812. Boredom was another culprit.[109] Other environmental causes for the disease were possible, such as physical exertion, warm weather and even the consumption of cold drinks.[110] Brühl-Cramer provided a scientifically sound theory that provided a direct causal link between the drink and the disease.

The treatment Brühl-Cramer proposed was simple, and logical. First and foremost, he prescribed vegetable acids, or sulfuric and nitric acids for the cure of the disease together with iron and a healthy diet. However, he insisted that the patient must genuinely desire to be cured. If the drunkard was happy with his state, he reasoned, why should anyone keep him from his pleasure?

Brühl-Cramer's liberal laissez-faire argument was also a matter of practicality. He claimed that if a patient did not wish to be cured, he would find ways to circumvent it. Thus, medicaments alone were not the sole methods for success, nor were chemical agents that rendered alcohol unpalatable.[111] He concluded by turning to his readers and asking:

> Imagine, if possible, a picture of the aftermath of this unnatural pleasure, and lament humankind for inventing such a seductive poison. Yet, keep hoping that a time will come, when a clear understanding of the sad outcome of this evil that affects the individual, family and the body politic will induce a practical legal measure that would at least reduce it.[112]

---

108 Kielhorn, "The History of Alcoholism," 126.
109 Brühl-Cramer, *Ueber die Trunksucht*, 10-11, 16, partially translated in Kielhorn, "The History of Alcoholism," 122-123.
110 Brühl-Cramer, *Ueber die Trunksucht*, 13-15.
111 Kielhorn, "The History of Alcoholism: Brühl-Cramer's Concepts and Observations," 125.
112 Brühl-Cramer, *Ueber die Trunksucht*, 92.

The drinking disease, like any other disease, was an unnatural evil that had to be overcome,[113] and this could only be achieved by implementing rational drinking laws. The gauntlet had been dropped, and German physicians and politicians were eager to pick it up. They worked incessantly to define, redefine and explain the disease as well as provide means to isolate the agent that caused it without attracting the ire of the people, who had been avid drinkers since time immemorial.

The identification of the drinking disease, free of moral condemnation and devoid of the devil's presence in the bottle, could be construed as a paradigm shift. But as with many medical developments in history, change came neither quickly nor smoothly, even among those identified with Brühl-Cramer's work.

In a guidebook to medicine first published in 1836, Hufeland retained a measure of moralizing in his definition of the drinking disease, which in addition to *Trunksucht* he referred to using the Greek term *polydipsia*:

> *Polydipsia.* Trunksucht
> Diagnosis: Insatiable thirst. Thirst, the necessity to drink, is like hunger; it is very relative and varies among individuals, appearing as a strong urge in some and weak in others. In this case also, habituation considerably takes effect.
> The morbid [*krankhafte*] thirst develops either due to inner heat (therefore it is a symptom of every fever, especially those caused by infections), or due to an increase in liquid evacuations (therefore in diarrhea, perspiration, diabetes), or also due to convulsive tightening of the inner exhalation of the mouth and throat (such as in hysteria, hypochondria and other nerve diseases). It can also be caused by jaundice.
> The treatment depends on the various causes. With special attention, one should consider it as a symptom of latent *diabetes mellitus*, of which it is often the only indication, and one should examine the urine. The same is true for liver diseases. I have cured it in one case, in which the patient had to drink more than 30 pounds of water a day, by a stay in Karlsbad [today Karlovy Vary] and also by dispensing pill No. 93. In nervous people I have seen a complete cure from a stay at the seacoast.
> More important and even sadder is the drinking disease caused by spirits, especially brandy wine [*Branntwein*]. It is always the result of a bad habituation, leading in the end to dropsy [*Wassersucht*], *delirium tremens*, hardening of the stomach, emaciation, and is difficult to heal.
> The means are: gradual withdrawal (with the gradual filling of the drinking glass with sealing wax), by switching to less harmful self-healing substitutes,

---

113 Gerald N. Grob, *The Deadly Truth: A History of Disease in America* (Cambridge MA: Harvard University Pree, 2002).

for example *Tinct. Absinth.*, by spoiling the brandy with the adverse usage of stimulating additives, such as tartar emetic; in addition benefits have been noted with mineral acids (*Elix. acid. Haller.*, 10, 20, drops 3 times a day) and *Quassia* (pills from *Extr. Quass.*, *Absinth*, *Cascarill.*)[114]

Although *polydipsia* is known today as an excessive consumption of liquids, usually among diabetics, it was understood differently in the 19th century. For Hufeland the drinking disease and *polydipsia* were related – both were caused by an insatiable desire to drink.[115] The habituation to either spirits or water was a symptom of the disease. The language of the text appears neutral at first glance, yet Hufeland's healing methods revealed a hint of moralizing, if not direct links to Galenic medicine. By suggesting that the sick should consume quassia extract, a bitter compound from the West Indies that was also used as an insecticide in the 19th century, one cannot escape the notion that he had hoped the drunkard would cleanse himself by self-flagellation. Perhaps this is an indication that the most famous physician in Prussia was not yet aware of the ever-elusive paradigm shift.

The two other suggested cures were also particularly bitter: cascarilla, or the extract from the croton eleutria plant, and the tincture of absinthe, or the legendary green fairy from which so many French Romantics and Impressionists hallucinated. In fact, absinthe was so bitter that the Romantics always consumed the drink with sugar and water to make it more palatable.

The tincture of absinthe contained alcohol, and might sound like a rather odd choice as a cure for the drinking disease to the modern reader. But using one drug to cure the habit caused by another is a recurring theme throughout history, with examples of treating morphinism with cocaine or alcoholism with ether. Incidentally – and presumably contrary to *Hufeland's* intentions – bitterness and alcohol were combined in the late 19th century by several distillers. Aside from gin and tonic, which was made of quinine: cascarilla added the bitter taste to Campari, and wormwood, the plant from which absinthe was produced, added the bitter taste to Vermouth.

---

114 Christoph Wilhelm Hufeland, *Enchiridion Medicum oder Anleitung zur medizinischen Praxis* (Berlin, 1842 [1836]), 198-199.

115 In later publications, the disease became known as *polydipsia ebriosa*. See "Oinomania; or the Mental Pathology of Intemperance" *The Journal of Psychological Medicine and Mental Pathology* 8 (1 April 1855), 176.

Hufeland was hardly the only follower of Brühl-Cramer for whom the lines separating vice from disease and physical illness from mental illness remained unclear. Carl Rösch (1807-1866), a physician who founded the Mariaberg asylum in the Western possessions of Prussia, claimed that habitual drunkenness was a product of external and internal conditions ranging from humanity's natural inclination for drunkenness to poverty.[116] By adopting parts of Brühl-Cramer's ideas, Rösch introduced a new one: The drinking disease was a mental illness, which caused physical degeneration.[117] He also claimed that the drinking disease was the number one cause of suicides in England, Germany and Russia in 1829. No less than a quarter of all suicides committed in Berlin between 1812 and 1821 could be attributed, he declared, in unmistakably morality-tinged terminology, to the "vice known as the drinking disease."[118]

Rösch distinguished between spirituous liquor and wine. The former was not a foodstuff and was the real cause of the ailment, whereas the latter was benign.[119] Consequently, only those who drank liquors and brandies were susceptible to contract the disease, which manifested itself in four mental conditions. The first of the conditions, the degeneration of morals and the temperament, manifested itself in two forms: Drunken savagery (*ferocitas ebriosa*), which occurred mostly with robust, uneducated people, primarily among the lower classes of society. With continued consumption of alcohol it led to imbecility. The other manifestation, which appeared primarily among the educated, was drunken discontentment. Expressed through the symptoms of unhappiness with the self and others, it caused, among other things, impotence and led to melancholia.

The second condition was the drinking disease (*Trunksucht*). Rösch directly acknowledged the struggle between morality and medicine, but left that debate to others with this combination of Thomas Trotter's (1760-1832) mental illness with Brühl-Cramer's physical disease: "I wish here only to note that the drinking disease begins as a vice and later turns

---

116 Carl Rösch, *Der Missbrauch geistiger Getränke in pathologischer, therapeutischer, medizinisch-polizeilicher und gerichtlicher Hinsicht* (Tübingen, 1839 [1838]), 154-157.

117 Sournia, *A History of Alcoholism*, 26-27.

118 Rösch, *Der Missbrauch geistiger Getränke*, 112.

119 Ibid., 8-9, 75-78.

into a disease."[120] There were three grades of the disease, separated by severity: a desire to drink more spirituous liquors, an almost uncontrollable desire for the drink, and an uncontrollable desire to drink which turned into a real monomania.

The third condition was drunken hallucination and drunken insanity (*sensuum fallacia* and *halucinatio ebriosa*). The manifestation of this condition was rarely among robust characters, and was often seen in persons with weak temperaments. The fourth and final of the mental disturbances caused by drunkenness (*vesania ebriosa*), such as *delirium tremens*, appeared only in those who misused spirituous drinks for a long period of time.[121] Rösch, notably, was not troubled by the fact that *delirium tremens* was identified in 1813 as a purely physical disease resulting in the withdrawal of alcohol from a person who was habituated to it.

For Rösch, "dypsomanie is therefore a disease of the nervous system. Similar to nymphomanie and other diseases, but it has deeper roots, and depends without a doubt, on the decomposition of the blood."[122] The drinking disease was a physical disease linked to mental weaknesses and social problems. It was, in a sense, a monomania with physical manifestations with pathologies in the stomach (constant inflammation), liver (cirrhosis of liver), lungs (thickening of the membrane surrounding the lungs), heart (flabby heart muscle) and brain (congestion of the veins).

Whether physical or not, Rösch considered the disease a vice, and the more rooted it was, the more severely the disease manifested itself.[123] As a social problem, drinking had to be controlled. He cited precedents for limiting drinking from ancient Greece and Rome, medieval edicts and even Muslim law. He believed in a series of legal measures against alcohol, including making intoxication a punishable offense.

Rösch proposed imposing higher taxes on ardent spirits, as well as forbidding the manufacture of spirits in times of crop failure. Alcohol production had to be controlled and limited, keeping prices up so as to make drinking prohibitive. He proposed that alcohol peddling be declared illegal, and that pubs be required both to be licensed and to serve food

---

120 Ibid., 8.
121 Ibid., 7-22.
122 Ibid., 37.
123 Ibid., 71.

with alcohol. These measures were to be enforced by the police.[124] Rösch's theories held wide sway until monomania as a mental disease fell out of grace in the 1840s. However, his ideas served as the basis for the comprehensive description of the alcohol disease by Magnus Huss and others.[125]

Magnus Huss (1807-1890), a Swedish physician, coined the term "Alcoholismus" in his treatise "*Chronische Alkoholskrankheit, oder Alcoholismus chronicus,*" which was first published in Swedish in 1849 but attained worldwide recognition after its appearance in German in 1852.[126] The term slowly percolated into English – as did other associated "isms," such as morphinism. Although it is noteworthy that heroinism and cocainism, which never gained much popularity. In German, however, *Morphinismus*, *Kokainismus* and *Heroinismus* remained the terms used to describe drug addiction until the mid 20th century, and *Alkoholismus* and *Trunksucht* were used interchangeably for the drinking disease.

The advent of alcoholism in the vocabulary of physicians did not necessarily imply that the disease was believed to be prevalent. As it is made clear in an anecdote recounted by several historians. One of Huss' nominators to the Prix Montyon of the *Acadèmie Française* reportedly stated: "Magnus Huss has collected a great deal of material relating to chronic alcoholism, a condition rarely seen in France."[127] Indeed, it took some time before addiction was recognized a problem in France and elsewhere.

Huss did not define alcoholism, but rather described it through clinical observation. He gave the disease its modern name, but also provided "the most sensitive clinical treatment of the 19th century."[128] He examined case

---

124 Ibid., 89-96, 99-106.

125 Bynum, "Chronic Alcoholism in the First Half of the 19th Century," 177, 180.

126 Magnus Huss, *Chronische Alkoholskrankheit, oder Alcoholismus chronicus; ein Beitrag zur Kenntniss der Vergiftungs-Krankheiten, nach eigener und anderer Erfahrung* (Stockholm and Leipzig, 1852 [1849]). In English: "the chronic alcohol disease, or chronic alcoholism."

127 Sournia, *A History of Alcoholism*, 49. For a different account, which Sournia discounts see Michael Marrus, "Social Drinking in the *Belle Epoque*," in *Journal of Social History* 7:4 (1974), 115-141: "At the time, Huss's work was crowned by the *Acadèmie Française* and given a special prize for its contribution to medical science. Alcoholism, however, was not seen as having any special significance for France. 'There may be a good many drunkards in France,' commented the *rapportuer* on awarding Huss the Prix Montyon, 'but happily there are no alcoholics.'"

128 Bynum, "Chronic Alcoholism in the First Half of the 19th Century," 185

after case of alcoholism, demonstrating how the disease affected his patients. If a death occurred, he provided a detailed report of the autopsy, a rarity at the time. He concluded that the illness manifested itself in two forms: chronic, and acute alcoholism (or alcohol poisoning.) Acute alcoholism affected the organism and manifested itself physically in the liver, spleen, blood and other organs. It could appear after a one-time poisoning, or after habitual drinking over a long period of time. Thus, *delirium tremens* was an acute disease resulting in chronic poisoning.[129] Like many physicians after him, Huss insisted that acute poisoning was different from chronic alcoholism, but had difficulties drawing a distinct division between the two.

The symptoms of chronic alcoholism affected the nervous system and were separated into three categories: motoric, sensory and mental. "This group of symptoms I wish to designate by the name *alcoholismus chronicus*, by which I understand those pathologic symptoms which develop in such persons who over a long period of time continually use wine or other alcoholic beverages in large quantities," Huss wrote in his treatise. "These symptoms do not [always] have a direct connection with organic changes of the nervous system."[130] In other words, no single straight line connected the symptoms. No physical cause was necessary, as a chronic alcoholic could appear healthy to an outside observer with no nerve or liver damage, even as the incessant appetite for alcohol made him sick. The alcoholic also suffered from nausea, vomiting, tremors, paralysis, vertigo, sensory loss and myriad other neurological problems, in addition to mental problems in the form of anxiety, dementia, hallucinations, melancholia and memory loss.[131]

As modern as Huss' conception of the disease might have been, his worldview was nonetheless trapped within the scientific thought of his day. In the final words of the introduction to his treatise, Huss mentioned "spontaneous combustion" as an independent form of alcoholism not related to either chronic or acute forms of the disease. Spontaneous combustion was a legendary disease in which a drunkard went up in flames after drinking alcohol. Huss was cautious. He suspected that the disease did not exist, yet he reported the experience of others. He

---

129 Huss, *Chronische Alkoholskrankheit*, 33-44.
130 Ibid, 3, translated in Bynum, "Chronic Alcoholism in the First Half of the 19th Century," 181.
131 Huss, *Chronische Alkoholskrankheit*.

described the color of the flame, blue, and the manner in which humans combusted due to the inner heat produced by brandy, first igniting in the respiratory system.[132]

Finally, Huss denied Brühl-Cramer's claim that alcoholism was hereditary, and attributed it to individual behavior or to the environment. Thus, he concluded, an alcoholic owed his disease to climate, place of residence, age, gender, temperament, constitution and occupation. Most alcoholics were poor, born into squalid conditions. The disease manifested among the middle aged, usually afflicting nervous people.[133] Perhaps the secret of Huss' success was the coinage of a simple term that was understood and which entered the tongues of the masses with ease. Although it took some time for his terminology to be adopted, particularly in English, once it did it became almost impossible to talk about the drinking disease without calling it alcoholism.

Drunkenness was believed to spread like an epidemic in the cities and countryside. As one popular medical text explained in 1867, the drunken father sets a bad example for his children, drawing them to a series of diseases, vices and criminal behavior: "The drinking disease becomes a local vice. And by turning into a local pest, it destroys the physical and the moral fiber of many generations… and makes a healthy, public life impossible."[134] Statistics from the neighboring Austrian Empire, meanwhile, reinforced belief in the concept of drinking disease, with data showing that habitual drinkers lived shorter lives.[135]

Cheap beer and wine attracted the poor to drink, and they in turn indulged in it, seeking their freedom in the bottle. However, alcoholism awaited them either as a physical or mental disease. Aside from harming the individual's health, the drinking disease was also perceived as a social problem. "A drunkard cannot be a good and honest father as much as he cannot be a useful citizen of a state," one medical text warned in 1867. "Either he becomes a tyrant to his children, or he teaches them all manners

---

132 Ibid., 44-46.
133 Ibid., 503-537.
134 Eduard Reich, *Die Ursachen der Krankheiten der physischen und der moralischen* (Leipzig, 1867), 188.
135 Sournia, *A History of Alcoholism*, 26. On Franz Wilhelm Lippich (1799-1845) statistic work, see Bynum, "Chronic Alcoholism in the First Half of the 19th Century," 175-176.

of vice to which they become habituated."[136] The conclusion was simple: he who poisoned the family with the drinking disease endangered society.[137]

Huss himself explicitly declared the socially-driven aims of his research:

> Allow me, therefore, to foster the hope that through this treatise of science a small contribution is delivered to the teacher of religion and to the friends of humanity, to be used as a weapon in the fight against the vice of the drinking disease; and more so, that it will provide the drunken sot himself a few warnings and frightful examples; then my goal is achieved, and the labor, which I herewith address, are heftily rewarded.[138]

Huss's translator, Gerhard van dem Busch of Bremen, was even more explicit in his criticism, claiming that the Germans had mistakenly ignored the efforts of the temperance societies and not taken the drinking disease seriously enough. Instead of fighting against the disease, the agitation against alcohol only declined, "giving inducement to all types of intemperance."[139] Echoing Huss' introductory remarks, the translator hoped the book would increase the understanding of the sins of drunkards – a development from which the temperance societies in Germany could only gain.[140]

More ammunition against the drink was exactly what the German temperance societies required, since the consumption of spirits increased at an alarming rate at the beginning of the 19th century. According to a contemporary estimate, Prussians' thirst for spirits trebled between 1806 and 1831, increasing from three to over nine liters of pure alcohol per person, per year. Spirits overshadowed both beers and wines, of which the production of the former was on the decline and the latter of little significance. In essence, Prussians not only drank more, they drank harder. The 1840s marked a temporary decline in alcohol consumption in Germany, probably due to the economic recession that culminated in the Revolution of 1848. With the restoration of law and order in Germany, consumption of both spirits and beer increased in the 1850s until they reached their

---

136 Reich, *Die Ursachen der Krankheiten der physischen und der moralischen.*, 191
137 Ibid., 192. See also Huss, *Chronische Alkoholskrankheit*, 508-509.
138 Ibid., v.
139 Ibid., viii.
140 Ibid., ix.

peak after unification in the 1870s, after which beer continued to increase and spirits began to decline.[141]

Beer remained a staple in German production, consumption and society. German beer consumption reached its highest level in 1909, at 118 liters per person, decreasing slightly to 102 liters in 1913. During World War I, consumption sank sharply, dropping to 39 liters in 1918.[142] After the war, consumption steadily rose. One estimate showed that 6.7 percent of an individual's salary was spent on alcohol in 1935.[143] Other estimates were higher. In 1933-1934, Germans spent 4 billion Reichsmark on alcohol.[144] An estimated 13.5 million bottles of Sekt (German champagne) were opened in 1936, comparable to the number of bottles opened before the outbreak of World War I.[145] Prosperity and peace brought with them alcohol and drunkenness, in turn fueling the temperance societies' cracking of their moral whips against the growing legion of evil sinners.

The great landowners of East Prussia, the Junkers, were also the great distillers. They converted the grain grown on their land by tenant farmers into spirits and beer sold in the cities, wielding extraordinary financial power. For example, the brewing industry alone was worth 718 million Marks in capital stocks in 1913-1914, second only to machine tools.[146] Their clout was enormous. In 1837, King Friedrich Wilhelm III

---

141 James S. Roberts, "Long-Term Trends in the Consumption of Alcoholic Beverages" in *The State of Humanity*, ed. Julian L. Simon (Oxford: Oxford University Press, 1995), 115-116.

142 Teich, "The Industrialization of Brewing in Germany (1800-1914)," 102-113.

143 Alexander Elster, *Das Konto des Alkohols in der deutschen Volkswirtschaft* (Berlin, 1935), reprinted in *Nazis on Speed*, Vol. 1, ed. Werner Pieper (Munich: Grüne Kraft, 2002), 42-44.

144 Gerhart Feuerstein, *Rauschgiftbekaempfung-ein wichtiges Interessengebiet der Gemeindverwaltung* (Berlin, 1936), p.8.

145 "Summary of the Stettin Conference (10 October 1937)," StA—München, Pol. Dir. 7582.

146 Mikuláš Teich, "The Industrialization of Brewing in Germany (1800-1914)," in *Production, Marketing and Consumption of Alcoholic Beverages since the Late Middle Ages*, ed. Erik Aerts et al. (Lueven: Leuven University Press, 1990), 102-113. Please note, 718 million Marks were roughly equivalent to 170 million dollars at the time (the average daily rate was 4.2 Marks per dollar.) A comparison between the two countries is difficult to recreate due to scanty data. The capital stock value of the beer industry in the United States was probably larger than in Germany, since the production value of beer reached about a quarter of a billion dollars in 1900. See Committee of Fifty, *The Liquor Problem: A Summary of Investigations Conducted, 1893-1903* (New York, 1970 [1905]), 128.

(1770-1840) – influenced by his personal physician, Hufeland – ordered a decrease in the consumption of spirits, but this early Prussian attempt at controlling the drinking disease did not succeed.[147] The farmers and great landowners had too great of an interest in the alcohol industry. They did not treat alcohol as a secondary source of income, but as their primary one. Unlike in the United States, where alcohol production remained mostly in the hands of small farms, alcohol production in Germany was a well-developed and profitable industry.[148]

In the 19th century, not all doctors agreed with physicians being recruited to the temperance warriors' cause. Friedrich Wilhelm Böcker (1818-1861) of the University of Bonn claimed in 1845, "The dipsomaniacs are insane. They belong in an asylum and not in the hands of priests and the medical laity."[149] Böcker's animosity against the German temperance movement was directed against priests and other men professing morality, since they beat on the moral drums against a vice while ignoring Brühl-Cramer's physical disease.[150]

Other physicians were distrustful of those who preached teetotalism. Johann Ludwig Casper (1796-1864) claimed that the rhetoric of the temperance societies, by advocating tea instead of alcohol, only resulted in increasing the consumption of opium; thus, people substituted one intoxicant for another.[151] His chief point, however, was that "it yet remains to be proven that cases of dipsomania (always isolated and rare) have been actually cured by purely voluntary abstinence."[152] Clearly, both Casper and Böcker wished to protect the prerogative of physicians to treat their patients from priests and moralists.

---

147 Alfred Heggen, *Alkohol und Bürgerliche Gesellschaft im 19. Jahrhundert* (Berlin: Colloquium Verlag, 1988), 96-109.

148 Edward Kremers, "Agricultural Alcohol: Studies of its Manufacture in Germany," in *Bulletin of the U.S. Department of Agriculture* 182 (2 February 1915).

149 Quoted in Spode, *Die Macht der Trunkenheit*, 131. Böcker used the word *Trunksüchtigen* in German, but the term 'dipsomaniacs' is used here for simplicity's sake.

150 Ibid., 129-131.

151 Johann Ludwig Casper, *A Handbook of the Practice of Forensic Medicine, based upon Personal Experience*, George William Balfour (tr.), (London, 1865 [1856]), 267-268.

152 Ibid.

Attacked by both drinkers and physicians, the German temperance societies realized that their goal could not be total abstention from alcohol, as had been pursued in the United States, but rather moderation. Abraham Adolf Baer (1857-1908), a district physician of Berlin and the chief physician of the Plötzensee prison as well as one of the leaders of the German temperance movement and an honorary member of the American Association for the Cure of Inebriates,[153] wrote in 1880 that the state had no choice but to regulate the drinking sin, which was responsible for social ailments including crime, insanity and poverty.

Baer recognized that prohibition, like the version enforced in Maine in 1851, was ineffective. Although he believed it a noble idea, he realized that a ban could not stand for long because of the political pressure exerted by drinkers. Thus, barring prohibition, "one of the most effective prophylactic measures against the increase of the drinking disease is the decrease of the number of bars with the full force of the law."[154] Baer was aware that such a measure would not stop those who already suffered from the disease, but it could prevent others from succumbing to it.[155] Taxation and licensing were imperative in reducing the number of bars, saloons and restaurants selling alcohol.

Any relaxation of the law would be disastrous. For example, the requirement for a liquor license was abolished in Bremen, leaving only a tax on alcohol. This caused the number of bars to rise from 521 in 1863 (when the licensing requirement was abolished) to 728. By 1867, no less than 829 bars were operating in the city. The numbers were so high that the city-state's Senate considered reinstating the need for licensing and concessions.[156] In Prussia, where the licensing system was lax,[157] the number of liquor stores rose from 116,811 in October 1869 to 129,672 in

---

153 In 1904, Baer was criticized by *Die Zeit am Montag* and *Vorwärts* for his cruelty towards mentally ill prisoners. The case was used as an example of the changing attitudes towards crimes committed by the insane. See Benjamin Carter Hett, *Death in the Tiergarten: Murder and Criminal Justice in the Kaiser's Berlin* (Cambridge MA: Harvard University Press, 2004), 197-198.

154 Abraham Adolph Baer, "Gesetzliche Maßregeln zur Bekämpfung der Trunksucht" *Preußische Jahrbücher* 46 (1880), 603.

155 Ibid., 604.

156 Ibid., 608

157 James S. Roberts, *Drink, Temperance and the Working Class in Nineteenth-Century Germany* (Boston: Allen & Unwin, 1984), 50.

January 1872, and the number of bars rose from 42,612 in 1868 to 69,305 in 1877.[158]

Fear of social unrest caused by the economic depression of 1878-1879 prompted the Reichstag to enact a law in July 1879 enabling the local authorities to limit – as they saw fit – the number of bars and their licenses. For a moment, the danger of alcohol was taken seriously in Berlin. Prompted by Baer, in 1881 the Reichstag discussed a bill, known as the *Trunksuchtgesetz*, on the punishment of drunkenness.[159] The provisions of the bill assessed fines and confinement to those found guilty, with repeat offenders forced to eat only bread and water, and in the most extreme cases sent to hard labor. The bill passed the first parliamentary reading and was sent to a committee for deliberation. But before a second reading could be arranged, election losses suffered by the National Liberals and Conservatives in 1881 shelved the bill.[160]

Ten years later, the government tried to pass a similar bill. Kaiser Wilhelm II (1859-1941) himself expressed an interest in the legislation, believing that effective controls on alcohol had to be imposed before wage increases, since more money in the workers' pockets would result in more drinking. Chancellor Otto von Bismarck (1815-1898) was reluctant to support the law, but when he was removed from office in 1890 his objections became moot. The new chancellor, Leo von Caprivi (1831-1899), who was in favor of the bill, could not push it through the newly elected Reichstag. The landowners of the East, despite claiming that they wanted controls over drinking, wished to protect their liquor production. The Socialists believed that there were more pressing bills than drinking controls, and the Liberals wished to curry favor with petit bourgeois pub owners. In the end, the 1891 bill on fighting the drinking disease was never signed into law.[161]

The failure of the *Trunksuchtgesetz* in 1881 gave new impetus to reformers, and brought about the formation of two temperance organizations in 1883. The first was the *Blaues Kreuz*, or Blue Cross, which was founded by a priest named Louis-Lucien Rochat (1849-1917) in Switzer-

---

158 Baer, "Gesetzliche Maßregeln zur Bekämpfung der Trunksucht," 609-610.
159 *Trunksuchtgesetz* literally translates as the Drinking Disease Law.
160 Heggen, *Alkohol und Bürgerliche Gesellschaft im 19. Jahrhundert*, 142-143; Roberts, *Drink, Temperance and the Working Class in Nineteenth-Century Germany*, 52-53.
161 Ibid., 74-77.

land and was to be modeled after the Red Cross, including its religious undertone. The second was the secular *Deutscher Verein gegen den Missbrauch geistiger Getränke* (DV), or German Association Against the Misuse of Spirits, which relied on science.[162] Membership was never high. The DV counted only 36,618 members in 1911. The Total Abstinence Societies, a confederation of 30 independent organization of a religious bent including the Good Templars and the Blue Cross, had 125,893 members.[163] There was also a German branch of the Woman's Christian Temperance Union, with about 2,600 members in 1912.[164]

The rivalry between the organizations often crippled their efforts. They could not agree whether their goal should be abstention or temperance. "Was there at least agreement, by the turn of the century, that chronic alcoholism was a disease that could be cured only by serious medical attention?" one historian rhetorically asked. "Not at all, for some church-related groups stressed the central importance of prayer in any cure. As late as 1927, the Protestant Blue Cross organization was still issuing pamphlets that talked of alcoholism as a sin that could never be healed by medicine alone."[165] Those undertaking the moral crusade refused to acknowledge the drinking disease, but their numbers were few and their infighting was too great to influence German politics or medicine.

Toward the end of the 19th century, political ideologues joined in the chorus against the drink; among the most vocal were the Socialists, who wanted to keep workers sober. In 1876, Friedrich Engels explained in "Prussian Schnapps in the German Reichstag" how the Junkers, the great landlords and military leaders of Prussia, could not have existed without their distilleries, where they turned their excess of potato yields into spirits: "With the collapse of the distilleries, Prussian militarism shall

---

162 Ibid., 52-54.
163 "How Germany is trying to solve her Temperance Problem" in *Current Literature* 50:6 (1911), 636-637. Between 1884 and 1913, the number of members grew from about 6,000 to 41,000. See Heggen, *Alkohol und Bürgerliche Gesellschaft im 19. Jahrhundert*, 143.
164 Ian Tyrrell, *Woman's World, Woman's Empire: The Woman's Christian Temperance Union in International Perspective, 1880-1930* (Chapel Hill: North Carolina University Press, 1991), 64.
165 Geoffrey J. Giles, "Drinking and Crime in Modern Germany" in *Criminals and Their Scientists: The History of Criminology in International Perspective*, ed. Peter Becker and Richard F. Wetzell (Cambridge: Cambridge University Press, 2006), 477.

collapse, and without it, Prussia is nothing."[166] Alcohol, in short, served as the financial lifeline of the political elite and German Imperialism. But alcohol also served to finance the German temperance movement as well. In July 1918, just before the end of the war, the government formed a liquor monopoly that spent four million Marks to mitigate the damage caused by the drink, and most temperance movements (save for the Blue Cross) were invited to make suggestions how to spend the money.[167]

German Socialists did not blame the drink for the inability of the masses to develop class-consciousness, as other temperance organizations had hoped they would. After all, the neighborhood pub was the only place where workers could meet unmolested.[168] The DV, though not a Socialist organization, also feared that drunkenness among laborers reduced productivity, among other malefic effects of alcohol.[169] Not surprisingly, abstinence was not popular among workers before or after the war attested by the dismal membership of the social-democratic *Arbeiter-Abstinenten-bund* (Workers' Abstinence Union), which boasted 3,300 members in 1924.[170]

When the issue of alcohol was raised in the Reichstag in 1891, the newly elected Socialist party fell on the far side of the fence. They argued that the government's attempts to enact laws against public drunkenness were nothing more than a smokescreen that was meant to dupe the public from debating the true causes of the workers' misery.[171] The ideological concerns raised by Engels were set aside for political considerations.

In general, attitudes toward alcohol at the time were more moderate in Germany than in the United States. The German abstainers did not share the American obsession against alcohol, and in fact feared that American fanaticism would spread in Germany. According to the observation of an American teacher in Germany, the abstainer in the "Empire of Beer" was

---

166 Quoted in Heggen, *Alkohol und Bürgerliche Gesellschaft im 19. Jahrhundert*, 22-23.
167 Claudius Torp, *Konsum und Politik in der Weimarer Republik* (Göttingen: Vandenhoeck & Ruprecht, 2011), 250.
168 Roberts, *Drink, Temperance and the Working Class in Nineteenth-Century Germany*, 83-88.
169 Ibid., 68.
170 Torp, *Konsum und Politik in der Weimarer Republik*, 249.
171 Roberts, *Drink, Temperance and the Working Class in Nineteenth-Century Germany*, 74-75. The Socialist party was banned in Germany in 1878, but was allowed back in the Reichstag in 1890.

molested and ridiculed. Whereas the Germans did not bother those who drank a little, they tended to make fun of those who abstained completely. In a small city of 150,000 people, the traveling American teacher found only four teetotalers, all of whom had bad experiences whenever they went to the local pub, or *Kneipe*.[172]

By the end of the 19th century, there were three types of non-political temperance societies in Germany: those which were espoused by the Catholic Church, those which were espoused by the Protestant Church (mostly Lutheran), and thirdly, lay organizations that relied on scientific research and physicians for guidance.

The temperance societies struggled against the deeply ingrained role of alcohol in society. At any gathering of any sort, alcohol had be consumed, a phenomenon they dubbed *Trinkzwang*, or drinking compulsion. The societies pushed for enacting laws against natives drinking alcohol in Germany's colonies, and attempted to revive the *Trunksuchtgesetz* in 1891, but to no avail.[173] In the end, these associations failed in their quest. Germans continued to drink, and physicians continued to treat the drinking disease.

Where the temperance movement failed, however, eugenicists succeeded. Racism and the fear of racial degeneration fueled the fears of alcohol through what appeared to be objective scientific facts. Specialists, whether physicians or racial anthropologists from varied political back-grounds, agreed that certain races were susceptible to different drugs, and that a continued consumption of alcohol by an individual caused the degeneration of his or her progeny.

Brühl-Cramer noted in 1819 that heredity might be a cause of the drinking disease, even skipping a generation, and thus a grandfather and a grandson might succumb to the disease without it affecting the father.[174] Alcohol, as the agent of the disease, not only affected the physical body of the patient, but also the bodies of his children. The idea that heredity caused the drinking disease remained unsettled for decades afterward (Huss, for example, rejected it), but by the end of the 19th century, most

---

172 W. A. Averill, "The Teetotaler in the Empire of Beer," in *The Independent* 68:3211 (16 June 1910), 1344-1345.

173 "How Germany is trying to solve her Temperance Problem" in *Current Literature* 50:6 (1911), 636-637.

174 Kielhorn, "The History of Alcoholism," 126.

German physicians believed that heredity played some role in the contraction of the disease.

In a report written by the Ministry of Justice in preparation for the *Trunksuchtgesetz* of 1881, the government justified the law by relying on science and medicine:

> It is sufficient to point out... a large proportion of suicides (8-16 percent in Germany) and a still greater proportion of mental illnesses derive from excessive alcohol abuse, and the latter also represents the most common source of pauperism, encourages prostitution, undermines the sense of public order and respect for law, and that its effects on physical and mental being are inherited by future generations, leading to degeneration.[175]

Eugenics and the degeneration of the German people had long troubled the government. It could rely on a long list of specialists who feared the degeneration of the German people. The 1881 law failed to pass, but the heredity aspect of the disease still received a legal hearing. In an explanation of the status of mental diseases in the rule of law in Germany, the Viennese psychiatrist Ludwig Schlager (1828-1885) wrote in 1882 that a court-appointed physician must investigate perpetrators' hereditary diseases – and the drinking disease was listed as one – before submitting his report to the judge.[176]

Abraham Adolf Baer, the Berlin physician and temperance movement leader, admitted in an 1893 study on the causes of crime that poverty drove most criminals, but noted in passing the role of degeneration caused by the drinking disease and vice in parents, which affected the criminal behavior of their children. No less than 41.7 percent of convicts imprisoned in 120 institutions in 1876 were drinkers, of which almost half suffered from the drinking disease.[177] The link between crime, heredity and disease was therefore established.

In 1903, the psychiatrist Gustav Aschaffenburg (1866-1944), one of the most influential criminologists in Germany until the Nazis forced him out of the country in 1933 because of his Jewish heritage, established the link between alcohol and criminality. Alcohol and alcoholism both contributed to crime, the former directly and the latter indirectly. In addition to the fact

---

175 Quoted in Giles, "Drinking and Crime in Modern Germany" 474.

176 Ludwig Schlager, "Die Bedeutung und die Aufgaben der Irrengesetzgebung im Rechtsstaate" in *Die gerichtliche Psychopathologie* (Tübingen, 1882), 86.

177 Abraham Adolph Baer, *Der Verbrecher in Anthropologischer Beziehung* (Leipzig, 1893), 155-156, 265-267.

that the descendents of alcoholics often suffered from hereditary diseases, Aschaffenburg claimed that they were also susceptible to commit crimes, either due to poor family life or an inability to succeed in life under lawful circumstances. Furthermore, the criminologist argued, the need to finance the habit of drinking forced many drunkards to commit petty theft. Alcoholics and occasional drunkards were over-represented in prisons and jails, and among them, the occasional drunkards seemed to have more problems with the law, especially on payday when a substantial portion of the workman's salary was spent on booze, leading to violence. Alcohol should therefore be restricted in Germany to save the future of the workmen, students and clerks who occasionally drank and consequently committed crimes.[178]

Physicians and psychiatrists often advocated temperance to deal with the German drinking problem. Perhaps the two most famous temperance psychiatrists were Emil Kraepelin (1856-1926) and Richard von Krafft-Ebing (1840-1902). The latter was particularly concerned with degeneration, but attributed alcohol excesses to poverty and occupation, rather than heredity.[179] Yet he conceded that heredity played a role in the "abnormal constitution" of the habitual drinker.[180] He wrote in 1879 that the first symptoms a chronic alcoholic manifested were poor ethics and morals. Alcoholism went hand in hand with emotional irritability and violence. In the mornings, depression and even suicidal tendencies could be identified among alcoholics, until they indulged in excessive drinking for which they were responsible: "An early manifestation in the psychic domain is a remarkable degree of weakness of the will toward the fulfillment of the duties of occupation, and especially those of citizenship." And "with these symptoms finally there is a progressive diminution of intellectual power *in*

---

178 Gustav Aschaffenburg, *Das Verbrechen und seine Bekämpfung* (Heidelberg, 1903), 55-72. Aschaffenburg was a specialist in alcohol diseases, writing his doctoral thesis on *delirium tremens*. He relied on Baer's statistics regarding alcoholics in prisons, upon which he based his conclusions. See 59-60. Aschaffenburg was also a student of Emil Kraepelin in Heidelberg, to whom the book was dedicated.

179 Richard von Krafft-Ebing, *Text-Book of Insanity based on Clinical Observation for Practitioners and Students of Medicine* (Philadelphia, 1905 [1879]), 154-155.

180 Idem, *Grundzüge der Criminalpsychologie auf Grundlage des Strafgesetzbuchs des deutschen Reichs für Aerzte und Juristen* (Erlangen, 1872), 110.

toto."[181] Finally, about 80 percent of male alcoholics suffered from a delusion of being sexually deceived by either their wives or mistresses.[182]

Aside from the mental disturbances in chronic alcoholics, there were also physical manifestations of the disease, such as circulatory disturbances in the brain that caused symptoms like headaches, dizziness, heaviness, confusion, mental embarrassment and restless sleep. In addition, alcoholics suffered from reduced motor functions and sensory disturbances, as well as a reduced libido. Krafft-Ebing stressed that chronic alcoholics could not be treated privately and ought to be treated in hospitals, or asylums. Forced confinement was justified because the patient was not in control of his mental faculties. Finally, treatments with quinine or other bitter substances employed in private practice, as advocated by Hufeland earlier in the century, were deemed useless.[183]

Contrary to Huss, who believed in mental and behavioral causes for alcoholism, a new wave of German or German-speaking clinicians sought the origins of alcoholism in heredity. In the 1880s, Emil Kraepelin, at the time one of the most influential psychiatrists in Germany, cited sources claiming that no less than 80 percent of chronic alcoholics suffered from defective heredity.[184] He quoted Tacitus, who had declared 1,800 years earlier that the Germanic race was prone to drink excessively, a habit that only became worse over the centuries until the average worker in Prussia spent 17-20 percent of his wages on alcohol.

Although Kraepelin conceded that alcohol misuse was also a sign of poverty, he was certain that it was a poison that affected the reproductive

---

181 Idem, *Text-Book of Insanity based on Clinical Observation for Practitioners and Students of Medicine*, 512-514.

182 Ibid.; See also A. Ross Diefendorf, ed. *Clinical Psychiatry: A Text-Book for Students and Physicians, Abstracted and Adapted from the seventh German edition of Kraepelin's 'Lehrbuch der Psychiatrie'* (New York, 1915 [1907]), 54.

183 Krafft-Ebing, *Text-Book of Insanity*, 514-519.

184 Emil Kraepelin, *Psychiatrie: Ein Lehrbuch für Studierende und Aerzte*, 6th ed., vol. 1 (Leipzig, 1899), 47-48; Ibid., Vol. 2, 70-72. See also Diefendorf (ed.), *Clinical Psychiatry*, 165. In the first edition of Kraepelin's textbook published in 1883 drug intoxication and drug addiction do not appear. Only in the third edition of his book published in 1887 do they appear as "chronic intoxications," "alcoholism" and "morphinism." In the fourth edition, "cocainism" was added. In the sixth edition published in 1899 "acute" and "chronic intoxications" were added as sub-groups. See Thomas Szasz, *Ceremonial Chemistry* (Garden City NJ: Doubleday, 1974), 6 - 7.

system, thereby afflicting generations to come.[185] He considered intoxication from alcohol as one of the most dangerous forms of mental disturbances, together with the effects of syphilis.[186]

Kraepelin may have been the more famous psychiatrist, but the most influential figure in the new field of abstinence medicine was arguably Swiss researcher August Forel (1848-1931).[187] He was a man of many contradictions. He was a member of the Church affiliated Blue Cross, but converted to the Bahai'i faith. He was a pacifist, but seemed to be content with the thought that whole races would disappear from the face of the Earth to fulfill their Darwinian destiny.[188] He was the first European physician to sterilize a patient on eugenic grounds, removing the regenerative organs of a hysterical woman at the Burghölzli clinic in Zurich in 1886.[189] And yet in 1908 he founded the International Order of Ethics and Culture, an organization whose purpose was to replace Christian morality with scientific truth.[190]

According to Forel, no less than half of all crimes and venereal diseases were caused by alcohol misuse, or while people were under the influence of alcohol. Excessive drinking was responsible for more than 10 percent

---

185 Kraepelin, *Psychiatrie*, Vol. 1, 44-45. Kraepelin often quoted Abraham Baer regarding alcohol.

186 Eric J. Engstrom, "Emil Kraepelin: Leben und Werk des Psychiaters im Spannungsfeld zwischen positivistischer Wissenschaft und Irrationalität," (MA thesis, Ludwig-Maximilians-Universität Munich, 1990), 106.

187 The Viennese neuroanatomist and professor of nervous diseases, Theodor Meynert taught August Forel and Sigmund Freud. See Otto M. Marx, "Nineteenth-Century Medical Psychology: Theoretical Problems in the Work of Griesinger, Meynert, and Wernicke," *Isis* 61:3 (1970), 356, 362.

188 Richard Weikart, "Progress through Racial Extermination: Social Darwinism, Eugenics, and Pacifism in Germany, 1860-1918," *German Studies Review* 26:2 (2003), 284.

189 Donald K. Pickens, "The Sterilization Movement: The Search for Purity in Mind and State," *Phylon*, vol. 28/1 (1967), 83; Hans Jakob Ritter and Volker Roelcke, "Psychiatric Genetics in Munich and Basel between 1925 and 1945: Programs-Practices-Cooperative Arrangements," *Osiris* 20 (2005), 276; Marie E. Kopp, "Surgical Treatment as Sex Crime Prevention Measure," *Journal of Criminal Law and Criminology* 28:5 (1938), 698.

190 Richard Weikart, "Darwinism and Death: Devaluing Human Life in Germany, 1859-1920," *Journal of the History of Ideas* 63:2 (2002), 326. Forel was also an active member of the *Monist League* founded by Ernst Haeckel in 1906, see Daniel Gasman, *The Scientific Origins of National Socialism* (New Brunswick NJ: Transaction Publishers, 2004 [1971]), 21.

of deaths in Swiss cities. He cited statistics compiled by English life insurance companies that showed that alcohol significantly reduced the life expectancy of the drinker.

Most importantly, Forel declared, alcohol degenerated the race. It poisoned the germ cells of the organism, thus resulting in the degeneration of subsequent generations.[191] Ethanol was not only a danger to heredity, but also poisoned the protoplasm, or the living content of the cell. It caused the deformation of the fat within the cell and the atrophy and contraction of the protoplasm. Temperate drinking was also ineffective, since drinking alcohol reduced motor activities, mental and physical faculties.[192] The conclusion, in Forel's eyes, was clear: Whereas drinking might loosen the tongue, the alcohol made it dumber. He stated that there was no real use for alcohol in social settings or in the practice of medicine. After all, there were more effective narcotics that did not cause the associated depressions and dangers to the human body. "The voices of the facts consistently demonstrate to us, to the individual, as well as to the public and to racial hygiene: Away with alcohol in the normal diet," Forel concluded. The Swiss researcher took to the road to spread his theories, traveling across Europe to convince university students to stop drinking, and in general delivering a message that alcohol should be banned.[193]

Three of Forel's students continued his teachings on alcohol: Alfred Ploetz (1860-1940), Eugen Bleuler (1857-1939) and Ernst Rüdin (1874-1952). Ploetz, one of the founders of racial hygiene as an academic discipline, was first introduced to questions of heredity after working with

---

191 August Forel, "Abstinenz oder Mäßigkeit?" *Grenzfragen des Nerven- und Seelenlebens* 74 (1910), 1-26. Forel relied on the German biologist August Weismann (1834-1914), who developed the Germ plasm theory (or *Keimplasma* in German). According to Weismann, an organism consisted of two types of cells: 'germ cells' (*Keimzellen* in German) and 'somatic cells.' The former, found in sperm and the egg, transmitted the inherited characteristics of the organism to the following generation. See August Weismann, *The Germ-Plasm: A Theory of Heredity* (New York, 1893 [1892]).

192 Forel, "Abstinenz oder Mäßigkeit?" Forel primarily uses here Emil Kraepelin's tests on alcohol's effect on mental faculties.

193 August Forel, "Die Trinksitten: Ihre Hygienische und Sociale Bedeutung, ihre Beziehungen zur Akademischen Jugend. Eine Ansprache an den Enthaltsamkeits-Verein der Studenten zu Christiana und zu Upsala am 7. und 13. September 1890," (Stuttgart, 1891) at HUJI-ML, IZAK 76D 8694.

Forel, who had sworn him to alcohol abstinence.[194] "The belief that alcoholism is a degenerative disease of the entire race reached an increasingly larger audience in England, North America, Scandinavia and recently in Switzerland," Ploetz wrote in 1893. "But more accurate evidence demonstrated that only a certain part of the race, not more than a 10th, would be harmed. Whether this is enough to bring forth the degeneration of the entire race in reality remains disputable."[195] And yet Ploetz quoted Baer in his estimate that each year more than 10,000 patients were sent to German hospitals for treatment of chronic alcoholism. In addition to these allegedly visible victims of alcohol misuse, the drinking disease caused an unknown number of cases of deaths, broken families, defective children, and crimes that result in incarceration.[196] Although not perceived as a danger to the entire race, alcohol and alcoholism clearly remained a problem.

Ploetz, aside from his avowed temperance, believed that sexual selection, or the idea that those with desired racial traits should be allowed to breed, was the key to save the race from oblivion. He viewed Socialism and its professed equality as a danger to the survival of the race, therefore linking his profession with politics. He also influenced his brother-in-law, Rüdin, a Swiss psychiatrist who moved to Munich to work in Kraepelin's clinic in 1909. In 1917, Rüdin became the director of the Genealogical-Demographic Department at the German Institute for Psychiatric Research, which Kraepelin had founded a decade earlier.[197] After a short hiatus, Rüdin enlarged his department in 1928 and in 1931 he was appointed as the head of the Institute for Psychiatric Research. After the Nazi rise to power in 1933, he secured even more financial support for his programs, among which was the sterilization of severe alcoholics.[198]

---

194 Sheila F. Weiss, "The Race Hygiene Movement in Germany," *Osiris* 3 (1987), 200.

195 Alfred Ploetz, *Die Tüchtigkeit unserer Rasse und der Schutz der Schwachen: Ein Verusch über Rassenhygiene und ihr Verhältniss zu den humanen Idealen, besonders zum Socialismus*, Vol. 1 (Berlin, 1895 [1893]), 190.

196 Ibid., 191-193.

197 The *Institute* was a part of the *Kaiser Wilhelm Society* and served as a model to other institutes around the world, see Ritter and Roelcke, "Psychiatric Genetics in Munich and Basel between 1925 and 1945," 263-264.

198 Matthias M. Weber, "Ernst Rüdin, 1874-1952: A German Psychiatrist and Geneticist" *American Journal of Medical Genetics. Part B, Neuropsychiatric Genetics* 67:4 (1996), 323-331.

Bleuler, Forel's successor at Burghölzli and another of Rüdin's teachers, believed that one-fifth of his patients suffered from a physical impairment of the nervous system, and that that physical impairment was responsible for their mental state. For the remaining majority of his patients, Bleuler employed Sigmund Freud's psychoanalysis as a means of treatment.[199] Whereas Bleuler was a supporter of psychoanalysis in psychiatry, he relied upon Kraepelin's theories regarding alcohol, claiming that although little was known about the origins of the disease, three pathologies caused chronic alcohol poisoning, two of which were due to hereditary disposition that spoiled, among other things, the ethics of the patient.[200]

Bleuler declared that alcohol misuse caused crime and ruined families. Only once the biological nature of the criminal was identified, as he was certain would be the case, and the causes of alcoholism were reduced, would it be possible to cure children from degenerated families and their criminality.[201]

Gustav Aschaffenburg, Emil Kraepelin, Richard von Krafft-Ebing, August Forel, Alfred Ploetz, Eugen Bleuler, Ernst Rüdin – these were hardly anonymous physicians practicing out in the hinterlands of Germany, Austria and Switzerland. They were the most influential psychiatrists in the German-speaking world. They were the heads of the most advanced clinics in Vienna, Zurich and Munich, and their books were read in all the medical faculties in Germany. They were translated into many languages, and psychiatrists and physicians in Britain, France and the United States were familiar with their work. American addiction specialists, in fact, continued to cite them well into the 1960s. And each and every one of these German-speaking figures believed that alcoholism was hereditary, or at least that the propensity to alcoholism was inherited – a view that would strongly influence the Third Reich's treatment of severe alcoholics.

---

199 Bernard Glueck, "Psychogenesis in the Psychoses of Prisoners," *Criminal Science Monographs* 2 (1916), 1-66. On the uneasy relationship between Bleuler and Freud, see Peter Gay, *Freud: Life for Our Time* (New York: Norton, 1988), 215-216.

200 Bernard Glueck , *Lehrbuch der Psychiatrie* (Berlin, 1916), 168-170, 176-178.

201 Eugen Bleuler, *Der geborene Verbrecher: Eine kritische Studie* (Munich, 1896), 31, 87.

Their theories did little to dent the public's appetite for the drink. Indeed, their efforts to sober the German national failed just as badly as those made a millennium earlier by morality-driven preachers. But their collective medical understandings undoubtedly influenced policy in Germany as the 20th century progressed. Perhaps most importantly, they established the primacy of medical science in the treatment of alcoholism. Henceforth, heavy and uncontrollable drinking became a disease to be treated by doctors, rather than the moral failure it had been perceived to be for ages.

2. The Birth of Drug Addiction

Going back at least two millennia, physicians warned that opium could, when consumed immoderately, turn from a medicinal panacea into a potentially fatal poison. In ancient Greece, doctors urged caution in the consumption of *opion*, declaring it to be a *pharmakon* that could be both medicinal and poisonous, depending on dosage, usage and other variables. Laudanum, Paracelsus' 16th-century precursor to Thomas Sydenham's tincture of opium, caused the death of more than one notable politician during its two centuries of widespread use.

Though opium was yet to be understood as a cause for a specific disease, there was growing awareness that its consumption was, at a minimum, a bad habit. The habitual use of opium, John Redman Coxe (1773-1864) wrote in his 1818 book, *American Dispensatory*, is difficult to relinquish.[202] And Felix von Niemeyer (1820-1871), the King of Württemberg's personal physician, claimed that opium could cause brain damage.[203] Yet despite the evident dangers, von Niemeyer often injected morphine into his patients, and even praised morphine and opium's ability to treat various diseases such as neuralgia.[204] Opium, in fact, was one of the three main ingredients in medicine that bears his name, the Niemeyer pill, along with quinine and digitalis.[205]

Von Niemeyer was hardly the only physician who, aware of its potential malefic effects, nonetheless prescribed opium. Christoph Wilhelm Hufeland recommended the administration of opium with mercury to treat syphilis in his 1829 enchiridion on medical practice. Since syphilis poisoned the reproductive system, which Hufeland believed to be connected to the nervous system, opium was the natural medical treatment, as it was the drug with the strongest effect on the nerves. He also

---

202 John R. Coxe, *The American Dispensatory* (Philadelphia, 1818), 410.
203 Felix von Niemeyer, *Lehrbuch der speciellen Pathologie und Therapie: mit besonderer Rücksicht an Physiologie und pathologische Anatomie*, Vol. 2 (Berlin, 1865), 150, 271.
204 Ibid.
205 Anton Sebastian, *A Dictionary of the History of Medicine*, (New York: Parthenon Publishing Group, 1999), 538; "Niemeyer Pill," *Journal of the American Medical Association*, vol. 56/3 (1911): 211.

recommended opium as an antidote to poisoning, be it from mercury, lead, arsenic or snake venom, and prescribed the versatile drug for treating, among other ailments, smallpox, polyps in the vagina, throat and ear tracts. That it also relieved pain and fear, he argued, made opium nothing less than a cure-all drug.[206]

Like his Greek predecessors, Hufeland qualified his praise for the drug with a stern warning about its potential dangers. Opium was so effective in alleviating pain, he cautioned, that it could deceive both patient and doctor into believing that a cure had been found. The medicine could also cause apoplexy in children, worsen inflammations, cause constipation and increase pollutants in the blood. Eventually, Hufeland warned, opium turned on the patient it had been helping:

> In chronic illness one can at least get so accustomed to the use of opium that it becomes a daily need, also if pains have been removed, in order to lift the general feeling to the point of well being, of liveliness, of physical and mental usefulness – just in the same way as the drinker of spirits finally gets accustomed to spirits and they become an indispensable need for him, but also with the same consequence, the need for ever higher doses. The opium disease [*Opiumsucht*] – completely in analogy to the drinking disease [*Trunksucht*] and its effects – [causes an] ever-increasing weakening of the nerves, trembling, destruction of the digestive and reproductive powers, in the end *Delirium tremens*, bluntness of the senses and the mind, hemorrhages, dissolution of the blood, *Tabes*.[207]

Hufeland, almost as an afterthought, described opium usage with wording borrowed from Brühl-Cramer's drinking disease. Though it was hardly recognized as a watershed moment at the time, Hufeland's drawing an analogy between the opium disease and the alcohol disease was without a doubt a milestone in the long road to understanding drug addiction.[208]

At the time, however, there was relatively little interest among physicians in further examination of the drug. After traditional German medicine reasserted its supremacy over Brunonianism by the beginning of

---

206 Hufeland, *Enchiridion Medicum oder Anleitung zur medizinischen Praxis*, 521-525.

207 Ibid., 526-527. Hufeland first published this passage in an essay on opium in the *Journal der Practischen Arzneykunde und Wunderarzneykunst* 59:1 (1829). The translation was primarily taken from Maehle, *Drugs on Trial*, 184-185, 219n with some modifications.

208 Margit Kreutel, *Die Opiumsucht* (Stuttgart: Deutscher Apotheker Verlag, 1988), 209.

the 19th century, opium was viewed as a medicine used by medical practitioners, and generally speaking, that is where debate on the drug ended. It was not until the German wars of unification that the opium disease again became a subject of discussion. Like opium, morphine received a warm welcome from physicians when it was discovered by Friedrich Sertürner (1783-1841) and then mass-produced by Merck in the 1830s. Its potential malefic effects were noted, but there was little interest in further examination of the drug.

The few Germans to show interest in the opium disease were mostly world travelers, with occasional attention from literary figure like Heinrich Heine (1797-1856). Heine, who took morphine for a mysterious ailment, penned a poem called "Morphium," but it was dedicated to lost health, rather than addiction, and was published only after his death.[209] Most German authors simply ignored drugs altogether. Those who did mention opium or morphine did so in passing, and then in only general terms as a medicine, sleep inducer and poison. Germany had no Baudelaire or de Quincey, a literary figure who catalogued his active and willing use of drugs in order to gain a better understanding of the world.

Perhaps one of the reasons why German romantics virtually ignored opium and its derivatives was lack of contact. No German soldiers returned to the Fatherland with hashish as did Napoleon's troops from Egypt, nor did German principalities hold any stakes in the opium trade as did many British merchants in India and China. Historically, Germany had little contact with the Orient and South America, in contrast to Britain, France, Spain and even the United States.

German principalities and kingdoms had virtually no colonies overseas, and very limited influence in the Asian opium trade. Before the Opium Wars in the mid-19th century, trade between Hamburg and China was negligible. The northern city-state's harbor, Germany's biggest and most important, only received 51 ships from China between 1816 and 1842.[210] And after the wars, German interests in China were concentrated on

---

209 Heinrich Heine "Morphine," (1849-1851), with a facsimile of the manuscript at: http://germa83.uni-trier.de/HHP/werkfaksimiles/D03/h/z/D03S0277_01hz.jpg (Last access, 19.12.2015).

210 Chunxiao Jing, *Mit Barbaren gegen Barbaren: Die chinesiche Selbststärkungsbewegung und das deutsche Rüstungsgeschäft in späten 19. Jahrhundert* (Berlin: LIT, 2002), 54.

weapons dealing, rather than opium.[211] Most Germans never met a Chinese person in their life, and opium smoking or coca chewing were just as foreign. The only source Germans had regarding the massive scale of opium smoking came from reports by travelers such as Baron Ernst von Bibra (1806-1878) in South America or Baron Ferdinand von Richthofen (1833-1905) in China.

The turning point came with the German wars of unification against Denmark in 1864, Austria in 1866 and France in 1870. During that decade of upheaval, interest spiked in the opium and morphine diseases. It is unclear whether this was primarily a result of morphine being widely used to treat wounded soldiers on the battlefield, or more because growing awareness of the drug among physicians led to its proliferation and, in turn, rising numbers of addicts. What is clear is that physicians began to recognize addiction to opium and morphine. J. Samter, a physician from Posen in West Prussia, was among the first doctors to describe treatment of a patient suffering from the opium disease. "That the pains of B. were, in general, self generated as a disease and his morphine consumption had developed into a real morphiophagie [morphine eating], should be of interest to many colleagues," he wrote in an 1864 article for medical journal.[212]

Three years earlier, Samter wrote, B., a construction worker, came to his clinic in Posen, complaining about stomachaches that might have been caused by an ulcer.[213] Samter, who was leaving for a neighboring city,

---

211 Mechthild Leutner and Klaus Mühlhahn, "Interkulturelle Handlungsmuster: Deutsche Wirtschaft und Mission in China in der Spätphase des Imperialismus," in *Deutsch-chinesische Beziehungen im 19. Jahrhundert: Mission und Wirtschaft in interkultureller Perspektive*, ed. Mechthild Leutner and Klaus Mühlhahn (Münster: LIT, 2001), 21-23; Peter Merker, "Der Kampf um Chinas Bodenschätze: Einheimische Erschließungsvorhaben und Bergbauaktivitäten der Firma Carlowitz & Co. im Widerstreit," in Ibid., 133-181. Hosea Ballou Morse, a British tax collector in China and an authority on the opium trade never mentioned Germany or German traders as a source of the opium trade, see Hosea Ballou Morse, *The Trade and Administration of the Chinese Empire* (Taipei: Ch'end Publishing, 1966 [1907]).

212 J. Samter, "Ein Morphiophagie" *Deutsche Klink. Zeitung für Beobachtungen aus Deutschen Kliniken und Krankenhäusern* 16:16 (16 April 1864), 157-158. Albrecht Erlenmeyer (1849-1926) identified this case as the first identification of the morphine disease. See Albrecht Erlenmeyer, *Die Morphiumsucht und ihre Behandlung* (Berlin, 1887 [1883]), 404.

213 Samter, "Ein Morphiophagie," 157-158.

referred B. to a Dr. Fink, who proceeded to treat the patient with increasing doses of morphine: 4-6 grains daily. Samter and Fink suspected abdominal cancer, and sent the patient to a local hospital. He was treated for eight days with tincture of iodine, chloroform and bismuth, but there was no improvement until he was treated again with morphine. After two months, the patient was released from the hospital in the same condition as he had entered.

Several months later, Samter recounted, B. surprisingly returned to the clinic in Posen, to report that he was healthy and pain-free. The patient told Samter that he had been taking 3 grains of morphine in the mornings and evenings. It was only when he stopped taking his medication, B. said, that he suffered the diarrhea, stomachaches and weakness in the legs that he had suffered earlier.[214] A week later, the physician received a letter from a Dr. Fuchs, who informed Samter that he had treated B. in the past months. Fuchs stated that he had supervised a steady increase in dosage of morphine, which eventually totaled a staggering 1,347 grains in 323 days. Fuchs wrote that he attempted to reduce the amount of morphine B. was taking, but to no avail.[215]

As similar case studies were recorded and shared by physicians in medical journals, it became increasingly apparent that something was amiss with morphine. In a lecture given in 1871 at the Psychiatric Association of Berlin, Heinrich Laehr (1820-1905), the director of the Schweizerhof mental asylum in Berlin, reported on what appeared to him to be a morphine disease, which was difficult to cure. It produced symptoms nearly identical to alcoholism that could eventually lead to suicide. Laehr also recounted his experiences with treating wounded soldiers in 1866, noting that they often vomited after being injected with morphine.[216] Laehr's claims were received cautiously. Many physicians were hesitant to condemn their panacea, and some suggested that the symptoms reported by Laehr might have been caused not by a disease, but by bad batches of morphine administered poorly by army surgeons.

---

214 Ibid., 158.
215 *Deutsche Klink. Zeitung für Beobachtungen aud deutschen Kliniken und Krankenhäusern* 16:17 (23 April 1864), 163-164.
216 Heinrich Laehr, "Ueber Missbrauch mit Morphium-Injectionen" *Allgemeine Zeitschrift für Psychiatrie und psychisch-gerichtliche Medicin* 28:3 (Berlin, 1872), 349-352.

It took five more years for the concept of morphine addiction to finally take root. In 1875, German Jewish psychiatrist Eduard Levinstein's (1832-1882) delivered a lecture in Graz on "*Die Morphiumsucht,*" marking the acceptance of drug addiction by the medical community. Levinstein sought the rehabilitation of patients both somatically and mentally, offering them a quiet place to recuperate at his Maison de Santé ("House of Health") in Berlin. The House, which had served in the past as a restaurant, was too small to be considered a full-fledged asylum.[217] Despite the modest size of his institution, Levinstein would go on to become the most prominent expert on drug addiction in Germany, and arguably in the entire world.

After delivering additional speeches on morphine addiction, Levinstein published "*Die Morphiumsucht*" in 1877.[218] The book was translated into several languages; the English edition appeared in 1878 under the title, "The Morbid Craving for Morphia,"[219] which brought him great renown in England and the United States. But the translated edition also corrupted his thesis ever so slightly, as can be discerned from the very title of the book. The German "*Sucht*" turned in English into a "morbid craving." Since the word "addiction" was not yet in popular use in English, and Levinstein's *Morphiumsucht* was more than just a habit (which hitherto had been the term used by physicians to describe opium and morphine dependency), the English translator invented a new term: "morbid craving."

The new terminology, as it turned out, did not catch on. Although a number of American and English doctors used "morbid craving" to explain the disease, "addiction" prevailed in the end, leaving the word "morbid" to be associated with death. But with Levinstein's writings still being read long after the terminology had been settled upon, more than a few 20th-century readers may have misunderstood the English edition of his book, because they were thinking that he viewed addiction as an inher-

---

217 W. Gehewe, "Reisebericht durch Irrenanstalten Deutschlands und der Schweiz in den Jahren 1869 und 1870" *Allgemeine Zeitschrift für Psychiatrie und psychisch-gerichtliche Medicin* 28:1 (Berlin, 1872), 65-66.

218 Eduard Levinstein, *Die Morphiumsucht: Eine Monographie nach eigenen Beobachtungen* (Berlin, 1877 [1883]).

219 Edward Levinstein, *The Morbid Craving for Morphia (die Morphiumsucht): A Monograph founded on Personal Observations*, translated by Charles Harrer (London, 1878).

ently life-threatening disease rather than one better understood by the original Latin word "*morbus.*"

Levinstein also introduced a new term to German, one that has stuck to this day. Until his time, "*Sucht*" was almost synonymous with "disease," but after Levinstein it came to designate a specific ailment: addiction. "One can disagree about names," Levinstein wrote in *Die Morphiumsucht*:

> And in some pages, morphinism, morphinomania and the morphine disease all share the same meaning. Yet none of the three truly describe the disease as I see it. An individual, who suffered from an acute and painful ache treated with months-long morphine injections, could fall under the description of morphinism; that is, a specific symptom of morphine poisoning. But he is in no way a morphine addict, if, after the pain was relieved, he had no desire for morphine. Furthermore, an individual can suffer from morphine disease for years, without the appearance of morphinism.[220]

The morphine disease, or "*Morphiumkrankheit*," was considered an unsuitable name to describe the condition,[221] as was "*Morphinomania*," since the latter implied that the disease was mental, rather than physical with mental symptoms.[222]

Levinstein, following Laehr's lead, blamed the development of addiction on the careless practice of physicians in the battlefield, claiming that since the war of 1866 the number of known cases of addiction in Germany had risen. Morphine should be used sparingly and with great care, he argued, and discontinued once the ailment for which it was prescribed was cured. Doctors should not teach their patients to inject morphine, and should keep the dosage to the bare minimum.

Morphine addiction was similar in symptoms and in nature to the drinking disease, with the main difference being that it appeared among members of wealthier classes, who, once addicted, often indulged in drinking as well.[223] Levinstein asserted that any drug user would become an addict, regardless of class, state of mind or strength of will. Drug addiction, he claimed, was first and foremost a physical disease. It would eventually afflict anyone who used drugs, a state that could be identified by

---

220 Levinstein, *Die Morphiumsucht*, 2.
221 *Morphiumkrankheit* was translated to the 'morphine evil,' probably because the 'morphine disease' was too close to the translator's 'morbid craving.' See Levinstein, *The Morbid Craving for Morphia*, 2.
222 Levinstein, *Die Morphiumsucht*, 2.
223 Ibid., 1-7, 10-11. See also Erlenmeyer, *Die Morphiumsucht und ihre Behandlung*, 406.

physical manifestations and tests, such as amenorrhea, impotence, the dilatation of the iris, or a urine analysis as well as the symptoms of withdrawal.

Morphine addicts were not mentally deformed, nor did they necessarily suffer from mental disturbances, at least until the drug was taken away from them. They did not suffer from psychoses, alienation or any other mental disease. The mental instability they displayed while experiencing withdrawal was temporary and lasted until the patient was fully cured. The only method of treatment was the immediate forced abstention of the patient, a process that could take up to six months. Despite the physical nature of addiction, the cure's success rate was low, with patients relapsing to morphine use more than 75 percent of the time.[224]

Despite Levinstein's warnings, morphine and opium remained a valued medicine for treating pain. In psychiatry, leading figures like Richard von Krafft-Ebing found opium and morphine useful for treating mental patients, especially those who suffered from melancholy and psychoses. An injectable solution was preferable to oral consumption, and was administered together with Spanish wine.[225] Krafft-Ebing, like many other proponents, was cautious in his praise, claiming that morphine was not only a narcotic used to calm the nerves, but also a stimulant and a luxury good, especially among those suffering from neuropathic disturbances. Morphine was in no way harmless, he warned, and could cause habituation resulting in a weakening of the will of the patient, even among those who wished to stop taking the drug. The chronic intoxication of morphine eventually devolved the user, who eventually stopped experiencing its euphoric effects and resorted to taking increasing doses to sustain normal life.[226]

Louis Lewin (1850-1929), perhaps the most famous toxicologist of his time, published a handbook on the side effects of drugs in 1881 in which he claimed that habituation to drugs or poisons was in fact caused by the body's gradual adaptation to the drug. Likely influenced by homeopathy, he concluded that this phenomenon was the reason why addicts required

---

224 Ibid., 12, 14-22.
225 Richard von Krafft-Ebing, *Lehrbuch der Psychiatrie auf klinischer Grundlage für Praktische Ärzte und Studierende* (Stuttgart, 1890 [1879]), 294-296.
226 Ibid., 630-631. On the neuropathic nature of addicts, Krafft-Ebing relied on Erlenmeyer's work on addiction, rather than Levinstein.

an increasing dosage of drugs in order to achieve the effects experienced previously.

Lewin also explained how addicts could consume large quantities of opium or other drugs that would otherwise poison and kill a non-addict. The explanation he provided was a mechanical one: drugs affect the cells of the body. Over-stimulation from using drugs caused exhaustion of cell tissue that rendered any lesser stimulation ineffective. The disease, he noted, was not irreversible. "If the drug be discontinued, complete recovery may take place and the same parts eventually react normally to medicines,"[227] he wrote. Since the drug affected the entire body, with-drawal would cause physical disturbances to digestive, respiratory and other functions, as the body became accustomed to the physical balance that existed before the addiction.[228] Tolerance to drugs, therefore, was a symptom of addiction.[229]

Lewin's explanation concentrated on the organism and its physical exis-tence, well in line with Levinstein's conclusions that the disease was, in fact, physical. The drug altered the mind as well, but a person of weak mind was not more or less susceptible to addiction or habituation. The opposite, in fact, was the case. A drug user would eventually develop a weak mind as a result of the effects of the drug on his body.[230] More than 40 years later, Lewin conceded that no cellular change among addicts was found that would indicate their addiction. Yet he remained an ardent supporter of the idea that habituation (*Gewöhnung* in German) was a phys-ical result of extensive drug use, and argued as much in his popular 1924 handbook *Phantastica*.[231]

A contemporary of Lewin, Albrecht Erlenmeyer (1849-1926), took Levinstein's findings in a somewhat different direction. An expert on drug addiction, Erlenmeyer published in 1883 a compilation of research on addiction as a disease. Drawing upon material in English, French, German

---

227 Louis Lewin, *The Incidental Effects of Drugs: A Pharmacological and Clinical Hand-book* (New York, 1882 [1881]), 18.

228 Ibid., 20.

229 Ibid., 142. In the German original, Lewin wrote about the *Morphiumsucht,* which was translated into English as the morphine habit. See for example the third edition of the book published in German: Idem, *Die Nebenwirkungen der Arzneimittel: Pharmakologisch-klinisches Handbuch* (Belin, 1898), 98.

230 Ibid., 99-106.

231 Idem, *Phantastica: Über die berauschenden, betäubenden und erregenden Genußmittel* (Cologne, 2000 [1926/4]), 20-36.

and other languages, Erlenmeyer found that in the 11 years between the 1864 war against Denmark and Levinstein's first lecture on morphine addiction in 1875, 24 articles and essays were written on the pathological symptoms resulting from drug use. In the 11 years after Levinstein's lecture, he demonstrated, more than 235 books, articles and essays were written on addiction – a 10-fold increase.[232]

Although Erlenmeyer recognized the importance of Levinstein's break-through, he disagreed with many of his predecessor's assertions. According to him, whether a drug user became an addict depended on an inherent predisposition to the drug – which was, in essence, a weakness of the will.[233] Therefore, he concluded, not all drug users would eventually develop an addiction. Furthermore, Erlenmeyer opposed Levinstein's prescription of immediate withdrawal. He also discounted the method of slow withdrawal popular at the time in the United States. Instead, Erlen-meyer advocated what he termed "quicker withdrawal," which he argued avoided the dangers inherent in Levinstein's method.[234]

The fear of sudden withdrawal of morphine was unquestionably based on concern for patient discomfort, but accepted wisdom at the time also warned of the risk of *delirium tremens*. Most physicians and psychiatrists of that era believed that alcoholism and addiction shared similar character-istics, and there was real fear that sudden withdrawal could lead to the agonizing death of the drug addict – as happened often enough with the sudden withdrawal of alcohol from alcoholics.

With growing awareness of morphine addiction came more pronounced questioning of the potential for addiction to other drugs, notably cocaine. The coca plant was first introduced to the wide German public in the writ-ings of Baron Ernst von Bibra, who travelled to South America soon after the failure of the 1848 revolution. In 1855 he published his book *The Narcotic Drugs and Man*, in which he described the intoxicants of the world.[235]

---

232 Erlenmeyer, *Die Morphiumsucht und Ihre Behandlung*, 404-436.
233 Ibid., 13-14.
234 Ibid., 16, 111-129.
235 The translation of the title is somewhat misleading, since the German word used by von Bibra was *Genußmittel*, or luxury good, rather than the German equiva-lent for drug. The meaning of '*Genußmittel*' was and remains neutral, if not posi-tive, and could refer to tea, coffee, chocolate as well as coca, hashish and opium. See Wolfgang Schivelbusch, *Tastes of Paradise: A Social History of Spices, Stim-ulants, and Intoxicants* (New York: Vintage Books, 1993), xiii.

In his account, Bibra relied on Eduard Friedrich Pöppig (1798-1868), who traveled in Peru between 1827 and 1832 and described how *coqueros* refused to give up the vice of chewing the coca leaves. The mystery of why the natives were so enamored with their coca leaves was revealed the moment Pöppig concluded that coca, just like opium, was a stimulant.[236] This odd insight that lumped a narcotic – a sleep-inducing drug – with a stimulant is a clear testimony to the lasting effect of Brunonianism in scientific thought. Pöppig stressed the malefic effects of the coca leaf. The habit was not only immoral and kept the heathens from espousing Christianity, but also dangerous to their health. Coca chewing caused bad breath and encouraged excessive drinking among the common people.[237] Addiction, however, was not mentioned.

In contrast, Bibra believed that Pöppig's assessment was too moralistic and harsh, recounting his own experience with the plant, which were mild.[238] He expressed a hope that one day; coca would enter the European pharmacopoeia as it promised many medicinal uses. In 1860, Albert Niemann (1834-1861), a German scientist, isolated cocaine and the promotion of the drug in medicine had begun.[239]

Cocaine, like morphine before it, was initially hailed as a panacea. Two Viennese physicians of Jewish descent were primarily responsible for popularizing this drug. At the time, the more influential of the two was Karl Koller (1857-1944), an ophthalmologist who immigrated to the United States in 1888. He introduced cocaine as a local anesthetic in eye surgery in September 1884, thus enabling the performance of complex eye surgery for the first time in history.[240] The second doctor was Sigmund Freud (1856-1939). Although he published an essay on cocaine in July 1884, several months before Koller's watershed use of cocaine in surgery, fame was initially bestowed on the ophthalmologist, not Freud. The two

---

236 Ernst von Bibra, *Die narkotischen Genußmittel und der Mensch* (Nuremberg, 1855), 156-157.

237 Ibid., 161.

238 Ibid., 171.

239 Albert Niemann, "Ueber eine neue organische Base in den Cocablättern: Mittheilung aus der Inaugural-Dissertation," *Archiv der Pharmacie*, vol. 153/2 (1860), 140; Paul Gootneberg, *Andean Cocaine: The Making of a Global Drug* (Chapel Hill: North Carolina University Press, 2008).

240 Joseph F. Spillane, *Cocaine: From Medical Marvel to Modern Menace in the United States, 1884-1920* (Baltimore: Johns Hopkins University Press, 2000), 12, 168n-169n.36.

doctors knew each other in Vienna, and Freud was, if only briefly, embittered by Koller's success.

After reading several favorable reports from the United States, as well as an article on the positive effects of cocaine in alleviating exhaustion among Bavarian soldiers during training maneuvers in 1883,[241] Freud decided to experiment with the drug and was in the process of writing a report on his findings when he administered the drug to a patient of his who was suffering from pain. Koller happened to be at the scene, and after witnessing Freud's treatment embarked upon further research.[242]

Freud, noting the analgesic effect of the drug, had himself wished to conduct a series of tests. But it had been a year since he had last seen his fiancée, who lived in Bohemia, and so he left town and entrusted the research to a colleague, who failed to produce any results. Koller, who conducted the necessary tests independently, proved the effectiveness of cocaine in eye surgery, and received credit for the breakthrough after demonstrating his findings in Heidelberg.

After missing his chance at fame, Freud turned to study the effects of cocaine on morphine addiction.[243] In May 1884, Freud administered cocaine to a colleague who suffered from morphine addiction. Cocaine, he noticed, helped his patient deal with the sudden withdrawal symptoms of morphine without suffering from depression, diarrhea or nausea. This led Freud to believe that cocaine was an antagonistic agent to morphine, a suspicion he published in an article that July.[244] The article was favorably received, earning Freud a modicum of fame and a translation into English, but it was quickly overshadowed by Koller's achievement.

---

241 W. H. Bentley, "Erythroxylon Coca in the Opium and Alcohol Habits," (1880) and W. H. Bentley, "Erythroxylon Coca as an Antidote to the Opium Habit," (1880) both reproduced in Robert Byck, ed. *Cocaine Papers* (New York: Stonehill, 1974), 15-21; Theodor Aschenbrandt, "The Physiological Effect and Significance of Cocaine Muriate on the Human Organism. Clinical Observations during the Fall Maneuvers of the Year 1883 of the Bavarian II. Artillery Company, 4 Division, 9. Regiment, 2. Battalion," reproduced and translated in, Byck, ed. *Cocaine Papers,* 21-26. Incidentally, Aschenbrandt also heavily relied on Bibra's account.

242 Ernest Jones, *The Life and Work of Sigmund Freud*, Vol. 1, (New York: Basic Books 1953), 85-86.

243 Ibid.

244 Siegmund Freud, "Über Coca," *Centralblatt für die gesammte Therapie* 2:7 (1884), 289-314.

Freud continued to research, write and talk about the effects of cocaine, claiming that it was not only an antagonist to morphine, but also to chloral hydrates.[245] He wrote on the physical effects of cocaine on the body, and expanded upon the use of cocaine for treating morphine addiction.[246]

Koller and Freud's research incited the imagination of doctors in Germany and around the world, helping spread the popularity of cocaine. In the winter of 1884, a Dr. Richter from the Berlin suburb of Pankow delivered a talk before the Berlin Society for Nervous Disease and Psychiatry where he claimed that cocaine produced by Merck in Darmstadt, as opposed to the one produced by Gehe in Dresden, effectively countered the effects of sudden morphine withdrawal.[247]

The next year, Albrecht Erlenmeyer – already an established authority on the morphine disease – began, following Freud's example, treating morphine users with cocaine. He observed 236 injections of cocaine, of which eight were administered to morphine addicts. Erlenmeyer discovered that cocaine reduced the patient's appetite for morphine for only a short period of time, approximately 10 to 15 minutes. Cocaine, he concluded, was useless in the cure of the morphine disease. Cocaine neither relaxed the patients nor soothed their withdrawal-induced sleeping disorders. Furthermore, cocaine was not antagonistic to morphine, but served as a substitute for the drug – in Erlenmeyer's words, replacing "the devil with Beelzebub."[248]

Erlenmeyer publicly chided Freud for advocating a dangerous drug, and provided proof that cocaine was indeed addictive. "Cocaine addiction joined the drinking disease and morphine addiction as a noteworthy third scourge of humanity," he wrote in 1886, in the first published article on

---

245 "Aus den Vereinen: Academie des Sciences zu Paris," *Centralblatt für Nervenheilkunde, Psychiatrie und gerichtliche Psychopathologie* 8:6 (1885), 142-143.

246 Sigmund Freud, "Contribution to the Knowledge of the Effect of Cocaine," (1885) and "On the General Effects of Cocaine. A Lecture given at the Psychiatric Union on March 5, 1885," both translated and reproduced in Byck, ed. *Cocaine Papers*, 97-104, 113-118.

247 Richter, "Ueber Cannabinon und Cocain," (8 December 1884) reproduced in Erlenmeyer, *Die Morphiumsucht und ihre Behandlung*, 158. Erlenmeyer, in a different article, claimed the talk took place in October.

248 Albrecht Erlenmeyer, "Ueber die Wirkung des Cocaïn bei der Morphiumentziehung," *Centralblatt für Nervenheilkunde, Psychiatrie und gerichtliche Psychopathologie* 8:13 (1885), 289-299. Erlenmeyer was the editor of this journal, a fact that Jones used against him.

cocaine addiction. "Anyone who took it was immediately inflicted with a considerable damage to the body, soul and morality."[249] The next year, Erlenmeyer updated his book on the morphine disease and included his conclusions regarding cocaine, nearly doubling the length of the new edition as a result. He cited no less than 12 articles, most published in German, in proving that cocaine did indeed cause addiction. He thus laid down the gauntlet, but there was still substantial business interest in cocaine, and the power of money was evident in his own book. On the back page of the 1889 English edition, Park, Davis & Co., the largest cocaine manufacturer in the United States at the time, published an advertisement for its pure Peruvian cocaine product.[250]

Cocaine also had support in America. A former United States surgeon general, William Alexander Hammond (1828-1900), declared in 1887 that the cocaine habit was no worse than drinking tea or coffee, and could be used to treat other forms of addiction.[251] Freud, facing tough criticism for endorsing cocaine, was glad to receive Hammond's support, and quoted him in his last paper on drugs, published in 1887. He also suggested that Erlenmeyer had erred in his experiment, since he injected minimal doses of cocaine to his patients, as opposed to the much larger oral doses Freud recommended. He acknowledged the dangers of the drug when used to treat morphine addiction, but refused to concede that cocaine caused addiction among healthy persons.[252]

Freud's protestations, however, had begun to ring hollow. In 1886, the *New York Medical Record* declared, in an article headlined "The Cocaine Habit," that "no other medicine with such a short history was responsible for so many victims as cocaine. The cocaine habit caused more damage to body and soul than morphine, as in the case of one medical doctor and his daughter who entered a hotel in New York City and behaved like maniacs

---

249 Albrecht Erlenmeyer, "Über Cocainsucht. Vorläufige Mitteilung," *Deutsche Medizinalzeitung* 7:44 (1886), 483-484.

250 Idem, *On the Treatment of the Morphine Habit* (Detroit, 1889), 114.

251 W. A. Hammond, "Coca: Its Preparations and their Therapeutical Qualities, with some Remarks on the So-Called 'Cocaine Habit'" (1887), in Robert Byck (ed.), *Cocaine Papers* (New York, 1974), 177-194.

252 Sigmund Freud, "Beiträge über die Anwendung des Cocaïn: Bemerkungen über Cocaïnsucht und Cocaïnfurcht mit Beziehung auf einen Vortrag W. A. Hammonds," *Wiener Medizinische Wochenschrift* 37:28 (1887), 929-932.

due to misuse of cocaine, which they [had] previously injected."[253]Over the next year, stories about the destructive effects of cocaine appeared regularly in The New York Times, and Freud's views on cocaine were generally disregarded by physicians.[254] Just months after Freud published his last paper on cocaine, Jansen B. Mattison (1845-?), a physician in New York, announced that he had discovered seven cases of cocaine addiction.[255]

Freud, bruised by the affair, kept silent. He thought he had lost his credibility as a researcher. To make matters worse, the patient he had been treating with cocaine – a friend and colleague – died in 1891 after suffering the symptoms of cocaine addiction.[256] Soon after, he moved to Paris to study under Jean-Martin Charcot (1825-1893) at the Salpêtrière. Although Freud continued to take cocaine privately, he distanced himself from his early claims. His cocaine articles were not included in his collected works in either German or English; and later in life, Freud himself claimed that his research on cocaine was but a diversion.[257]

Freud's cocaine episode, odd and perhaps embarrassing to his adherents, is best understood through the German understanding of addiction. Freud believed addiction to be a disease like any other. When his friend became addicted to morphine, and after reading favorable results from America and Bavaria, he concluded that he could use cocaine as a cure. To justify his treatment, it was necessary for cocaine to counteract morphine, hence the importance and debate over whether cocaine was an antagonistic agent. Even Freud, who would become the preeminent analyst of the mind, believed as late as the 1880s that addiction was a purely physical phenomenon.

253 "The Cocaine Habit," *New York Medical Record* (29 May 1886), reproduced and translated to German in Erlenmeyer, *Die Morphiumsucht und ihre Behandlung*, 461.

254 Spillane, *Cocaine*, 32-33, 70-71.

255 David T. Courtwright, "The Rise and Fall and Rise of Cocaine in the United States," in *Consuming Habits: Drugs in History and Anthropology*, ed. Jordan Goodman, Paul E. Lovejoy and Andrew Sherratt (London: Routledge, 1995), 207-208.

256 Jones, *The Life and Work of Sigmund Freud*, 91-92.

257 Lawrence V. Driscoll, *Reconsidering Drugs: Mapping Victorian and Modern Drug Discourses* (New York: Palgrave, 2000), 73-74. See also Paul Roazen, *Encountering Freud: The Politics and Histories of Psychoanalysis* (New Brunswick NJ: Transaction Publishers, 1990), 7-8, 77.

What was a professional aberration for the father of psychotherapy was career-defining for Erlenmeyer and Levinstein, whose research influenced the understanding of addiction in Germany for years to come. Indeed, their conclusions served as the starting point for psychiatric research on addiction. Emil Kraepelin, for one, relied on Erlenmeyer and Levinstein's work while developing his own model of addiction. He included their theories in his textbook *Clinical Psychiatry*.[258] Alcoholism, however, remained the primary focus of his investigation, with only limited space devoted to developing his ideas regarding addiction.

Ether drinking, morphinism and cocainism were all syndromes of chronic poisoning of the brain, Kraepelin declared. The diseases manifested themselves as mental disorders that changed the character of the patient, resulting in a weakening of the will and impairment of mental faculties.[259] Morphinism and cocainism shared a common origin, and many cocaine addicts were previously morphine addicts.[260] Other drugs, whether benzene, chloroform, ether, hashish, lead, mercury or tobacco, could potentially have similar effects on the brain.[261]

According to Kraepelin, doctors were not only a main cause of the spread of morphine addiction, they were also its primary victims. Doctors, he warned, were freely handing out syringes to patients and teaching them how to inject themselves, clearly unaware of the difficulties of curing the newly acquired morphine habit:

> The intolerance of pain among people of this age, together with the laxity of the physicians in dispensing analgesics, accounts in part for the extensive use of this drug. Being an expensive drug, its victims are limited to the better classes. Considerably over one-half of the patients are those who are best acquainted with its ill effects – physicians, dentists and professional nurses. At least one-half of these patients are men. On the Continent it is claimed that 75 percent are men.[262]

Notably, in the German edition, Kraepelin made no mention of the people of that era having a noticeable intolerance for pain. The editor of the

---

258 Kraepelin, *Psychiatrie*, Vol. 2, 101.
259 Ibid., vol. 1, 49-51.
260 Diefendorf, ed. *Clinical Psychiatry*, 210.
261 Kraepelin, *Psychiatrie*, Vol. 1, 50-51.
262 Diefendorf, ed. *Clinical Psychiatry*, 202. Aside from the English editor's complaint of the men of his day, this section is an almost exact translation of the passage found in Kraepelin, *Psychiatrie*, vol.2, 107.

English edition of his textbook took some liberties in his translation from the original, a practice not entirely uncommon at the time.

Kraepelin insisted that only carefully treated abstention could restore the health of the patient. Echoing Levinstein's sentiment, he blamed physicians for recklessly causing addiction in patients and called for more conservative dispensing of the drug.[263] Wars and militaries also produced addicts, Kraepelin noted, citing the example of one of his patients who, while serving as an officer in a Russian regiment, received morphine injections for pleasure from the regiment's doctor, as did most of his comrades.[264]

Kraepelin, following Magnus Huss' model for alcoholism, divided the morphine diseases into two types, acute and chronic. Acute poisoning was usually pleasurable, enticing the habitué to continue consuming the drug. The continued consumption of morphine, he concluded, usually resulted in the chronic manifestation of the disease. He also noted that not all patients were susceptible to the pleasurable effects of the drug, thus rendering them immune to the disease. He added that many cases of morphinism developed in patients who suffered from earlier neuroses, such as hysteria.[265]

The editor of Kraepelin's English edition mentioned the hereditary disposition of those who suffered from neuroses that led to addiction.[266] Kraepelin himself, however, shared Levinstein's views on the physical origins to the disease, believing it was caused by contact with the drug. At the time, morphine was usually prescribed to treat pains, neuralgia, sciatica, rheumatism, headache, dysmenorrhoea and different forms of colic. The majority of cases developed in patients between the ages of 25 and 40. Kraepelin noted that one of his patients contracted morphinism after being given morphine by his physician to treat alcoholism.[267]

The beneficial effects of the drug diminished with usage, requiring an increase in dosage. Some patients developed ill side effects, while others did not. There were cases of patients who lived their lives with a morphine habit without a single ill side effect; others experienced memory and cognitive problems. Kraepelin was explicit in warning of the malefic

---

263 Ibid., 103-104.
264 Ibid., 107-108.
265 Ibid.
266 Diefendorf (ed.), *Clinical Psychiatry*, 202.
267 Kraepelin, *Psychiatrie*, vol. 2, 103.

effects of the drug. "Difficult and exhausting work becomes impossible without its administration," he wrote. "Consequently, the patients are either in a condition of exhilaration, stupidity or nervous irritability, none of which are compatible with mental work."[268]

The only successful treatment was complete abstinence. Two methods were available: rapid and gradual withdrawal. The former required great skill, but was also better for the patient. It was the method Kraepelin recommended, but even he conceded that success was seldom achieved.[269] In pushing for rapid withdrawal, he again followed in Levinstein's footsteps.

Much like Kraepelin, Swiss psychiatrist Ernst Bleuler spared few words on the morphine and cocaine diseases, sharing the view that those suffering from the disease often suffered from a weakness of will. "Most morphinists are essentially psychopaths," Bleuler stated. "Even extremely gifted and famous men succumb to addiction."[270] He noted that morphine addicts were not naturally drawn to the drug, as was the case with alcoholics. They were given the drug to treat pain, and therefore their psychopathic behaviour was acquired rather than innate.[271] He reported that when checked into hospitals for treatment, addicts reverted to lies that would allow them to keep up their morphine habit.

Using similar terminology as Freud, Bleuler believed that the disease was physical, and the increase in dosage was a result of the body's antagonism to the poison. "Fast or slow, depending on the individual constitution, the body finds a way to destroy the poison, which explains the need of the addict to increase dosage," Bleuler explained.[272] Echoing Kraepelin, Bleuler argued that only complete abstention could cure the disease, and therefore required the withdrawal of morphine from the system. He, unlike Kraepelin and Levinstein, believed that rapid withdrawal could be dangerous to some patients, and therefore he recommended the gradual withdrawal of morphine within a manner of weeks, a view in line with Erlenmeyer's teachings.

Bleuler stated unequivocally that there were no known chemicals that could make withdrawal easier on the patient, and that the remedies being

---

268 Diefendorf (ed.), *Clinical Psychiatry*, 203-204.
269 Kraepelin, *Psychiatrie*, vol. 2, 111-117.
270 Ernst Bleuler, *Lehrbuch der Psychiatrie* (Berlin, 1916) 209.
271 Ibid.
272 Ibid., 207-208.

offered at the time by physicians and chemists were simply fraudulent. And withdrawal was only the beginning of the process of curing the disease. Once the body was cleansed of the poison, the more difficult task began: rehabilitating the character of the patient, the success of which determined the ultimate outcome of the treatment.[273]

Cocainism was considered a more difficult affliction to cure than morphinism, with a higher chance of relapse. The disease also caused hallucination in addicts, such as of their legs being eaten by parasites. In a departure from Kraepelin's course of treatment, Bleuler recommended the sudden withdrawal of the drug.[274] He wasted little space on discussion of the opium disease, summarizing his views as follows: "Akin to the morphinism is opiophagie and opium smoking. Both do not play a great role with us. The appearances and treatment of opiophagie does not considerably differ from morphinism. Regarding opium smoking, we know very little."[275]

Bleuler's suggestion that addiction might also be connected to the psyche found scant reception among German physicians and psychiatrists. The medical wisdom of the day espoused a purely physical approach to addiction, in accordance with Levinstein and Kraepelin's views. Indeed, in 1933 – more than 50 years after the publication of Levinstein's book – psychoanalyst Sándor Radó (1890-1972), a student of Freud who settled in Berlin before fleeing to the United States, criticized German psychiatrists for following the disease model with too much zeal. He accused them of treating addiction as if it were the common flu, in the process ignoring the mental instability, which caused the patient to turn to drugs in the first place.[276] Radó's criticism exemplifies just how ingrained Levinstein's model became in German medical thinking.

In the late 19th century and early 20th century, German medical journals led the way in clarifying and expanding the understanding of drug addiction. The superiority of German medicine, and its identification and treatment of drug addiction, was undisputed.

German physicians were the first to identify the addictive potential of amphetamines as well as of over-the-counter sleeping pills, reporting 30

---

273 Ibid., 209-210.
274 Ibid., 210-211.
275 Ibid., 210.
276 Sándor Radó, "The Psychoanalysis of Pharmacothymia (Drug Addiction)," *Psychoanalytic Quarterly* 11 (1933), 1-23.

cases between 1920 and 1938. German physicians also identified the tendency of addicts to switch from one drug to another, depending on availability. Many opiate addicts, a psychiatrist at Breslau University Hospital noted in 1940, especially those addicted to eukodal and acedicon, take sleeping pills such as phanodorm when opiates became unavailable due to international treaties and laws against drugs.[277]

In Germany, physicians and later psychiatrists were viewed as those with the most authority on the subject of addiction, given their track record in identifying and treating the disease. However, with the advent of psychoanalysis arose a new field of expertise in the treatment of addiction: Psychoanalysis first appeared in the German-speaking world, but failed to break through as a practice into mainstream treatment in Germany, since it was not only perceived as a Jewish science, but it originated in Vienna. Instead, the new method took hold in the United States. The transition from Europe to the United States served as a conduit to transfer older German ideas to the New World.

The father of psychoanalysis himself was an occasional cocaine user and well-known lover of cigars (smoking as many as 20 per day), but Freud did not tolerate alcohol.[278] He had no such reservations, however, about drugs. In *Civilization and its Discontents*, he approved of the use of intoxicants to keep misery away.[279] In recent years some historians have tried to find a hint of psychoanalysis in Freud's early writings on cocaine. According to Rik Loose, a modern scholar of psychoanalysis, Freud betrayed a glimpse of his views on addiction in his final paper on cocaine in 1887, when he claimed that cocaine was dangerous to morphine addicts since they were apt to replace one drug with another due to their weakened will.[280] "The implication of this statement was that it was not cocaine itself which caused addiction, but a factor in the person which made them susceptible to any addiction," Loose concluded. "This is a conception of addiction which is more advanced than some contemporary theories on addiction."[281]

---

277 Diez Sacher, "Über Suchte mit rezeptfreien Schlafmitteln," *Archiv für Psychiatrie und Nervenkrankheiten*, 112:4 (1940), 552-561.

278 Roazen, *Encountering Freud*, 8.

279 Sigmund Freud, *Civilization and its Discontents* (New York, 1961 [1930]), 28.

280 Idem, "Bemerkungen über Cocaïnsucht und Cocaïnfurcht," 929-932.

281 Rik Loose, *The Subject of Addiction: Psychoanalysis and the Administration of Enjoyment* (London: Karnac Books, 2002), 20.

Was it indeed an advanced theory first developed in 1887? Freud's warning against treating morphine addicts with cocaine, however, was not innovative nor was connected to psychoanalysis. By pointing out that some people were more susceptible than others to addiction, Freud was simply borrowing from theories published by Erlenmeyer in 1883 and Krafft-Ebing in 1878 – nearly nine years before Freud's last article on cocaine.

It was only after leaving Vienna and studying under Charcot in Paris that Freud began to break free from the notion of addiction as a physical disease, or as an affliction of specific character types. Only in 1891 did he claim that hypnosis could be used for "purely functional, nervous disorders, for ailments of psychical origin, and for toxic as well as other addictions, and that in general it should be avoided for symptoms with an organic cause."[282] A hint – a mere sidenote to another topic – suggested that Freud changed his mind regarding addiction, and that he had come to believe that addiction was also a psychological problem.

After his cocaine episode, Freud rarely commented about drugs or addiction. In a rare comment, Freud, now careful with the prescription of drugs, warned against the use of narcotics to treat hysteria, since he believed intoxicants could be one of its causes. Thus the prescription of morphine for a hysteria patient was "nothing less than a serious technical mistake."[283] Experience from the 1880s lead Freud to caution.

A few years later, Freud claimed that the drinking disease, or dipsomania, could become a source of denial and jealousy. The drinker, he explained, would never accuse himself or his drink for his impotence, but would instead point the finger at his wife. Then, in 1897, Freud wrote that the drinking disease was a secondary symptom caused when the compulsions of obsessional neurosis turned into a motor impulse against the obsession. He also claimed that the drinking disease was merely an attempt to numb the mind against obsessions. In a letter written that January, Freud claimed that the drinking disease, like gambling, was due

---

282 Sigmund Freud, "Hypnosis," (1891) in *The Standard Edition of the Complete Psychological Works of Sigmund Freud*, Vol. 1, (London: Hogarth Press, 1953), 106.

283 Sigmund Freud, "Hysteria," (1888) in *The Standard Edition of the Complete Psychological Works of Sigmund Freud*, Vol. 1, (London: Hogarth Press, 1953), 50.

to the substitution of a repressed sexual impulse with drinking.[284] Freud's transformation, therefore, occurred only after his chastising experience in Vienna and after his stint in Paris.

Karl Abraham (1877-1925), the first psychoanalyst to thoroughly treat alcoholism and addiction, also drew a link between sexuality and alcoholism. "Men turn to alcohol," he wrote in 1908, "because it gives them an increased feeling of manliness and flatters their complex of masculinity."[285] He suggested that it might explain why men drank alcohol more than women. But alcohol proved to be a "false friend," since acute attacks of alcoholism caused impotence. Furthermore, Abraham argued, there was a much deeper psychological problem among alcoholics: homosexuality. Since chronic drinkers lost their sense of shame, drinking allowed them to withstand their own deviance.[286]

Once alcoholism and homosexuality were linked with one another, it was only a matter of time for addiction to other drugs to be associated with homosexuality. Abraham explained that, for example, a pre-oedipal trauma led the patient to homosexuality, but to cope with this deviance the patient sought cocaine.

Drug addiction followed alcoholism in psychoanalytical circles. The sexual roots of the two diseases were explored, and the latter was used to explain the former. Psychiatrist Otto Juliusburger (1867-1952), a follower of August Forel and a member of the German lodge of the Good Templars who would later join Abraham's Psychoanalytical Institute in Berlin,[287] conceded that alcohol indulgence was somewhat rooted in culture and social customs, but insisted that alcoholism was caused by sexual deviance – namely, homosexuality:

> Homosexuality seems to be one of the important unconscious causes of alcoholism. One prominent action of the alcohol is the abolition of repression, deadening of the higher nature, allowing the lower repressed instincts free play and satisfaction. This is especially plain in many criminal acts committed

---

284 Loose, *The Subject of Addiction*, 24-25.
285 Karl Abraham, "The Psychological Relations between Sexuality and Alcoholism," (1908) in *Selected Papers of Karl Abraham* (London: Hogarth Press, 1942), 86.
286 Ibid., 87-89.
287 Hanns Sachs in Viktor Tausk, "On the Psychology of Alcoholic Occupational Delirium," (31 May 1915) in *Minutes of the Vienna Psychoanalytical Society, 1912-1918*, Vol. 4 (New York, 1962), 289.

under the influence of alcohol in which the sadistic instinct can be distinctly seen. Although the article is of considerable length, it does not shed much new light on the problem under discussion.[288]

Viktor Tausk (1879-1919), a student of Freud's, claimed in a talk before the Viennese Psychoanalytical Society in 1915 that "occupational delirium" among social drinkers who expressed fear of not finishing a task was in fact a fear of impotence that might betray homosexual tendencies, even among women. Freud replied by distinguishing between two types of alcoholics: those who did not work and tried to deflect reproach in their dreams, and those who were anxious to finish their tasks before their inebriety inhibited them.[289] Abraham noted that many hysterical patients – who, by definition, were suffering from a sexual disorder – sought out morphine to alleviate their mental pains. But the sexual connection to drug addiction and use was even stronger than the mere desire of hysterics. He also mentioned how his insane patients viewed morphine injections as a sexual assault, the syringe being a sharp, long phallus pricking their skin with a liquid.[290]

Sándor Radó, who as mentioned earlier criticized German psychiatrists for treating addiction as if it were the common flu, believed that addiction or pharmacothymia was symptomatic of a more serious disorder. Radó argued that the disorder had to be explored and dealt with through analysis, without which the patient would relapse time and again into drug use. He also took on the conventional wisdom among his fellow psycho-analysts, arguing for a framework of addiction that did not resort to psychosexual explanations.[291]

The last of Freud's students to deal with addiction was not herself a major author on the phenomenon, but gained renown because she suffered from it. Ruth Mack Brunswick (1897-1946), an American by birth who traveled to Vienna to be treated by Freud in the 1920s, was the most analyzed of Freud's students. She had a tendency to hypochondria and

---

288 C. R. Payne, "Psychology of Alcoholism" *Psychoanalytic Review* 3:1 (1914), 469-471.
289 Tausk, "On the Psychology of Alcoholic Occupational Delirium," 288, 290-291.
290 Karl Abraham, "The Psychological Relations between Sexuality and Alco-holism" (1908) in Jones (ed.), *Selected papers of Karl Abraham,* 89
291 Rik Loose, "The Addicted Subject Caught between the Ego and the Drive: The Post-Freudian Reduction and Simplification of a Complex Clinical Problem," *Psychoanalytische Perspectieven* 41:24 (2000), 56-81.

addiction. Taking morphine for an alleged pain in the gall bladder, Brunswick was a confirmed addict, a fact that repulsed Freud at a later stage in life.[292]

Brunswick was also the teacher of Karl Menninger (1893-1990), who, together with his brother William and their father, founded a psychiatric clinic in Topeka, Kansas in the 1920s.[293] The Menningers would go on to leave an indelible mark on the American understanding of addiction. Karl Menninger, in the 1938 book "Man Against Him Self," explained why psychiatrists stopped reporting on cases of *delirium tremens* and other effects of alcohol: because they were no longer interested in the effects of drinking, but rather in why people drank in the first place. As a follower of psychoanalysis, his answer was that men and women were willing to destroy their own lives by drinking time and again, addicting themselves to the drink, because alcohol was a means to escape a mental disturbance, or anxieties, and alcohol served as self-medication to an affliction that might otherwise lead to suicide.

Alcoholism, therefore, was not a disease at all, but a symptom of something much deeper.[294] Or, as another American psychiatrist described it, alcohol addiction appeared either as a reactive symptom to a neurosis, or from a deformed character developed in childhood.[295]

Freudian ideas soon percolated into psychiatry in America. William Menninger (1899-1966), Karl's brother, served as the head of the US Army's psychiatric division. In 1943 he presided over a committee that wrote "War Department Technical Bulletin, Medical 203." The document, which classified mental disorders into distinct categories, was heavily

---

292 Paul Roazen, *Freud and His Followers* (New York: Knopf, 1979), 425-430. She was not the only member of Freud's circle who succumbed to addiction. Otto Gross, the rebellious psychoanalyst turned anarchist and one of Freud's earlier defenders, became addicted to morphine while on a voyage as a ship's surgeon to South America early in 1899. He went in and out of treatment for the rest of his life, even while practicing medicine. While in treatment at the Burghölzli clinic, he met Carl Jung, who recruited him to Freud's psychoanalytical circle.

293 A. C. Houts, "Fifty Years of Psychiatric Nomenclature: Reflections on the 1943 War Department Technical Bulletin, Medical 203," *Journal of Clinical Psychology*, vol. 56/7 (2000), 935-967.

294 Karl A. Menninger, *Man Against Him Self* (New York: Harcourt, Brace, 1938), 160-169.

295 Robert Knight, "The Psychodynamic of Chronic Alcoholism," *Journal of Nervous and Mental Diseases* 86:5 (1937), 538-548.

influenced by psychoanalysis. It presumed that mental disorders were not necessarily biologically inherent, and in fact were often acquired as a mechanism to cope with life experiences. The impact of what came to be known simply as "Medical 203" was not immediate, but over the coming decades it continued to resonate, as successive diagnostic manuals continued to adopt its classifications.[296]

Addiction was defined in "Medical 203," under "Character and Behavior Disorder," as follows:

> This diagnosis usually implies antisocial behavior, while the individual is under the influence of alcohol or drug, such as pugnaciousness, deception, stealing, sexual assault, etc. It represents a much deeper character disturbance than cases where the usage of alcohol or drug represents a symptom of some more extensive psychiatric illness. This term should not include excessive symptomatic utilization of alcohol, which is a symptom of depression or psychoneurosis; nor should it include acute alcoholic intoxication. The term includes cases formerly classed merely as 'drug addiction' and also some cases which were formerly classified as 'constitutional psychopathic state.' The diagnosis should specify whether the addiction is to alcohol or drug.[297]

In many ways, addiction was but a secondary diagnosis caused by other mental disorders – namely, anti-social behavior. It was not until the publication in 1968 of the second edition of the "Diagnostic and Statistical Manual of Mental Disorders" (DSM-II), the authoritative source for classifying mental illnesses, that addiction became a mental condition on its own right, without requiring a "recognizable underlying disorder."[298]

The definition of addiction reflected American laws. Drugs were separated from alcohol, tobacco and medically prescribed drugs as long as "the

---

296 Houts, "Fifty Years of Psychiatric Nomenclature: Reflections on the 1943 War Department Technical Bulletin, Medical 203," 935-938, 940, 942-944. Proposals to categorize mental diseases existed throughout the 20th century. For example, the *American Medico-Psychological Association* tried to categorize mental diseases in 1917, with limited success. Alcoholism and drug addiction without psychoses were to be classified under the 'not insane' category, as opposed to psychoses caused by toxins such as alcohol, morphine, cocaine, chloral and other drugs. See *Proceedings of the American Medico-Psychological Association at the Seventy-Third Annual Meeting* (Baltimore, 1917), 129-130, 138.

297 Office of the Surgeon General, Army Service Forces, "War Department Technical Bulletin, Medical 203," reproduced as "Nomenclature of Psychiatric Disorders and Reactions," *Journal of Clinical Psychology* 56:7 (2000 [1943, 1946]), 930.

298 *Diagnostic and Statistical Manual of Mental Disorders*, 2nd ed. (Washington DC, 1968), 2.

intake is proportionate to the medical need." The use of alcohol and tobacco could turn into a disorder, whereas the use of medically prescribed drugs could not.[299]

The Menningers, Ruth Mack Brunswick and Sigmund Freud's many other followers in the United States faithfully propagated what they believed to be a new understanding of addiction. In point of fact, however, the insights that they reached were but an evolution of the theories developed by Freud's nemesis, Albrecht Erlenmeyer. Once Erlenmeyer's ideas found their way across the Atlantic, where the understanding of addiction had taken a far different trajectory, they were regarded as new and revolutionary. Psychoanalysis, in effect, resurrected Erlenmeyer's old ideas and presented them in America as a new approach to addiction. Among psychiatrists and psychologists, the imported ideas would hold sway until well into the 1960s, and in some medical circles even beyond.

---

299 Ibid., 45.

3. Diminished Responsibility

The evolving debate in Germany over the nature of alcohol and drug addiction had far-reaching implications, perhaps nowhere as much as in the realm of criminal law. After the drinking disease was identified in the 19th century, drunkenness turned from a moral sin into a physical disease, thereby allowing for diminished criminal responsibility for acts committed while under the influence.

The concept of "diminished responsibility" was hardly a new one. In ancient Rome, the law allowed for limiting the drunkard's culpability in committing a crime and provided for either immunity from prosecution or a reduced sentence – no small matter, given that drunkards in Rome were condemned to either prison or hell. Roman views on the culpability of drunkards found their way, centuries later, into *Zurechnungsfähigkeit*, Germany's legal conception of criminal responsibility. One had to be of sound mind to bear such a responsibility. Therefore, soon after Brühl-Cramer's definition of habitual drunkenness as a physical disease, law courts began considering cases of the drinking diseased and *Zurechnungsfähigkeit*. By the mid-19th century, German judges were known to have accepted physicians' prognoses as expert testimony regarding dipsomaniacs' inability to stand trial.[300] Since the disease was involuntary, judges increasingly ruled, those suffering from it bore no criminal liability.

Germany's legal tradition, it ought to be pointed out, was far from uniform. Numerous cities, states and kingdoms dotted the country, each with their own tradition regarding drunkenness, criminal responsibility and expert testimony. Laws regarding criminal responsibility existed in Baden, Bavaria, Saxony and the Prussian possessions in the Rhineland, but they often differed from place to place. Prussia itself, in fact, was not

---

300 F. Hergt, "Bericht über die Leistungen in der gerchitlichen Medicin" in *Jahres-bericht ueber die Fortschritte der gesammten Medicin in allen Laendern im Jahre 1845*, Vol. 7, ed. Canstatt and Eisenmann (Erlangen, 1846), 101. According to the revision of § 280 of the Prussian Criminal Code (*Kriminalordnung*) on 11 December 1805, judges required asking physicians for their opinion regarding a person's mental ability to stand trial; but they did not have to accept the assessment.

subject to the laws on drunkenness that it imposed on its Western posses-sions. In addition, in more than one case, the authorities elected to main-tain public order rather than debate the finer points of Roman law and defendants rights.[301]

Despite the confusion and disorder, physicians and jurists tried throughout the 19th century to form a coherent sense of diminished crim-inal responsibility. They endeavored to form objective definitions of crime, looking to rational philosophy and the French penal code for guid-ance as a way around the legal differences among Germany's principali-ties.[302] As a result, physicians from all around Germany rigorously debated the legal definition of the drinking disease.

Not all of them agreed with Brühl-Cramer. The question of whether the law should protect what many perceived as the vice of drunkenness troubled some specialists in forensic medicine. It became clear that unscrupulous criminals could use drunkenness as an excuse to commit crimes.[303] Critics of the drinking disease continued to beat on the morality drum, pointing at what they construed as loopholes in the theory of dimin-ished responsibility.[304]

"Every disease of a person is both physical and mental, but it will not stand out as one or the other," declared a Saxon physician specializing in mental illnesses, Johann Christian August Heinroth of Leipzig (1773-1843), in 1825. "In other words, it will not appear as either organic or moral disease. Instead, it will depend on the character of the person-

---

301 Beverly Ann Tlusty, *Bacchus and Civic Order: The Culture of Drink in Early Modern Germany* (Charlottesville: University Press of Virginia, 2001), 80-84, 90-91, 96-102.

302 Franz von Liszt, *Lehrbuch des deutschen Strafrechts* (Berlin, 1908), 49-52. On the role of psychiatry in the French Penal Code devised by Napoleon, see Jan Ellen Goldstein, *Console and Classify: The French Psychiatric Profession in the Nineteenth Century* (Chicago: Chicago University Press, 2001), 162-169. Napoleon occupied the Rhineland and had given it as the Kingdom of Westphalia to his younger brother, Jérôme Bonaparte. Perhaps the French influence over the region was the reason why Prussia instated articles pertaining criminal responsi-bility after it had assumed its control over the region in 1815.

303 Diez, "Bemerkungen über Zurechnungsfähigkeit und Todesstrafe, in Beziehung auf den neuen Strafgesetzentwurf für Baden" in *Annalen der Staatsarzneikunde*, Vol. 3:2, ed. J. Schneider, J. H. Schürmayer and F. Hergt (Tübingen, 1838), 503-506.

304 Bynum, "Chronic Alcoholism in the First Half of the 19th Century," 164.

ality."[305] Consequently, he argued, drunkenness might at first seem to be "a cause for diminished responsibility, but [it] does not in a more inquisitive glance. The same is true for the drinking disease, which brings about uncontrollable anger."[306]

Heinroth distinguished between three grades of drunkenness: intoxication (*Rausch*), drunkenness and complete inebriation. Unless the consumption of alcohol (or opium) was unwitting, it did not excuse a person's actions. In fact, the more serious the crime, the more liable the perpetrator for his actions. After all, Heinroth wrote, in an echo of G. E. Lessing's *Nathan the Wise*, "no person has to have to" drink.[307]

Although the symptoms of drunkenness and insanity were often similar, he argued, their origins were not. A person chose to drink, whereas insanity was uncontrollable. Nor was drunkenness a disease like insanity. Heinroth insisted, despite the identification of *delirium tremens* in 1813 and the association of alcohol with death, that the drinking disease was not physical in nature:

> That one makes the drinking disease and its subsequent complications a pure physical evil proves that one sees only the physical level of people; one should say, only the body. As if mental degeneration does not proceed in the same pace as physical ruin into an ever-increasing constraint and passivity.... In fact, physical ruin is only a companion, a necessary result of the permanent continued mental (moral) offence. Every step towards passivity, every new surrender of the will and freedom (self control) to the slavery of desire, every step of sinking into the nefarious state, is noticeable in... the body; or in other words, by a grade of organic disorder and gradual ruin, so that at last it brings about an organic disease, which is usually untreatable.[308]

Physical ruin was caused by moral ruin; therefore, the drinking disease was only an extension of drunkenness, and as a result inexcusable. Yet despite Heinroth's position in Saxon medical, legal and royal circles, most Germans declined to adopt his view. It was only among moralists and clerics across the Atlantic that his sentiments found support.

A fellow Saxon royal physician, Johann Christian August Clarus (1774-1854), perhaps most famous for his role in a murder case that

305 Johann Christian August Heinroth, *System der psychisch-gerichlichen Medicine* (Leipzig, 1825), 166.
306 Ibid., 258.
307 Ibid., 258-261n.1-3, 5.
308 Ibid., 263-264n.6.

became the subject of an opera a century later,[309] adopted Brühl-Cramer's drinking disease as grounds for an inability to stand trial. Clarus maintained in 1828 that not every habitual drunkard, or *Trunkfällig*, was ill, and that not every form of drunkenness ought to be excused in the court of law.[310]

The need to distinguish between types of drunkenness was clear: To preempt criticism from those claiming that alcohol could serve as a loophole for getting away with committing crimes. Like Heinroth, Clarus divided drunkenness into three separate types. The first could be best described as common drunkenness, in which drunkards "have such a mastery over their vice as never to be altogether overcome by it. They drink daily, without ever being actually drunken; weakening thereby their digestion and their mental energy more and more, and, finally, fall victims to bodily diseases arising from chronic alcoholic poisoning."[311]

The second type was temporary insanity caused by drunkenness, in which drunkards "fall into that form of periodic insanity which is only too

---

309 See Johann Christian August Clarus, "Die Zurechnungsfähigkeit des Mörders Johann Christian Woyzeck, nach Grundsätzen der Staatsarzneikunde aktenmäßig erwiesen" (Leipzig, 16 September 1821 and 1 August 1824) in C. M. Marc, *War der am 27ten August 1824 zu Leipzig hingerichtete Mörder Johann Christian Woyzeck zurechnungsfähig?* (Bamberg, 1825). In June 1821, J. C. Woyzeck murdered a widow and was brought before a judge, who ordered an assessment regarding his ability to stand trial. Dr. Clarus, after meeting Woyzeck five times, declared the man healthy and the trial continued. Woyzeck was sentenced to death in 1822. Shortly before the execution date, Dr. Clarus composed a second report reinforcing the first assessment, and Woyzeck was executed in 1824. After the report was published it caught the attention of the public, since it was attested to by others that Woyzeck had been mentally ill. An unfinished play by Georg Büchner published posthumously in 1879 focused on the trial, and was later adapted into the opera "Wozzeck" by Alban Berg in 1925.) See Maurice B. Benn, *The Drama of Revolt: A Critical Study of Georg Büchner* (Cambridge: Cambridge University Press, 1976), 217-222; Otto Friedrich, *Before the Deluge: A Portrait of Berlin in the 1920's* (New York: Fromm International, 1972), 180-183. Heinroth disagreed with Clarus' report. In effect, he acted more leniently than his colleague, even though in theory he appeared more dogmatic by his refusal to acknowledge the drinking disease as grounds for diminished criminal liability.

310 See Johann Christian August Clarus, *Beiträge zur Erkenntniß und Beurtheilung zweifelhafter Seelenzustände*, (Leipzig, 1828), 130; Friedrich Eduard Oehler, "Erstes Gutachten" in *Magazin für die Staatsarzneikunde*, Vol. 3, ed. Friedrich Julius Siebenhaar and Rudolph Julius Albert Martini (Leipzig, 1844), 47-48.

311 Casper, *A Handbook of the Practice of Forensic Medicine*, 262.

well known as the delirium of drunkards (*delirium potatorum, del. Tremens*), and which possess no more specific interest for forensic medicine than any other form of insanity that may arise from drunkenness, which is so frequent a cause of mental diseases in general. Because the estimation of illegal deeds done committed during a fit of delirium tremens differs in no respect from that of any other deed committed through insanity."[312] The third, and rarest, form of drunkenness was the drinking disease, as described by Brühl-Cramer.[313]

Of the three forms of drunkenness, temporary insanity held the most interest for legal scholars. Anselm von Feuerbach (1775-1833), a jurist from Jena who authored the Bavarian penal code of 1813, published the proceedings of a case of a petty landowner killed by his farmhand in Erlangen. The killing took place on the night of August 3, 1828, after both master and farmhand were drunk. When the local police arrived at the scene, they found the farmhand, known as Pürner, fast asleep and unable to wake up. They were forced to transport the suspect on a makeshift stretcher to jail, where he continued to sleep as if he were dead.

The forensic report on Pürner's mental health asserted that the farmhand was known to be a congenial drunkard, but on that fateful night he was so completely drunk as to have reached the second stage of drunkenness, causing him to think that his master was a weasel. The court recognized the farmhand as the perpetrator, but nonetheless set him free, arguing that he was not criminally culpable under Article 121 of the Bavarian Criminal Law because he was not consciousness while committing the crime.[314] Because he was found to be temporarily insane, Pürner was ruled to be unfit to stand trial.

By the mid-19th century, a growing number of jurists and physicians supported the argument that drunkenness could cause temporary insanity, rendering a defendant immune to punishment. Adolph Henke (1775-1843), a professor of medicine in Erlangen and privy councilor in

---

312 Ibid., 266.
313 Ibid.; Steegmann, "Zur Lehre von der gerichtsärztlichen Beurtheilung der Trunkenheit und der Trunkfälligkeit" *Zeitschrift für die Staatsarzneikunde* 15:4 (1835), 245-318.
314 Anselm von Feuerbach, "Johann Pürner oder Beispiel einer Tötung in höchster Trunkenheit" (1828?) in *Anselm Ritter von Feuerbach: Merkwürdige Verbrechen in aktenmäßiger Darstellung*, ed. R. A. Stemmle (Munich: Bruckmann, 1963), 182-199.

the Bavarian royal court, explained in an 1841 textbook on forensic medicine that there were various grades of intoxication – notably, from both wines and other narcotics – that resulted in differing degrees of impairment of the psyche. Depending on its degree of severity, intoxication reduced or completely removed a perpetrator's criminal liability, provided that the drunkenness or intoxication was not self-imposed.[315] Although the drinking disease might be caused by immoral behavior, Henke argued, it was a physical disease and therefore could not be considered a moral failure. Thus, a person ill with the drinking disease was not accountable for his actions, and had to be accorded either diminished criminal responsibility or complete acquittal.[316]

In 1856, Johann Ludwig Casper, a professor of forensic medicine in Berlin, wrote that the drinking disease, though rare, was in essence a periodic loss of sanity caused by a physical urge to drink. A person might rarely drink, but fall sick every so often by drinking uncontrollably. As such, the person suffering from the disease bore no criminal liability for his actions while under such a sickly bout of drinking.[317] Two decades later Albert Dalcke (1828?-1900), a senior Prussian state attorney, drew a finer distinction regarding culpability, arguing in 1879 that "drunkenness, which has not degenerated into unconsciousness, does not exclude criminal liability." Thus, it was not enough for a person to be unaware of his actions; he must not have desired those actions to begin with.[318]

By the mid 19th century Henke and Brühl-Cramer's theories on the diminished responsibility of those suffering from the drinking disease had gained preeminence in Germany, and it became a matter of practice in German courts to recognize the disease and its implications on criminal liability.[319] Recognition by the courts, however, hardly translated into a clear and uniform understanding of the legal status of intoxication, since no direct mention of liability under intoxication was made in the Prussian

---

315 Adolph Henke, *Lehrbuch der gerichtlichen Medicin* (Berlin, 1841), 204; idem, *Abhandlungen aus dem Gebiete der gerichtlichen Medizin* vol. 4/4, (Bamberg, 1840), 299.

316 Ibid., 205.

317 Casper, *A Handbook of the Practice of Forensic Medicine*, 266-267.

318 Albert Dalcke, *Strafrecht und Strafprozeß: Eine Sammlung der wichtigsten das Strafrecht und das Strafverfahren betreffenden Gesetze* (Berlin, 1929 [1879]), 30-31.

319 Hergt, "Bericht über die Leistungen in der gerchitlichen Medicin," 101-102.

Penal Code of 1851.[320] There was a Prussian law on the books that dealt with the diminished responsibility of those suffering from intoxication, but it was only in force in the western possessions of the kingdom. The General Law for the Prussian States, passed in 1794, directed that "persons who are deprived of the use of their reason by drunkenness are, so long as this drunkenness lasts, to be regarded insane."[321]

In Prussia proper, the penal code was the law of the land, and paragraph 40 directed that a person declared *non compos mentis* (of unsound mind) could not stand trial, but it did not define the terms by which a person's mental competency should be judged.[322] In other words, the law did not describe who or how a defendant could be declared of unsound mind.

Due to the fractured political situation in Germany, laws in other German principalities differed from those in Prussia in their recognition of gradations of limited responsibility for criminal action. Some principalities recognized diminished criminal responsibility; others adopted the *non compos mentis* clause fully. In theory, however, all laws shared some things in common: physicians and medical experts were recognized as the authoritative profession with the power to determine whether a person was of sound mind.[323] In practice, however, judges rarely consulted specialists in cases involving crimes committed under intoxication. Instead, the defendant's capacity to stand trial was usually determined based on witness testimony.

The question that concerned judges at the time was whether the perpetrator's drunkenness left him with his senses, or in fact deprived him of them. The latter condition would render him unable to stand trial.[324] The role of doctors in the courtroom, however, was not lost completely. Under the Code for Criminal Procedure promulgated after the unification of Germany, prosecutors were also permitted to send an accused for mental evaluation as part of the pre-trial procedure.[325] Soon, German physicians, psychiatrists and criminologists had become increasingly active in legal matters, exerting their influence on policy and pressing for changes in the

---

320 Casper, *A Handbook of the Practice of Forensic Medicine*, 262.
321 *Das Allgemeine Landrecht für die preußischen Staaten* (ALR), 5 February 1794, Tit. 4, § 28.
322 Ibid., § 40.
323 Casper, *A Handbook of the Practice of Forensic Medicine*, 262.
324 Ibid., 262-263.
325 Hett, *Death in the Tiergarten*, 197.

legal codes regarding diminished criminal responsibility. Their influence was great, especially when it suited the law courts and the ruling class, as to excuse a would-be assassin of royalty.

On 22 May 1850, a sergeant named Maximilian Joseph Sefolge attempted to assassinate Prussian King Friedrich Wilhelm IV (1795-1861). Sefolge managed to only lightly wound the king and was apprehended. Under custody, three psychiatrists – Carl Wilhelm Ideler of the Charité (1795-1860), Moritz Gustav Martini of the Leubus mental asylum (1794-1875), and Johann Ludwig Casper – examined the man and declared him mentally unfit to stand trial. Instead of receiving the death sentence for his capital crime, Sefolge was sent to a mental asylum in Halle, where he died nine years later of tuberculosis.

To be sure, medical intervention in the courtroom was not without political support. After the revolution of 1848, the Prussian monarch had no interest in admitting that the attempt on his life was political; he was rather content with the notion that it was the act of a deranged man. Yet, political considerations notwithstanding, the judge's reliance on the opinion of Ideler, Martini and Casper proved to be a legal watershed in Germany. And an unintended consequence of the Sefolge case was the ensuing rise in influence of forensic specialists and psychiatrists.[326] The law soon came to reflect their growing role in defining the legal parameters of diminished responsibility.

When the German Penal Code was passed in 1871, it incorporated elements of Paragraph 40 of the 1851 Prussian Penal Code – the section of the code dealing with criminal responsibility – into the following wording:

> 51. A criminal act is not existent if the perpetrator is deemed to be in a state of unconsciousness or is in a state of pathological disturbance of his mental faculties, through which his free will was suspended at the time of committing the act.[327]

The 1871 code marked a shift in the balance of power in the courtroom. Physicians had successfully broadened the term mental illness, replacing it with a "sickly disturbance of mental activity" and thereby opening debate

---

326 Kathleen Haack et al., "Der 'Fall Sefeloge': Ein Beitrag zur Geschichte der forensischen Psychiatrie," *Der Nervenarzt* 5 (2007), 586-593.

327 *Strafgesetzbuch für das Deutsche Reich* (15 May 1871), § 51.

on how drunk a person needed to be in order "to have himself declared not responsible for his actions."[328]

Physicians, psychiatrists and criminologists had hoped they would be the ones to decide on a person's mental fitness, in effect demanding that their expert testimony be the basis for judges' rulings. German judges, however, never entirely relinquished their preeminence in the courtroom, allowing medical and mental experts to testify but not outright determine a person's fitness for trial.[329] Buoyed by their inroads into criminal law, penal code reformers pushed even further, demanding almost immediately after the promulgation of the code that the state abandon morality-driven punitive justice and turn instead to empirical science and the causes of crime. Their new understanding of criminal responsibility was to be reflected in penal reform that would allow for reforming criminals and eventually reintegrating them back into society.[330]

Such penal reforms, however, were not realized in the 19th century. It was only with the Nazis' rise to power in the 1930s that such notions were codified into law – albeit in a highly distorted manner. Despite the eventual adoption of their ideas by the Nazis, the reformers' sway should not easily be dismissed or necessarily tainted. Their work influenced countless jurists and physicians, and they left an indelible mark on German courts.

Richard von Krafft-Ebing, who believed in the connection between crime and degeneration, wrote in 1872 that an intoxicated person in a state of *delirium tremens* could not bear criminal responsibility under any circumstances. Any person experiencing hallucinations caused by drugs or alcohol, in fact, could be excused for his actions. As for drunkenness and criminal liability, Krafft-Ebing claimed that it depended on several variables: when the alcohol was consumed, the type of company the drinker kept, how the witnesses understood the drinker's actions, and the physical condition of the drinker.

Krafft-Ebing admitted that, to his disappointment, final judgment rested with the judge, since Paragraph 51 of the Penal Code did not stipulate any specific guidelines regarding intoxication and crime. He believed there

---

328 Quoted in Geoffrey J. Giles, "Drinking and Crime in Modern Germany," 471-472.

329 Eric J. Engstrom, "Forensic Psychiatry in Imperial Germany," *Tabur* 2 (2009), 25-40. [Hebrew]

330 Richard F. Wetzell, "Psychiatry and Criminal Justice in Modern Germany, 1880-1933" *Journal of European Studies* 39:3 (2009), 270-289.

was scientific proof that maniac reactions to alcohol had physical symptoms. Similar to brain damage and meningitis, even though the alcohol disease could in some instances be inherited. Despite Krafft-Ebing's efforts, however, German courts did not automatically recognize the disease.[331]

On the question of diminished responsibility due to intoxication, the leader of the penal reform movement in Germany was unquestionably Franz von Liszt (1851-1919). The criminologist identified blackouts, sleep, delirium, sleepwalking and drunkenness as sickly disturbances of the mental faculties, disturbances he declared to be of sufficient severity to render the perpetrator unfit for trial. As others did before him, von Liszt issued a caveat, arguing that the motives of the drinker had to be benign.[332]

Other jurists, such as Reinhard Frank (1860-1934), a law professor in Tübingen and one of von Liszt's students, limited the idea of unconsciousness to include severe drunkenness (in German, *hohe Grade der Trunkenheit*). Needless to say, both the sickly manifestation of drunkenness and acute alcohol poisoning were grounds for diminished criminal responsibility. Frank, however, rejected monomania as a defense.[333] But by the beginning of the 20th century, monomania as a mental disease was discredited, and alcoholism attained a status of a disease on its own.

The possibility of drunkards getting off on technicalities worried the German government. After reading about a case in which a drunkard was set free even though he had bitten off a policeman's finger, Chancellor Otto von Bismarck asked his minister of justice to mend the situation. The minister replied with the *Trunksuchtgesetz*, a bill which would have enabled the incarceration of drunkards despite their status as lunatics. The matter was brought before the Reichstag in 1881, but failed to pass.[334]

Not all Germans enjoyed the wide interpretations of the laws that were on the books. Wealthy persons caught committing crimes while drunk

---

331 Krafft-Ebing, *Grundzüge der Criminalpsychologie auf Grundlage des Strafgesetzbuchs des Deutschen Reichs für Aerzte und Juristen*, 108-111.

332 Franz von Liszt and Ernst Delaquis (eds.), *Strafgesetzbuch für das Deutsche Reich* (Berlin, 1914), 83n3; Franz von Liszt, *Lehrbuch des deutschen Strafrechts* (Berlin, 1888), 153-154, 160.

333 Reinhard Frank (ed.), *Das Strafgesetzbuch für das Deutsche Reich* (Tübingen, 1908), 109-110.

334 Roberts, *Drink, Temperance and the Working Class in Nineteenth Century Germany*, 52-53.

usually had easy access to physicians who could attest to their temporary insanity, whereas the poor had no such recourse and were often incarcerated for their crimes. One byproduct of this uneven application of the law was the strengthening of the notion among reformers and temperance societies that alcohol consumption and drunkenness go hand in hand with crime.[335]

Complaints about the leniency of the law courts were raised time and again. Public outrage, however, did not translate into penal reform, and Paragraph 51 of the Penal Code – the section dealing with criminal responsibility – remained on the books into the 20th century. That attempts at reform met with so little success was particularly glaring given the frequency with which the diminished responsibility plea was raised in the courtroom. According to one police report, out of a total of 77 murder cases in Berlin in 1889-1900, 10 perpetrators were found insane and consequently were unable to stand trial. Between 1901 and 1904, no less than 17 of 58 perpetrators were unable to stand trial – roughly one-third.[336] In 1907-1908, it was 10 out of 48.[337] The steady number of murder cases being dismissed because the perpetrator was found unfit for trial was all the more worrisome for Germany, one of the few countries in Europe and North America that was experiencing an increase in crime.[338]

Such figures, it should be noted, must be taken with a grain of salt. The police were known to doctor their reports when political expediency so demanded. For example, in a report compiled for the German Ministry of Foreign Affairs at the request of the British embassy, the number of defendants in capital cases found unable to stand trial shrank to 11 out of 120 in the years 1904-1908, dropping to just six cases of 48 in 1907-1908.[339] In a

---

335 Giles, "Drinking and Crime in Modern Germany," 472-485.

336 "Regierungsassessor Dr. Lindenau (Polizei Präsidium Abteilung IV) to Minister of Interior: Capital Crimes According to Paragraphs 211-215 of the Reich Criminal Code in Berlin" (Berlin, 10 November 1905) in GSa. PKb. I.HA Re77 Tit. 235 No. 1 vol. 13, ff. 126-128.

337 "Regierungsassessor Dr. von Schmidt (Polizei Präsedium Abteilung IV) to Minister of Interior: Statistics from the Berlin Criminal Police, 1907-1908" (Berlin, 30 October 1908) in GSa. PKb. I.HA Re77 Tit. 235 No. 1 vol. 13, ff. 243-244.

338 Arthur MacDonald, "Criminal Statistics in Germany, France and England," *Journal of the American Institute of Criminal Law and Criminology* 1:2 (1910), 59-70.

339 "Minister of Foreign Affairs to Minister of Interior: British Embassy Criminal Statistics Request" (Berlin, 22 January 1909) and "The Criminal Statistics of

different report on 1903-1908, however, the figures given were 14 cases out of 120, with 11 of 64 in 1907-1908.[340]

When it was time to gain popular support by appearing to be tough against criminals, the police depicted a picture in which its hands were tied behind its back. But when it was time to demonstrate successes to the Foreign Ministry and to other countries, the police provided statistics that gave the appearance of a strong hand.

During the Second Reich and the republic that followed, German courts could only hand down sentences to drug users and addicts for violating Paragraph 367 of the Reich Penal Code, which primarily dealt with prescriptions. There were also cases in which a person under intoxication was found guilty of breaking Paragraph 230, which prohibited a person from causing harm to himself. And occasionally physicians were found guilty of prescribing too many drugs for themselves and their patients, thus harming their own or their patients' health.[341] Otherwise, however, drug use generally remained legal in Germany. No law was ever passed explicitly forbidding the use of a drug.

Pressure came from all directions, and dissatisfaction from the German criminal code and procedure were apparent to all, especially in regards to criminal responsibility and the place of alcohol in the law. Occasional public uproars filled the press. For example, in 1932, a farmer named Gustav Loose was accused of raping and killing a four-year-old girl, but the reporter of the newspaper, *Berliner Tageblatt*, did not blame the culprit. Instead, the reporter focused on Loose's deterioration caused by his alcoholism, blaming the 'devil alcohol' for the crime. Before committing his crime, Loose requested to be hospitalized for his alcoholism, but was met with indifference. The article blamed the health authorities for allowing such a case of alcoholism go untreated; after all, if Loose were in treatment for his disease, he would not have committed the crime. The

---

Berlin" (Berlin, ca. January 1909) in GSa. PKb. I.HA Re77 Tit. 235 No. 1 vol. 13, ff. 250, 240.

340 "Oberregierungsrat Hoppe (Polizei Präsidium Abteilung IV) to Minister of Interior" (Berlin, 8 February 1909) in GSa. PKb. I.HA Re77 Tit. 235 No. 1 vol. 13, ff. 258-261.

341 Louis Lewin and Wenzel Goldbaum, *Opiumgesetz: Nebst Internationalen Opiumabkommen und Ausführungs bestimmungen* (Berlin, 1928), 19. For examples, see the appendices of the book.

authorities were therefore the true culprits, and their incompetence was responsible for the crime.[342]

It was only with the National Socialists' rise to power that Germany finally enacted reforms to its criminal law.[343] In 1933, the Nazi-led Reichstag passed the Law Against Dangerous Habitual Criminals, which allowed for the indefinite incarceration of habitual criminals even after their sentences had been served. And, in a complete departure from the rule of law, the police were allowed to incarcerate professional or habitual criminals in concentration camps without a court order.[344]

There is nothing more habitual than addicts consuming their drug of choice, so it would stand to reason that drug addicts were sent to concentration camps in droves. Yet despite that fact that the Nazis were meticulous record keepers, no record of such deportations has even been found. Nor were there reports of drug addiction inside the concentration camps and prisons.

The police seemed to have received carte blanche to dispose of addicts, yet refrained from doing so. Why? An answer can be found in what may now appear to be a rather semantic argument: Drug use was never a crime in Germany, and therefore habitual drug users – drug addicts – were not criminals. And because they were not considered habitual criminals, they could not be sent to a concentration camp.

The Law Against Dangerous Habitual Criminals also included several modifications to Paragraph 42 of the Penal Code. It granted judges the ability to forcibly send those protected by Paragraph 51 to a sanitarium, and to forcibly enroll alcoholics in a detoxification program.[345] The law was not specifically written against drug addicts, but since Paragraph 51 also absolved them of criminal liability, they could find themselves in a sanitarium, or *Heil- und Pflegeanstalt* (either a regular or mental hospital).

The Nazi government was given the credit for reforming the lenient penal code. In the minds of many Germans, the court's inability before

342 August Hermann Zeiz, "Teufel Alkohol. Ein Mann kämpft vergeblich gegen seine Laster," *Berliner Tageblatt*, (7 October 1932). I would like to thank Daniel Siemens of Bielefeld University for this article.

343 Richard F. Wetzell, *Inventing the Criminal: A History of German Criminology, 1880-1945* (Chapel Hill: North Carolina University Press, 2000), 234-235.

344 "Gesetz gegen gefährliche Gewohnheitsverbrecher und über Massregeln der Sicherung und Besserung, 24 November 1933," *Reichsgesetzblatt* I, 995.

345 Ibid.

1933 to forcibly send addicts to sanatoria was the fault of the weak Weimar Republic during the 1920s.[346] The pushback against drug addiction was credited to the strong measures of the National Socialist state, and the Nazis made sure to remind the public of it later, as attested to by a 1942 speech by *Kriminalkommissar* Erwin Kosmehl.[347]

The Law Against Dangerous Habitual Criminals was used often against political opponents and others whom the Nazis found undesirable. Concentration camps filled, and so did the prisons. However, not every person who was forcibly dealt with under this law was indeed a political opponent, an undesirable, or even poorly treated. It was simply in the nature of the Nazi regime to have such a measure for all elements of society.

---

346 "Summary of the Stettin Conference, 10 October 1937" StA. München, Pol. Dir. 7582.

347 Erwin Kosmehl, *Der sicherheitspolizeiliche Einsatz bei der Bekämpfung der Betäubungsmittelsucht* (14 October 1942), BArch RD 19/30.

4. "Gay Weimar" and the Third Reich

Today the Weimar Republic is mostly remembered as a morally depraved Sodom and Gomorra, a time when Berlin was intoxicated with cabarets, champagne and cocaine. To the modern observer, no figure better symbolizes that era of German history than dancer Anita Berber (1899-1928).

Berber, along with her second husband Sebastian Droste (1898-1927), performed onstage either nude or barely clothed, with a repertoire of drug-induced dances including "Kokain," "Morphium" and "Absinthe."[348] "Kokain," the highlight of the couple's Viennese program in 1922, was based on a poem written by Droste to the sounds of Camille Saint-Saëns' "La danse macabre," opus 40.[349] Saint-Saëns was a fitting choice for Droste, who was himself a morphine and cocaine addict. A self-proclaimed pederast, Saint-Saëns had already established his reputation with "Songe d'opium" and "La princess jaune," an opera in which opium leads a man to believe that his wife is a Japanese princess.[350]

Berber was a particularly lewd dancer, and incorporated drugs and sex into her performances in ways few had done before. Her performances indeed drew the attention of the German authorities, but tellingly, it was not for her blatant public abuse of cocaine, morphine or absinthe. What troubled the law was her immoral dancing, with its sacrilegious undertones and pornographic displays, as well as the substantial debts she took on over the years.[351] Similar police indifference was exhibited toward the drug of choice in Celly de Rheydt's (1890-1924) dance "Opium Intoxication,"[352] which garnered outrage only for the dancer's reputation of using a cross as a dildo.[353]

---

348 Lothar Fischer, *Anita Berber: Göttin der Nacht* (Berlin: Edition Ebersbach, 2006), 99.
349 Ibid., 100.
350 Charles Camille Saint-Saëns, *La princess jaune* (Opus 30, 1872); idem, "Tournoiement (Songe d'opium)" *Mélodies persanes* (Opus 26 No. 6, 1870).
351 Erika Hughes, "Art and Illegality on the Weimar Stage: The Dances of Celly de Rheydt, Anita Berber and Valeska Gert," *Journal of European Studies* 39:3 (2009), 320-335.
352 Peter Jelavich, *Berlin Cabaret* (Cambridge MA: Harvard University Press, 1993), 156.

To the relative few who attended one of Berber or de Rheydt's shows, the Weimar years were indeed gay and depraved. But whether the 1920s was a time of rampant drug use in Germany, as has generally been assumed, is far from certain. Recent scholarship, in fact, has suggested that the country's sensationalist press fabricated the drug panic.[354] What is clear, however, is that Weimar officials' attitudes and policies toward drugs stood in stark contrast to their American counterparts at the time. Simply put, the German police were mostly disinterested in drugs, and German politicians hardly employed the drug issue to pursue their legislative agendas. When concerns were raised, they were done in a manner far more subdued than in Washington.

When Hamburg senator Alexander Zinn (1880-1941) expressed concern about the city's opium dens, for example, it was mostly in regard to projecting a positive image for Hamburg that would help promote the city's position as an international center of finance and trade. Notably, he did not introduce any effective measures for combating the perceived drug. He had little reason to do so, as there was little public demand for action.[355]

On the face of it, Hamburg would have seemed an ideal place for the drug plague to fester. As a major port, Hamburg was home to countless characters of questionable repute, from alcoholics and prostitutes to smugglers and wealthy merchants. And multiple overlapping jurisdictions made Hamburg a legal anomaly. The port city was also a recognized state of the German Republic. And further complicating matters, a small part of its harbor was leased to Czechoslovakia under the terms of the post-World War I Treaty of Versailles.

Declared a free port in 1888, Hamburg harbor operated for the most part free of control by the German customs office, which exercised only limited jurisdiction over imports and exports passing through the world's fourth largest port.[356] The city was a true haven for drug smuggling opera-

---

353 Hughes, "Art and Illegality on the Weimar Stage."

354 Annika Hoffmann, "Von Morphiumpralinees und Opiumzigaretten: Zur beginnenden Problematisierung des Betäubungsmittelkonsums im Deutschland der 1920er Jahre," in *Sozialwissenschaftliche Suchtforschung*, ed. Bernd Dollinger and Henning Schmidt-Semisch (Wiesbaden: Springer Verlag, 2007), 251-276.

355 Alexander Zinn (Head of the State Press Station), "Hamburgische Werbeprobleme," (1929) *Hamburger Wirtschafts-Chronik* 6 (2006), 134.

356 Lars Amenda, "'Welthafen' Hamburg-Kultur- und technikgeschichtliche Perspektiven," in *Hamburgs Geschichte einmal anders: Entwicklung der Natur-*

tions, serving as a hub for drugs in transit from their points of origin in French or German factories to the United States and other large illicit drug markets around the world.[357] It would be nearly impossible to determine what percentage of the drugs that passed through the city actually stayed there, but it can safely be assumed that at least some remained to satisfy local demand.

That demand, however, was limited. Germany's own encounter with the "Chinaman" and his nefarious opium offers a telling example. There were Chinese sailors in Hamburg who were known to smoke opium, including some who were also involved in the illegal drug trade.[358] As might be expected, there was the occasional illicit tale. In October 1922, for example, police discovered and raided an opium den on Schmuckstraße, in the center of Hamburg's Chinatown, where they found a stash of the drug and several weapons.[359] The opium dens of one of the city's rougher neighborhoods, to cite another example, were exposed in a local newspaper article headlined "The 'Yellow Peril' in St. Pauli."[360]

Such tales, however, were generally few and far between. Hamburg saw little need for anything more than the occasional police raid, and the city-state had no equivalent to the seclusion laws and opium den laws California had on its books from the 1870s through the 1930s. Germany never forbade Chinese nationals from entering its borders, though admittedly few actually seriously considered settling in Germany. When it came to enacting laws banning opium or Chinese immigrants, the governments in Hamburg and in Berlin showed lethargy more than anything else.

The absence of a nationwide drug panic was likely due less to German tolerance of drugs than to the limited number of foreigners on whom the scourge could be blamed. In the 1920s, a few Chinese sailors of Cantonese origin settled in the St. Pauli neighborhood, which was known even back then as a place of ill repute. With the Chinese sailors came the accompa-

---

wissenschaften, Medizin und Technik, Vol. 2, ed. Gudrun Wolfschmidt (Norderstedt: Books on Demand, 2009), 239-250.

357 Idem, *Fremde-Hafen-Stadt: Chinesische Migration und ihre Wahrnehmung in Hamburg, 1897-1972* (Hamburg: Dölling und Galitz Verlag, 2006), 151-152.

358 Ibid.

359 Ralf Nehmzow, "Mitten in Hamburg-eine Zeitreise nach Chinatown," *Hamburger Abendblatt* (28 July 2008), at: http://www.abendblatt.de/hamburg/arti cle930097/Mitten-in-Hamburg-eine-Zeitreise-nach-Chinatown.html (Last access, 20.12.2015)

360 Amenda, *Fremde-Hafen-Stadt*, 153-154.

nying fear of their opium dens, but with just 111 Chinese residents permanently registered in Hamburg in 1925, warnings of a "yellow peril" found little resonance.

During the interwar period, as many as 2,000 to 3,000 Chinese sailors temporarily took up residence in Hamburg.[361] Stories of labyrinths under the city streets filled with opium-smoking Chinese appeared in popular books, but in reality, the few Chinese who lived in town kept to themselves, often in cellars, working in laundries, vegetable retail and restaurants. Raids rarely produced evidence of foul play, a fact that the German police attributed more to Chinese cunning than to the absence of opium. Several novels were published in the 1930s about vile Chinese opium smokers who kidnapped white women to fulfill their sexual desires, but still no full-fledged racist panic ensued.[362]

During the Third Reich, the Criminal Police kept a closer tab on the Chinese in Hamburg. They occasionally discovered small quantities of opium during raids, but even the police themselves admitted that the drug peddlers they caught were nothing more than "small fry."[363] Indeed, by the time the Gestapo decided to liquidate Hamburg's Chinatown in 1944, there were no more than 130 Chinese to be deported to labor camps and apparently no opium to confiscate.[364]

The masses showed little inclination to use drugs, but lax drug laws and eager drug manufacturers made the country a haven for those who did wish to indulge in the habit. Drugs were readily available in Germany, and they were cheap. One heroin addict who picked up the habit at the age of 16 recounted just how easy drugs were acquired:

> I started using heroin in Hamburg around 1925. I heard about it by hanging out with fellows my own age down on the waterfront. I didn't even know

---

361 Nehmzow, "Mitten in Hamburg-eine Zeitreise nach Chinatown."

362 Amenda, *Fremde-Hafen-Stadt*, 73-74. This is not to say that there were no racial biases, but in comparison to the United States they were few and far between. What seemed to trouble the German authorities the most was the insular world in which the Chinese lived.

363 Ibid., 231-232. Regarding the case of Choy Loy, who was regarded as the most dangerous smuggler in Hamburg, see Ibid., 232-234. Needless to say, he was never caught with opium and only sat one year in jail for a different charge.

364 Idem, "Geheime Tunnel unter St. Pauli? Gerüchte über das 'Chinesenviertel' in den 1920er Jahren," originally published in *Die Tageszeitung* (1 September 2002), but can be found with documentation at: http://www.unter-hamburg.de/tunnel_unter_st__pauli.344.0.html (Last access, 20.12.2015)

what it was at first. We used to get a little package – we used to chip in. It came to about a quarter apiece for the four of us. We used to sniff and throw the rest away, instead of getting caught with it. It didn't cost anything.[365]

Germans, known for their organizational skills, were apt in organizing crime as well. But unlike their American colleagues, the crime rings did not evolve through ethnic or familial ties, but came to resemble trade unions or social clubs where thieves traded tips and formed alliances.[366] No German Arnold Rothstein or Lucky Luciano ever set the stage for large drug-smuggling operations in Germany. When American criminals sought drugs from Germany, they sent their own representatives to procure drugs directly from the manufacturers.[367]

When a large drug ring was finally caught in Germany in 1933, it was, not surprisingly, foreign. The smuggling racket was led by two Greek brothers, George and Elie Eliopoulos (1894-?), and focused on the American drug market. Originally operating in Paris, the brothers moved their morphine and heroin factories to Istanbul, from where American smugglers bought the drugs and shipped them to the United States via Hamburg.[368] When Turkey proved unfriendly to the illicit drug trade, the brothers moved to Sofia, keeping Germany as their preferred transit point.

According to contemporary press and police reports, the brothers owned no less than nine factories in Bulgaria, producing 1.5 tons of heroin every two months – all of it destined for the American market. After Elie Eliopoulos was caught in Mannheim in March 1933, he served five months in a Greek jail, where he confessed to Egyptian and American narcotic agents the extent of his smuggling operations.[369] None of the

---

365 David Courtwright, Herman Joseph and Don Des Jarlais, *Addicts who Survived: An Oral History of Narcotic Use in America, 1923-1965* (Knoxville: University of Tennessee Press, 1989), 109.

366 Hsi-huey Liang, *The Berlin Police Force in the Weimar Republic* (Berkeley: University of California Press, 1970), 145-147.

367 Jill Jonnes, *Hep-Cats, Narcs, and Pipe Dreams: A History of America's Romance with Illegal Drugs* (New York: Scribner, 1996), 79.

368 Ibid., 100. See also Kathryn Meyer & Terry Parssinen, *Webs of Smoke: Smugglers, Warlords, Spies and the History of the International Drug Trade* (Lanham: Rowman & Littlefield, 1998), 117-121; Ryan Gingeras, *Heroin, Organized Crime, and the Making of Modern Turkey* (Oxford: Oxford University Press, 2014), 68-71. In the adventures of Tin Tin and the Blue Lotus, the opium smuggler Rastapopoulos is modeled after Eliopoulos.

369 "Balkan Products, Ltd.," *Time Magazine* (3 April 1933).

heroin produced by the Eliopoulos brothers was ever meant for the German market.

How, then, did the Weimar Republic became synonymous with drug-driven debauchery? One answer may be that among the relatively small number of drug users in Germany, there were more than a few literary figures, and their chronicling of that era helped define it. Stories of Berlin as a hedonistic, drug-crazed city were repeated time and again. "Cocaine was the basic drug of Berlin in the 1920s, and it was everywhere," journalist Otto Friedrich (1929-1995) wrote in 1972. "Girls pushed it in night-clubs, one-legged war veterans sold it on street corners, and if one were going on a trip, everybody knew of foreign contacts. 'When I was going to Paris,' says one old Berliner, 'they told me before I left that you could get all you wanted right outside Maxim's. There was a man there who wore a yellow hat, and he could always provide it.'"[370]

Berlin became known as a powder city, and traveling American writers rarely failed to mention the immoral squalor and drug use found on visits to Berlin. Robert McAlmon (1895-1956) depicted the city as the home of homosexual prostitutes and cocaine addicts in his 1925 book *Distinguished Air: Grim Fairy Tales*. Ernest Hemmingway, who visited Berlin in 1923, "described the nocturnal entertainment in Berlin as repulsively vulgar in comparison to those in Paris or Constantinople, noting that in boring Berlin nightclubs cocaine was consumed instead of French champagne."[371]

Drugs were certainly common, but did they attract clients? Carl Zuckmeyer (1896-1977), the playwright who adapted Heinrich Mann's *Professor Unrat* to the script of the *Blue Angel*, recalled in his memoirs how as a struggling young man in Berlin, he was asked by a hustler to peddle cocaine on a street corner just off the famous department store *Ka-De-We*. It was a sham. The cocaine was nothing more than sugar and crushed aspirin; regardless, no one showed an interest in the drug. In the end, a Polish prostitute helped Zuckmeyer shake off a policeman and warned him that if he continued on to harass people offering them drugs, he would be reprimanded. This experience was enough for the playwright. His career as a drug peddler lasted only a day.[372]

---

370 Friedrich, *Before the Deluge*, 342.
371 Waldemar Zacharasiewicz, *Images of Germany in American Literature* (Iowa City: University of Iowa Press, 2007), 102.
372 Carl Zuckmayer, *Als Wär's ein Stück von Mir* (Frankfurt: Fischer, 1967), 411.

While the literati focused on the rampant drug use in the country's houses of ill repute, a more refined type of drug use was taking place in physicians' offices. Weimar Germany, in fact, proved to be a particularly good time for drug experimentations by doctors. No legal or ethical restrictions were imposed on drug research until well after World War II, leaving leading medicals minds free to expand themselves with mind-altering substances.

The attending physician at the Heidelberg university hospital, Kurt Behringer, conducted experiments with hallucinogens on junior physicians at the institution. In his autobiography, psychiatrist Hans Bürger-Prinz (1897-1976) recalled how, as a young assistant under Behringer, he was given mescaline while on duty, resulting in him hallucinating that his patients were squirming giant worms and the head nurse a skeleton.[373]

Drug experiments on humans were relatively common. Some were carried out in an attempt to better understand the human organism, while others were aimed more at self-discovery. Some, like Walter Benjamin (1892-1940), arguably the best-known drug experimenter of that era, combined both motives. In the late 1920s, Benjamin embarked on a series of tests with drugs. He first tried hashish under the supervision of Ernst Joël (1893-1929), a rival turned colleague who had become addicted to morphine during an internment in a British prisoner of war camp in World War I.[374] Beginning in December 1927, Joël, together with Fritz Fränkel (1892-1944) and Ernst Bloch (1885-1977), used Benjamin as a test subject for drug experiments.[375] Benjamin continued with the tests until 1934, hoping to write a book on hashish while under the influence of the drug.[376] The book never materialized, however, and only fragments of his drug-induced writing survived, among them two articles published in the early 1930s.[377] Aside from hashish and mescaline, Benjamin tried other drugs

---

373 Hans Bürger-Prinz, *Ein Psychiater berichtet* (Hamburg: Hoffmann & Campe, 1971), 70.
374 Scott J.Thompson, "Walter Benjamin, Dr. Ernst Joël and Hashish," (1997) at: http://www.wbenjamin.org/joel_frankel.html#wbjf_hash (Last access, 20.12.20015).
375 Ibid.
376 Walter Benjamin, *On Hashish*, edited by Howard Eiland, (Cambridge MA, Harvard University Press, 2006), for a complete translation of the fragments.
377 Walter Benjamin, "Haschisch in Marseilles," *Frankfurter Zeitung* (4 December 1932), and idem, "Myslowitz-Braunschweig-Marseilles," *Uhu* 7:2 (1930), 90. translated in Benjamin, *On Hashish*, 105-128.

as well, smoking opium with his friend Jean Selz (1904-1997) during a stay on Ibiza in 1933,[378] and taking eukodal as part of Joël and Fränkel's experiments in 1931.[379]

Benjamin was hardly the only German to write about his experiences under the influence. The number of literary figures who regularly used drugs was long and distinguished, ranging in political beliefs from the communist Johannes R. Becher (1891-1958) to the nationalist Ernst Jünger (1895-1998). Others, among them nihilist Godfried Benn (1886-1956), Austrian poet Georg Trakl (1887-1914) and Swiss writer Friedrich Glauser (1896-1938), also wrote shortly after the war about their experimentation with morphine and cocaine.[380] Jünger, unlike the others, would only write about his drug experimentation years later.[381]

Most of the addicted literati were either physicians like Benn, had access to pharmacies like Trakl, or had become addicted to morphine from war wounds like Glauser and Becher. Jünger and Benjamin, who were anomalies for seeking out drugs even though they did not always have easy access to them, may have been motivated by boredom. Or perhaps they were attempting to imitate Charles Baudelaire's *Artificial Paradise*.[382]

Benn admitted to experimenting with drugs out of boredom in occupied Belgium, but he did not fit the mold of the average drug user. He shied away from intoxication; or so he claimed. Instead, he took drugs "solely for the personal experience." How that differed from others, his readers are left guessing. In 1951 he wrote to Jünger that he never took drugs save for the brief period he was stationed in Brussels in 1916, which is when he wrote his two drug-laced poems, "Kokain" and "O Nacht."[383]

---

378 Lorenz Jäger, "Ceci n'est pas une pipe à opium: Wie Kommissar Maigret: Walter Benjamin Experimente," *Frankfurter Allgemeine Zeitung* (6 October 1998) 43; Tillman Rexroth, "Editorial Note," and Jean Selz, "An Experiment by Walter Benjamin," both in Benjamin, *On Hashish*, 13-14, 147-158.
379 Ibid.
380 Friedrich Glauser, "Morphium-eine Beichte (1932)" in *Morphium, Erzählungen* (Zurich: Arche, 1988).
381 Ernst Jünger, *Annäherungen: Drogen und Rausch* (Stuttgart: Klett, 1970].
382 Marcus Boon, "Walter Benjamin and Drug Literature," in Benjamin, *On Hashish*, 1-12; see also Marcus Boon, *The Road of Excess: A History of Writers on Drugs* (Cambridge MA: Harvard University Press, 2002), 140-142, 148-151.
383 Gunnar Decker, *Gottfried Benn: Genie und Barbar* (Berlin: Aufbau-Verlag, 2008), 101-105.

But perhaps no impressionist better exemplified the Weimar literati's experience with drugs than Rudolf Ditzen (1893-1947), better known by his pen name Hans Fallada. Ditzen's lifelong problems with the law had their roots in 1912, when he stood trial for murder in a suicide pact with a friend that went wrong. Ditzen got off on an insanity plea, and was subsequently sent off to be treated by Otto Binswanger (1852-1929), the same doctor who treated Friedrich Nietzsche (1844-1900) and would later treat Johannes Becher for his own addiction.[384] He was treated afterward at Arthur Tecklenburg's Tannenfeld exclusive mental asylum near Jena, a luxury paid for by his father who had arranged the insanity plea.[385]

In 1916 or 1917, a lover introduced Ditzen, by then an aspiring novelist in Berlin, to the effects of morphine; though not yet to the drug itself. One night she came to his apartment with a physician friend who had injected her with morphine. "Yes, such... such is life," Ditzen recorded her as saying that night, in what was clearly a moment that left an indelible impression on the young writer. "Life is so beautiful. It is so soft, a happy current flows through my limbs. It mellows all the small nerves and turns them gently like water lilies in a lake. I have seen rose petals – and I immediately know how beautiful a single, small tree in the meadow is. Do the bells in a church ring? Oh, life is so beautiful."[386]

Several months later Ditzen met an older woman whose son, Wolfgang Parsenow, had been treated in a military hospital with morphine for wounds suffered during the war. Upon his release from service Parsenow had received a block of blank prescriptions for morphine, and he is believed to have encouraged Ditzen to sample his treatment.[387] The drug very much appealed to Ditzen's taste. Indeed, as he later wrote, "I will only need to laugh, because morphine fulfills every wish of mine. I need only to close my eyes, and the whole world belongs to me."[388]

As long as Parsenow's prescriptions were available, Ditzen was able to supply himself from military stockpiles. But when his drug pipeline dried out, he turned to doctors, faking illnesses and pains to obtain the drug.

384 Jenny Williams, *More Lives than One: A Biography of Hans Fallada* (London: Libris, 1998), 9.
385 Ibid., 26-32.
386 Tom Crepon, *Leben und Tode des Hans Fallada* (Leipzig: Mitteldeutscher Verlag, 1992), 101.
387 Ibid., 103.
388 Ibid., 102.

And when, like many other addicts, he could not obtain morphine in a clinic or a pharmacy, he turned to the black market, often settling for cocaine, which was easier to obtain.[389] To support his addiction, Ditzen even went so far as to sell his library of some 3,000 books.[390]

In August 1919, Ditzen returned to Tannenfeld for treatment under Tecklenburg, the same physician who had treated him seven years earlier. After four weeks in the sanatorium without drugs, Ditzen resorted to lying, stealing and using falsified prescriptions to procure morphine. Tecklenburg, admitting failure, released him from Tannenfeld.[391] Half a year later, Ditzen published his first novel under the pseudonym Hans Fallada. As his success grew, Fallada's addiction continued unabated, and in fact became a key theme in his writing. At some point during the summer of 1920, shortly after completing his first rehabilitation tour, he wrote an autobiographical essay, "An Objective Report on the Bliss of Being a Morphine Addict." The essay, which he subsequently edited in the 1930s and which was only published after his death in 1955, laid aside any pretenses to a life without the drug: "Oh, life is soft and beautiful – even when I think of you, my sweet girl, that I have lost long ago, my only love is now morphine. She is evil, she agonizes me immeasurably, but she rewards me way beyond understanding."[392]

In 1923 a friend introduced Fallada to alcohol in an attempt to cure him of his morphine addiction, but the result was only the replacement of one habit for another. He consumed whatever he could acquire, be it cocaine, whiskey or morphine.[393] He was arrested twice for crimes committed to satisfy his morphine and alcohol cravings, the first time in 1924 for embezzlement and theft. In his memoirs, Fallada expressed his fear of morphine withdrawal, but in the end he overcame his morphine craving much faster than his need to smoke tobacco.[394] In a later account, Fallada

---

389 Crepon, *Leben und Tode des Hans Fallada*, 104.

390 Williams, *More Lives than One*, 47.

391 Ibid., 48.

392 Hans Fallada "Sachlicher Bericht über das Glück, ein Morphinist zu sein," (1925?) in Günter Caspar (ed.), *Drei Jahre kein Mensch* (Berlin: Aufbau-Verlag, 1997), 5-24; Carsten Gansel and Werner Liersch, ed. *Hans Fallada und die literarische Moderne* (Göttingen: V&R Uni Press, 2009), 52.

393 Crepon, *Leben und Tode des Hans Fallada*, 110-111.

394 Hans Fallada, *Strafgefangener, Zelle 32: Tagebuch, 22. Juni-2. September 1924*, edited by Günter Caspar (Berlin: Aufbau-Verlag, 1998), 9.

remembered how he collected cigarette butts from the ground "to satisfy yet another addiction."[395]

After his second arrest for stealing 12,000 Reichsmarks from his employer in 1926, Fallada insisted on his sanity in court, fearing what he considered to be a worse punishment than prison: commitment to a mental asylum.[396] A few months under the strict watch of prison guards changed his mind, and while in jail he attempted to change his plea to insanity, claiming that he had embezzled the money under the influence of drugs. Fallada's judge informed him that a plea could not be changed after a sentence had been delivered, and he served out the rest of his prison term.

Fallada, who would go on to become a successful and well-known writer, continued to struggle with addictions for the rest of his life. At one point he was so despondent about his habits that he even joined the International Order of Good Templars, which advocated complete abstinence. Membership in the Templars did not lead him to stay dry for long, but he did meet his first wife during his time in the order.[397] Incidentally, right before their divorce was finalized in 1944, he fired a gun at her and missed. Luckily for him, he was sent to a mental asylum for three and a half months because he was deemed unfit to stand trial because of his drunkenness. During his stay, he wrote his novel, *The Drinker*, which was published posthumously.

Fallada's long and tortured experience with addiction is instructive for understanding drug use in Germany during the interwar period, for several reasons. First, as evidenced by Wolfgang Parsenow's blank prescriptions, there was easy access to drugs, particularly for wounded veterans and their friends. Second, there were little to no drugs in German prisons, a reality that led to his change of heart about being declared sane. German prisoners, quite simply, did not have reliable access to morphine. Even smoking cigarettes was officially barred in prison, although in practice it was somewhat tolerated.[398] Third, Fallada's morphine addiction, which

---

395 Idem, "Drei Jahre kein Mensch" (1930?) in *Drei Jahre kein Mensch*, ed. Günter Caspar, 47.

396 Benjamin Robinson, "'Ist Knastschieben denn schön?' Hans Fallada und die Krise des Willens in der Weimarer Republik" in *Die Krise der Weimarer Republik: Zur Kritik eines Deutungsmusters*, ed. Moritz Föllmer and Rüdiger Graf (Frankfurt a.M: Campus, 2005), 359.

397 Williams, *More Lives than One*, 82.

398 Fallada, *Strafgefangener, Zelle 32.*

was known to the authorities, could have bought him freedom from imprisonment. And fourth, Fallada's addiction did not, for the most part, affect his public reputation. When the Nazis took power, they sought out Fallada and supported his work as long as it was politically viable for them – even as he continued to struggle with his addictions.

The drug-filled world depicted by Anita Berber, Fallada and other leading figures of the Weimar literati was misleading. Both morphine and heroin were consumed during the Weimar years and the Third Reich, with morphine proving far more popular than its more potent cousin. The exact number of addicts in Germany, however, is difficult to ascertain. Like many drug statistics today, the reported numbers of addicts were mere guesstimates rather than reliable figures, mainly because it was next to impossible to differentiate between addicts and users.

Figures on drug addiction provided by Oberregierungsrat Erich Hesse, a high-ranking official in the Reich Health Office in the 1930s and 1940s, offer a telling example. Hesse reported that from 1913 to 1922 the number of known opiate addicts in Prussia rose from 282 to 682. The increase was attributed to the wave of wounded veterans returning from the frontlines of World War I. For 1928, the Reich official put the number of morphine addicts in Germany at 6,356, among them 560 physicians.[399] Yet startlingly, in 1931 Hesse estimated Germany had 0.3 addicts per 10,000 males and 0.1 addicts per 10,000 females,[400] an estimate that yielded a total of roughly 1,200 addicts in Germany. No explanation was provided for how more than 80 percent of Germany's addicts disappeared in just three years.

Kurt Pohlisch (1893-1955), a psychiatrist at Bonn University who later actively participated in the sterilization of patients suffering from heredi-tary diseases such as severe alcoholism,[401] posited in 1931 that the number of opiate addicts in Germany who consumed more than 0.1 gram of morphine a day was exactly 3,500. Of these, only 237 consumed more than 1 gram; roughly one-third consumed an average of 0.2 gram a day.

---

399 Quoting *Oberregierungsrat* Hesse's 1953 study in Detlef Briesen, *Drogenkonsum und Drogenpolitik in Deutschland und den USA: Ein historischer Vergleich* (Frankfurt a.M:Campus, 2005), 73.

400 Albert Wissler, *Die Opiumfrage* (Berlin, 1931), 139.

401 Pohlisch served as the head of a provincial sanatorium under the terms of the "Sterilization Law," or the Law for the Prevention of Hereditarily Diseased Offspring.

Addiction was greatest in Berlin, where Pohlisch found 1.91 opiate addicts per 10,000 people.[402] Pohlisch's and Hesse's number clearly did not match up, and the authorities, realizing the discrepancy, preferred Pohlisch's estimates to be the reliable figures, and continued to use them until at least 1937.[403]

Other statistics on drug use in Germany appeared over the course of the decade, but they did little to clarify the exact extent of addiction in the country. Kriminalkommissar Werner Thomas, the head of the Reich police's drug unit, reported in 1932 that morphine addiction was on the rise, noting that there were roughly 1,500 registered morphine addicts.[404] How Thomas arrived at that figure just one year after Pohlisch arrived at an estimate that was well more than double remains an open question.

Unreliable statistics and guesswork found their way also into Nazi wartime records. In 1942, Oberregierungsrat Linz of the Health Office stated that the exact number of drug addicts in Germany was not known, and that from 1918 to 1925 no records had been kept. He then went about trying to ascertain a more exact picture of drug addiction in the Third Reich. Linz attempted to estimate the number of addicts in the general population by examining annual drug consumption in Germany. In doing so, he was operating on the assumption that Germany's legal drug industry was the source of illegal drug use in the country.[405] In 1926, Germans consumed 1.6 tons of morphine; by 1941, it was only 400 kilograms. According to Linz's calculation, 2.3 kilograms of morphine were consumed per 100,000 people in 1926, whereas in 1941 the rate was down to 435 grams per 100,000. In 1929, German opium consumption reached a peak of 2.9 tons. By 1932, the consumption dropped to 1.2 tons, where it stayed until 1939, when the outbreak of war marked a sudden increase in opium consumption.

---

402 Kurt Pohlisch, "Die Verbreitungs des chronischen Opiatmissbrauchs in Deutschland," *Monatsschrift für Psychiatrie und Neurologie* 79:1 (1931), 1-32. See also Tilmann Holzer, *Die Geburt der Drogenpolitik aus dem Geist der Rassenhygiene: Deutsche Drogenpolitik von 1933-1972* (Norderstedt: Books on Demand, 2007), 36-37.

403 "Summary of the Stettin Conference, 10 October 1937" StA. München, Pol. Dir. 7582.

404 Ibid., Thomas used old statistics in his presentation.

405 Linz, "Behoerdliche Durchfuehrung des Opiumgesetzes: Ziele und Ergebnisse" in *Suchtgiftbekämpfung*, ed. Gerhart Feuerstein (Berlin, 1944), 24-32.

While morphine remained an enduring attraction, Linz found, heroin and cocaine increasingly fell out of favor. Heroin consumption decreased from 50 kilograms in 1925 to just 1 kilogram in 1941, a drop attributed to an absence of any accepted medical use. Cocaine use, meanwhile, had declined by 1942 to one-ninth of its 1925 peak of 450 kilograms. The drug that most worried Linz was dolantin. Known in the United States as pethidine or demerol, dolantin was developed in 1937 by Hoechst, a pharmaceutical company then part of I. G. Farben, as a non-addictive analgesic alternative to morphine. When mass production of dolantin began in 1939, it was advertised as a non-addictive drug, but just two years later it was declared to be addictive.[406] In the interim many physicians prescribed the drug, in the process creating a new wave of addiction.

The drugs that came out of Germany were industrially produced preparates and derivatives, not naturally-grown drug crops, so tracing German drug imports should have been a fairly straightforward task for Nazi officials. In calculating the amount of drugs legally consumed in Germany, Linz relied on the annual reports sent to the League of Nations. These figures, however, can hardly be considered authoritative. Germany's drug companies were known to circumvent the international drug control regime overseen by the League of Nations, rendering suspect the statistics used by Linz.

For all their inexactness, the surveys of drug use in Germany during the first half of the 20th century have all been conspicuously constant in counting the numbers of addicts in the country. Through all the turmoil that roiled Germany in the Weimar era and the Nazi years that followed, the number of addicts never exceeded more than a few thousand. One need only look at the American experience during that era to call into question the likelihood that drug use ever grew beyond a relatively small number of addicts.

In 1931, the Federal Bureau of Narcotics chief Harry Anslinger stated that there were between 120,000 to 140,000 addicts in the United

---

406 Wilhelm Bartmann, *Zwischen Tradition und Fortschritt: Aus der Geschichte der Pharmabereiche von Bayer, Hoechst und Schering von 1935-1975* (Stuttgart: Franz Steiner Verlag, 2003), 171-172; Michel Rosenzweig, *Les drogues dans l'histoire entre remède et poison: Archéologie d'un savoir oublié* (Brussels: De Boeck & Belin, 1998), 151-152.

States.[407] The number was even higher according to others, ranging from 250,000 to as many as 1 million by the late 1920s.[408] The population of the United States at the time was roughly 122 million, which, if one takes Anslinger's "conservative" estimate, would imply that the addiction rate was roughly 1.4 addicts per 1,000 people. In Germany, if one were to take Hesse's "liberal" estimate of 6,356 addicts, the addiction rate was 0.09 per 1,000 people. If one were to rely on such numbers, Germany had 15 times less of an opium problem than the United States.

Similar caution deserves to be exercised in regard to statistics on cocaine use. In the wake of World War I, as military stockpiles found their way into the civilian market, cocaine consumption spiked. According to one estimate, "cocaine-related admissions to university health clinics rose from an average of 1.75 percent of admissions in 1913 to 3 percent in 1918, 7.5 percent in 1920, to fully 10 percent in 1921."[409]

Yet despite claims during the 1920s of a cocaine epidemic in Berlin, the number of addicts is unlikely to have been very high. According to contemporary estimates, in fact, cocaine consumption in Germany was highest in Karlsruhe, not Berlin: at 1.44 grams per 1,000 people in Karlsruhe and 1 gram per 1,000 in Berlin. Cocaine was clearly not consumed with abandon, even if one gram could be split into one to four doses.[410]

Figures compiled by the Nazis in the late 1930s also shed light on cocaine use prior to their rise to power. In 1937 Kriminalkommissar Thomas stated that there were a grand total of 300 registered cocaine addicts in Germany, and that their number had not risen since 1932.[411] Another Nazi official, Kriminalkommissar Erwin Kosmehl, later asserted that in 1942 there were just 465 known cocaine addicts. Assuming that the thousands of drug addicts found by Pohlisch and Hesse had not been miraculously cured in less than a decade, one may conclude that despite the cocaine craze in the mid-1920s, addiction to the drug remained low.

---

407 Treasury Department, *Traffic in Opium and Other Dangerous Drugs* (Washington DC, 1931) quoted in Meyer & Parssinen, *Webs of Smoke*, 3.

408 David T. Courtwright, *Dark Paradise: A History of Opiate Addiction in America* (Cambridge MA: Harvard University Press, 2001), 31.

409 H. Richard Friman, "Germany and the Transformation of Cocaine, 1860-1920" in *Cocaine: Global Histories*, ed. Paul Gootenberg (London: Routledge, 1999), 83-104.

410 Holzer, *Die Geburt der Drogenpolitik aus dem Geist der Rassenhygiene*, 37.

411 "Summary of the Stettin Conference, 10 October 1937" StA. München, Pol. Dir. 7582.

Notably absent from such reports, as well as those from the Weimar years, is any mention of either marijuana or hashish. Cannabis was rare in Germany at the time, as a 1945 letter from the intelligence branch of the German secret police (SD) to the Munich police attests. After noting that a Bulgarian worker had been caught with 15 grams of hashish in Halle, the SD inspector asked if a trend of hashish use among foreign workers had been noticed.[412] The Munich police, while dutifully stating that the police post in Berchtesgaden would investigate the matter, made clear to the secret police that hashish had never been a problem in Bavaria.[413]

The Munich police's lack of concern about hashish was, by all appearances, indicative of an overall confidence among German officials that the drug scourge did not particularly plague the Third Reich. Indeed, to judge by the official journal of the Reich Committee for the Health Service of the Volk and the Society of German Physicians of the Public Service,[414] *Der öffentliche Gesundheitsdienst*, drug addiction hardly troubled the German authorities. Of the 12 articles and book reviews on drug addiction and alcoholism the journal published in 1936-1937, just two dealt with substances other than alcohol and tobacco, and even then the two substances figured prominently in writing. In 1937-1938, the number was down to four, with two on alcohol and two on morphine. In 1938-1939, three of the six were devoted to alcohol, and another to tobacco.

War induced addiction was the sole concern of German health officials, as they based their assessment on a study conducted on World War veterans in 1931 describing, among other things, the treatment of war-addicts. Despite the assertion that users could consume drugs for years without becoming addicted, the paradigm was clear: wars created drug addicts, either because of wounded soldiers who received treatment with opiates, or due to low morale.[415]

---

412 The SD (*Sicherheitsdients*), acted upon the following order of the Reich criminal police office: *"Bekämpfung des Hashischhandels und Missbrauches* VB3c Nr. 1103/44." 5 November 1944.

413 *"Inspekteur der Sicherheitspolizei und des SD* to the Munich Police, 22 January 1945" StA. München, Pol. Dir. 7582.

414 *"Reichsausschuß für Volksgesundheitsdienst within the Staatsmedizinischen Akademie Berlin"* and the *"wissenschaftliche Gesellschaft der deutschen Ärzte des öffentlichen Gesundheitsdienstes."*

415 Friedrich Dansauer and Adolf Rieth, ed. *Über Morphinismus bei Kriegs-beschädigten*, (Berlin, 1931).

The fear of war induced addiction continued into World War II. On 12 November 1941 the Ministry of Interior instructed army surgeons to report addicted soldiers to their home medical districts.[416] Eleven months later, on 14 October 1942, Leonardo Conti (1900-1945), the Physicians' Leader of the Reich, declared that Germany did not have a drug problem, but that it had to prepare for one should it rise again after the war's end. Conti attributed the successes of the Nazi regime in combating the addiction phenomenon after World War I to various drug laws that were promulgated and to the various welfare workers.[417] He neglected to mention, however, that the main German drug law, the *Opiumgesetz* was enacted in 1929, four years before the Nazi takeover of power.

On the list of popular drugs, morphine and cocaine were ranked at the top of the pyramid, but they were not the only available drugs in Germany. In 1942, Kosmehl noted there were 84 pervitin addicts registered in the police rolls.[418] Pervitin, commonly known as crystal meth today, hardly caused a drug epidemic in the streets of the Reich, but it was a source of some concern among some officials, namely Leonardo Conti. As a result, Nazi Germany was probably the first country to regulate methamphetamines, but never banned them altogether. On 7 November 1939, the Ministry of Interior issued a police ordinance requiring a prescription for the sale of benzedrine (phenylaminopropane) and pervitin.[419]

On 21 June 1941, benzedrine, dolantin and pervitin were included in the sixth amendment of the German drug law. The reason, according to *Oberregierungsrat* G. Kärber, the head of the drugs division in the Reich Health Office, was their addictiveness. The ordinance and amendment did not constitute a ban, but rather dictated a prescription requirement for the administration and sale of the drugs. If a prescription was given for a long period of time, a record had to be sent to the proper authorities.[420] Despite these control measures, production of pervitin increased; from about seven

---

416 "Bekämpfung des Mißbrauchs von Betäubungsmitteln," *Ministerialblatt des Reichs- und Preußischen Ministeriums des Innern* (12 Novemner 1941).

417 Leonard Conti, "Begrüssungsansprache des Reichsgesundheitsführer" (1942) in Gerhard Feuerstein (ed.), *Suchtgiftbekämpfung* (Berlin, 1944), 5-6.

418 Kosmehl, *Der sicherheitspolizeiliche Einsatz bei der Bekämpfung der Betäubungsmittelsucht,* BArch. RD 19/30.

419 "Polizeiverordnung über die Abgabe von Leberpräparaten und anderen Arzneimitteln in den Apotheken, 7 November 1939" *Reichsgesetzblatt* I (1939), 2176.

420 G. Kärber, "Unterstellung von Dolantin, Pervitin und Benzedrin unter das Opiumgesetz," *Deutsches Ärzteblatt* 71:27 (5 July 1941), 260-262.

and a half million tablets in 1941, to nine million tablets in 1942 and a similar amount the following year, to eight million tablets in 1944. As a rule, military production was about half of the civilian production.[421]

Since 1938, the Wehrmacht researched pervitin and caffeine pills as effective means to counter sleep deprivation. The results were promising albeit problematic. Subjects who took pervitin were eager to solve problems and showed less signs of fatigue, but were prone to making more mistakes than the control group. The drug became operational during the invasion of Poland on a limited scale, with mixed results.[422] Troops, especially pilots and tank crews, received pervitin in various forms to enhance their performance under duress, in the campaign against France in 1940, the time period in which Heinrich Böll (1917-1985) was famously introduced to the drug while he was in uniform. In fact, he asked from his family to send him more pervitin to his post in the front.[423]

In 1939-40, the high point of German drug use in the war, the Wehrmacht and the Luftwaffe received about 35 million pervitin tablets.[424] How many of them were actually consumed is anyone's guess; but for the argument's sake, one may assume they were all consumed by combat soldiers. The German military at the time consisted of about 6.6 million soldiers. Assuming that about 15 percent were in the front line (though probably the percentage was higher) one gets about 35 tablets per head for the invasions of Denmark, Norway, the Low Countries and France. On average, German soldiers could expect half a tablet a day for the entire campaign. Certainly, this amount is not enough to support anyone's habit. This bigger picture turns Heinrich Böll's letter to his family on its head; after all, if pervitin were so common in the front lines, would he have required his family's help to obtain it?

In military operations, pervitin was used as a confidence booster, intended to improve soldier's morale similar to the use of alcohol for 'Dutch Courage.' There was no order from Berlin to use Pervitin in

---

421 Holzer, *Die Geburt der Drogenpolitik aus dem Geist der Rassenhygiene*, 244-249.

422 Norman Ohler, *Der totale Rausch: Drogen im Dritten Reich* (Cologne: Kiepenheuer & Witsch, 2015), 71-81.

423 Jochen Schubert, ed. *Heinrich Böll: Briefe aus dem Krieg 1939-1945*, Vol. 1 (Cologne: Kiepenheuer & Witsch, 2001), 22, 62, 81.

424 The exact figures are unknown. These estimates are mentioned in Ohler, *Der totale Rausch*, 136, even though production reports from Temmler, the company that produced the drug, were much lower.

combat, but rather local commanders and physicians dispensed the drug as they saw fit. As the war raged on, the German authorities realized the potential dangers of the drug. Experts debated over the malefic effects of pervitin,[425] and on 25 October 1941, the medical service of the *Luftwaffe* ordered pervitin to be among the drugs "kept under lock and key."[426] The Wehrmacht soon followed. Consequently, the preposterous claim some journalists have raised that drug-crazed soldiers lost all sense of morality because of pervitin is unfounded,[427] because most of the atrocities were committed after the summer of 1941.

What of the Allies? In the early stages of the war, Britain and the US were shocked by the German abilities and attributed the Wehrmacht's success to Pervitin. Consequently, British and later American scientists experimented with the properties of benzedrine sulfate (pervitin's brother in the West) to enhance performance among soldiers. Scientists from both sides of the Atlantic, like their German counterparts, quickly realized that the drug did not enhance performance at all, but rather bolstered confidence. Any improvements in test results were not attributed to the drug itself.[428]

To the dismay of many RAF pilots who wished to believe otherwise, benzedrine was not proven to be more effective than the old and trusted caffeine pill. Or, in the words of one English researcher who commented about his test subjects: "Individuals were disposed to try to make greater efforts; they thought they were working harder, whereas they were doing exactly the same amount of work."[429] In the end, benzedrine was given to soldiers in the field for morale reasons, and because it was believed that it

---

425 E. Speer, "Das Pervetinproblem" *Deutsches Ärzteblatt* 71 (1941), 4-6, 15-19; F. Dittmar, "Pervitinsucht und acute Pervitinintoxikation," *Deutsche Medizinische Wochenschrift* 68:11 (1942), 266-268; F. Kalus, I. Kucher, and J. Zutt, "Über Psychosen bei chronischem Pervitinmissbrauch," *Nervenarzt* 15 (1942), 313-324.

426 Geoffrey Cocks, *Psychotherapy in the Third Reich: The Göring Institute* (New Brunswick NJ: Transaction Publishers, 1997) 312-313.

427 See for example: Ohler *Der totale Rausch*, or Andreas Ulrich, "The Nazi Death Machine: Hitler's Drugged Soldiers" _*Spiegel Online* (6 May 2005) at: http://www.spiegel.de/international/the-nazi-death-machine-hitler-s-drugged-soldiers-a-354606.html (Last access: 25.1.2016).

428 Nicolas Rasmussen, *On Speed: The Many Lives of Amphetamine* (New York: New York University Press, 2008), 58.

429 Quoted in ibid., 63.

made them more aggressive. Both of which are extremely important in combat.

Whether a soldier's performance improved or not, is anyone's guess; but British officers were pleased with the results. A slight boost in confidence is all that takes to make a difference, or so thought General Bernard Montgomery (1887-1976) before the battle of Al Alamein, as he ordered his troops to take the drugs in preparation for battle: the standing order of the Army Group Middle East was to allow 20 mg of amphetamines per day for up to five days straight.[430]

RAF experiments reported: "In some people [amphetamines] may increase determination in circumstances of acute anxiety." This was of particular interest to bomber command, which had to deal with bomber crews suffering emotional breakdowns on their way back home from missions over Germany. By 1942, the RAF adopted the recommendation of administering 5 mg of Benzedrine for each pilot before every mission.[431] Curiously, this happened almost a year after Luftwaffe pilots virtually stopped taking pervitin.

The United States, entering the war after the Germans placed restrictions on the drug, also toyed with the idea of drugging its own soldiers. After studies had shown that benzedrine was as effective as caffeine, civilian and military researchers insisted that benzedrine's morale boost was vital for soldiers in the field, and so the United States administered government issued pep pills. As a result, from February 1943 on, the United States supplied its armed forces with 5 mg Benzedrine pep pills wrapped together in a six-pack to be dispensed whenever command saw fit. According to one estimate, the American military bought no less than 500 million tablets by the war's end, which it dispensed rather liberally in practice despite restrictions on paper.[432] In contrast, German troops never had the same access to pervitin for so long.

Towards the end of the war, the Wehrmacht reissued the tablets with a combination of other drugs in naval operations, hoping to find a way for the final victory.[433] But by that time it was clear the Third Reich was coming to an end, and every trick in the book had to be exploited. Even so, use among soldiers did not go without concerns. *Oberregierungsrat*

---

430 Ibid., 70-71.
431 Ibid., 61.
432 Ibid., 84.
433 Ohler, *Der totale Rausch*, 256-265.

Linz of the of Health Office predicted that more extreme measures would have to be taken against the drug after the war's end,[434] but nothing ever came of it.

Pervitin became infamous because the SS used it in experiments in concentration camps, as was recorded at the Nuremberg Trials. The catalyst for the experiment was the death from poisoning of an SS officer. The police believed that the death might have resulted from the reaction of pervitin with another narcotic drug. A conference took place in the Main Office of Reich Security to discuss the matter; the Gestapo chief *Gruppenfuehrer* Heinrich Müller (1900-?) presided. *Gruppenfuehrer* Arthur Nebe (1894-1945) of the Reich Criminal Police was also present as well as Dr. Joachim Mrugowsky (1905-1948). The latter erroneously pointed out that pervitin was not a poison and that it could be obtained without a prescription. He recalled that "one of the gentlemen present pointed out that in America experiments were carried out where up to 100 tablets of pervitin were administered and the effects were not fatal. But no one present could answer the question of whether a combination of pervitin and a soporific would be harmless, or whether it would lead to an increased reaction to any one direction. The latter appeared improbable to the experts."[435] To settle the question Mueller ordered Dr. Ding of the concentration camp in Buchenwald to conduct experiments on human subjects.

In conclusion, the great drug epidemic of the Weimar years was but a sensation kept in the minds of Bohemians, journalists, historians, literary figures, or even Conti's boastful comments. The government was not impressed and therefore was slow to react. The drug laws in Germany, compared to those in the United States, were lax. Even the health authorities under Nazi rule did not express a great concern. They were only bothered by the possibility of an increase in addiction once the World War would come to an end. Yet, the massive influx of addicted soldiers

---

434 Linz, "Behoerdliche Durchfuehrung des Opiumgesetzes: Ziele und Ergebinsses" in Gerhart Feuerstein (ed.), *Suchtgiftbekaempfung* (Berlin, 1944), 24-32.

435 Nuernberg Military Tribunal "Green" Series, "The Medical Case; Military Tribunals No. I, Case 1" in *Trials of War Criminals Before the Nuernberg Military Tribunals under Control Council Law No. 10*, vol. 1, pp. 690-692, http://www.mazal.org/archive/nmt/01/NMT01-T691.htm.

returning home failed to materialize; the addiction rates remained low even after Germany's defeat.[436]

---

436 Robert Stephens, *Germans on Drugs: The Complications of Modernization in Hamburg* (Ann Arbor: University of Michigan Press, 2007), 18-23.

5. German Drug Laws and Enforcement

Efforts by German authorities to control the trade and use of psychoactive substances began far earlier than in the United States, albeit on a rather limited scale. On September 27, 1725, King Friedrich-Wilhelm I of Prussia (1688-1740) codified the nation's first ordinance on medicines, delineating how they were to be prescribed, sold and acquired.[437] The ordinance treated opium no differently than any other medicine.

By the turn of the century, however, opium had been singled out for its malefic effects. In a royal directive issued on December 10, 1800, opium and its preparations were listed by name and banned from open sale. They were added to a list of known poisons including aconite, better known as the legendary wolfsbane; belladonna, which contains atropine; and other substances. These poisons could only be acquired with a legal prescription.[438] The law did not forbid drug use, limiting its mandate to regulating poisons.

As Germany grew as a colonial power during the 19th century, Berlin imposed stringent regulations on the narcotics trade in its territorial possessions in China. In 1898, the German authorities began taxing opium imported into Tsingtao. Only physicians and chemists, all of whom were German, could order morphine and other drugs from Germany, and then only with the approval of the colonial government. Morphine production was forbidden in the Shantung peninsula, and opium cultivation was only allowed under state monopoly.[439]

The drug laws governing Germany itself during the 19th century were divided into two categories, those that governed the traffic in drugs and those that governed the prescription of drugs. The former were usually

---

437 "Allgemeines und neugeschaerfftes Medicinal-Edict und Verordnung vom 27ten September, 1725" in *Corpus Constitotiunum Marchicarum*, Vol. 5, 219ff. Larch. Berlin 5-50z 723.

438 For a historical explanations, see Eduard Levinstein, *Die Morphiumsucht: Eine Monographie nach eigenen Beobachtungen* (Berlin, 1877), 150-151; *Allerhoechste Verordnung vom 25. Maerz 1872, betreffend den Verkehr mit Apothekerwaaren* [sic].

439 Feng Djen Djang, *The Diplomatic Relations between China and Germany Since 1898* (Shanghai, 1936), 77, 89.

employed against smugglers or to regulate wholesale production, while the latter were employed against drug users or regulating retail sales. Consumption of any drug was legal, but possession without a prescription was forbidden – a distinction that, as semantic as it may seem, had considerable bearing on the legal status of drug users and addicts in Germany for decades to come, particularly during the Third Reich.

Typical of the laws governing the prescription of drugs was an 1873 ministerial order that forbade the sale of poisonous drugs to the public.[440] The newly united German Reich allowed only pharmacists to sell and prescribe drugs, thereby safeguarding their monopoly, as long as a physician provided a prescription. In the process, the ministerial order ensured that both pharmacists and doctors remained an integral part of the drug control system.

It was in the pharmacists' interest to keep tight control over the trade, as they wished to preserve their professional monopoly. To comply with the law, pharmacists were required to record both customers' names and the prescriptions according to which the drugs were dispensed. Their records, however, were anything but immaculately kept.[441]

Prescriptions nevertheless remained a favored tool for exerting control over the drug trade. In 1887, the cities of Braunschweig (Brunswick) and Meiningen mandated that the consumption of cocaine be subject to a prescription because of its uncontrollable use by actors and musicians. In 1890 the drug was included in the laws governing the dispensing of medicine, and by 1896, a prescription was required throughout the Reich for the dispensing of cocaine.[442] Certain drugs were regulated by apothecary laws, while others were controlled by laws for poisons and yet others by laws for the medicine industry. This complicated legal system survived in Germany until World War I, making it all the more telling that despite its incoherence, the drug control regime worked fairly well.[443] The country had no drug epidemics. Pharmacists and physicians, instead of

---

440 *Allerhoechste Verordnung vom 25. Maerz 1872, betreffend den Verkehr mit Apothekerwaaren* [sic]. See also Eduard Levinstein, *Die Morphiumsucht: Eine Monographie nach eigenen Beobachtungen*, (Berlin, 1877) 150-160.
441 Ibid.
442 Wolf-Reinhard Kemper, *Kokain in der Musik: Bestandsaufnahme und Analyse aus kriminologischer Sicht* (Munich: LIT, 2001), 10.
443 Holzer, *Die Geburt der Drogenpolitik aus dem Geist der Rassenhygiene*, 41-42.

being hunted down by the authorities, became highly professional, while the German drug industry prospered.

During the Kaiserreich and the Republic that followed, the courts had limited means to put drug users and alcoholics in jail. The Reich Penal Code allowed German courts to sentence drug users and addicts for possessing drugs in excess of the amount prescribed, for falsifying or stealing prescriptions, for possessing drugs without a prescription, and for a several other narrow offenses.[444] Otherwise, drug use was legal in Germany.

German internal policy was reflected diplomatically. The German delegation to the International Opium Commission in Shanghai in 1909 showed little interest in the proceedings, generally brushing off the commission as a matter of significance only to those countries with possessions in the Far East.[445] Germany's intransigence extended to the talks for the 1912 International Opium Convention in the Hague, the first international treaty concerning the limitation of trade in psychoactive substances. Germany frustrated any measure that threatened its control over the global drug trade, explicitly declaring that it would protect its drug industry.[446] Germany eventually signed the treaty, but refused to ratify it and imposed other difficulties on getting the treaty to enter into effect.[447]

German diplomats insisted that their country's pharmaceutical industry depended on morphine, and by extension the raw product from which it is produced: opium. Germany's efforts in the Hague and other international drug talks were accordingly focused on protecting Germany's access to opium – specifically, from its rivals in the industrialized drug trade, like Britain, France and Switzerland. The diplomatic dealings before the Hague treaty and the conferences that followed in large part revolved around the German-British trade rivalry. After the Indian government

444 Louis Lewin & Wenzel Goldbaum, *Opiumgesetz: Nebst Internationalen Opium-abkommen und Ausführungs bestimmungen*, (Berlin, 1928) 19; for the examples, see the appendices of the book.

445 Sebastian Scheerer, *Die Genese der Betaeubungsmittelgesetze in der Bundesre-publik Deutschland und in den Niederlanden* (Göttingen: Otto Schwartz, 1982), 38.

446 Wissler, *Die Opiumfrage*, 185.

447 *International Opium Convention* signed at the Hague, 23 January 1912. See William B. McAllister, *Drug Diplomacy in the Twentieth Century: An Interna-tional History* (London: Routledge, 2000), 24-35.

promised in 1906 to reduce the amount of opium exported to China, Britain grew increasingly concerned that Germany would take over the Chinese market with its industrialized products, particularly morphine and heroin.[448] And indeed, as opium became scarcer in China, morphine and heroin became more popular.

It was only with Germany's defeat in World War I that the United Kingdom and the United States had sufficient leverage to compel Germany to meet its international obligations in regard to drug control. The Allies inserted Article 295 into the Treaty of Versailles, requiring Germany to ratify the Hague Convention without delay.[449] It was clear to both London and Washington that Germany's accession was essential if the treaty were ever to have any effect on the international drug trade.[450] Left with little choice, Germany eventually ratified the Hague Convention.

From a commercial perspective, Germany no longer had reason to object to the implementation of the Convention, since all major drug-manufacturing countries had ratified the treaty after the war, thereby preserving, at least theoretically, Germany's primacy in the industry.[451] But in point of fact, Germany started losing control over the international market during the war, when German companies operating in the United States, such as Bayer and Merck, were nationalized in 1917.

The inclusion of Article 295 in the Treaty of Versailles has led many historians to conclude that external pressure alone forced Germany to act against its own industrial interests. Such a view, however, does not sufficiently account for increased intervention by the German government while the war was still being fought. On March 22, 1917, new regulations were imposed restricting the traffic in drugs. Opium, morphine, cocaine and their derivatives could only be procured as medicine from pharmacies.

---

448 Scheerer, *Die Genese der Betaeubungsmittelgesetze*, 39-40.

449 Virginia Berridge, *Opium and the People: Opiate Use and Drug Control Policy in Nineteenth and Early Twentieth Century England* (London: Free Association Books, 1999), 259. See also Hans Joachim Jungblut, "Drogenrecht und Drogenpolitik. Internationale Vorgaben und nationale Spielräume," in *Sozialwissenschaftliche Suchtforschung*, ed. Bernd Dollinger and Henning Schmidt-Semisch (Wiesebaden: VS, Verlag für Sozialwissenschaften, 2007), 277-288.

450 Arnold H. Taylor, *American Diplomacy and the Narcotics Traffic, 1900-1939: A Study in International Humanitarian Reform* (Durham, NC: Duke University Press, 1969), 144.

451 H. Richard Friman, *NarcoDiplomacy: Exporting the U.S. War on Drugs* (Ithaca: Cornell University Press, 1996), 22-23.

Wholesale distribution of drugs was permissible only when sold to pharmacies with approval from the central state office. Those caught breaking the law faced up to one year in prison and a fine of 10,000 Marks.[452] Although the newly strengthened laws were passed in Berlin, enforcement was left in the hands of the individual states.[453] Throughout the regulation process, industrial representatives were rarely consulted when actions were taken against the industry,[454] further calling into question the accepted wisdom that the German government catered to the wishes of its powerful pharmaceutical companies.[455]

A few days before the cease-fire agreement was signed with Germany in 1918, the Ministry of War declared a confiscation of coca leaves and cocaine.[456] That December, with Germany in postwar revolutionary turmoil, the central government reinforced its drug regulations and required permits from the Ministry of War for the wholesale distribution of opiates. Failure to follow the regulations earned six months imprisonment, a fine or both.[457]

For the first time in the country's history, the Reich authorities imposed restrictions on the drug trade. The crackdown was driven by the government's concern that the industry would sell off its wartime drug stockpiles, thereby leading to shortages.[458] The German authorities certainly had good reason to be wary of the profit-driven pharmaceutical companies. During the war, the German branch of the Swiss-based company Hoffmann-LaRoche tried to sell pantopon, morphine in pill form, to the French; an act of treason, for which the German owner of the company sat in jail for a few months.[459] And yet in less than half a year, Germany's

---

452 "Verordnung, betreffend den Handel mit Opium und anderen Betäubungsmitteln, 22 March 1917" *Reichsgesetzblatt*, 256.
453 Briesen, *Drogenkonsum und Drogenpolitik in Deutschland und den USA*, 49.
454 Friman, *NarcoDiplomacy*, 22.
455 Holzer, *Globalisierte Drogenpolitik*.
456 *Bekanntmachung des Preussischen Kriegsministeriums, betreffend Beschlagnahme und Bestandserhebung von Cocablättern und Cocain*, 2 November 1918, No. 1/11 12, 2.
457 "Verordnung über den Verkehr mit Opium, 15 December 1918," *Reichsgesetzblatt*, 1447.
458 Friman, *NarcoDiplomacy*, 22-23.
459 Hans Conrad Peyer, *Roche: Geschichte eines Unternehmens* (Basel: Edition Roche, 1996), 68-69.

newly stringent regulations were relaxed for intrastate commerce.[460] The lifting of the Allied blockade in 1919 and subsequent replenishing of supplies after the long wartime shortage was the decisive factor.[461]

A closer look at the regulations enacted in 1917 reveals that enforcement was anything but strict. Between June 5, 1917 and August 14, 1919, for example 48 persons and companies received licenses to buy and sell opium and other drugs in Berlin. Among the 48 were several who applied for multiple licenses within a period of months.[462] Furthermore, the licenses did not dictate exact amounts. The companies were required to report the number of containers they filled with their drug products, but since the size of tubes, pills and tablets varied from one manufacturer to another, it would have been nearly impossible to calculate the real amount of drugs being sold. This lax policy allowed manufacturers, dealers and smugglers alike to exercise considerable leeway in meeting the demands of their customers.

Many licenses were effectively limitless. To cite one example, Dr. Heinrich Byck of Chemische Werke in Berlin received the following license: "The opium preparations (holopon) which are produced in the factory are only allowed to be sold to pharmacies or people to whom the sale is permitted by the authorities."[463] Chemische Werke's license granted it the ability to produce any number of holopon tablets, without anyone but the company bookkeeper being the wiser. Licenses for larger companies such as Schering had even more permissible wording: "For the sale of opium and other drugs in any suitable amount."[464] What exactly constituted a suitable amount was presumably left to the company's discretion. Such hands-off enforcement of drug laws was also found elsewhere in the country, including in Düsseldorf, where the local health

---

460 "Verordnung betreffend Abänderung der Verordnung über den Verkehr mit Opium vom 15. Dezember 1918, 20 August 1919," *Reichsgesetzblatt* II, 1474.

461 Briesen, *Drogenkonsum und Drogenpolitik in Deutschland und den USA,* 50.

462 "Berlin Police President to Minister of Welfare: Information regarding people and companies…with permission to trade in opium and other drugs according to the laws of 1917 and 1920" (Berlin, 6 December 1920) in GSa. PKb. I.HA Re76 VIII B Nr. 1246.

463 Ibid.

464 Ibid.

office gave the Leverkusen-based Bayer carte blanche to produce as much drugs as the company deemed necessary.[465]

In July 1920, Germany' disjointed drug regulations were reorganized into a single ordinance, with only minor modifications introduced. Authority over the drug control regime was transferred from the Ministry of War to the Reich Health Office.[466] But because the ordinance did not address the regulation of the export and import of drugs, as required by Article 295 of the Treaty of Versailles, a new law was brought into force on July 1, 1921. Finally, after almost two years delay, Germany ratified the terms of the Hague Convention.[467]

It would be another five years before Germany's highest court considered its first drug-related case. In October 1926, the German Supreme Court in Leipzig declared that it was illegal for a physician to prescribe cocaine for recreational purposes, overturning an earlier ruling by a lower court in Dresden. The recreational use of cocaine had clearly been declared illegal, but it remained legal to prescribe drugs to treat addiction – in other words, drug maintenance was still legal in Germany.[468]

In the wake of World War I, Germany suffered from serious inflation and a shortage of material goods. Pharmaceutical companies, however, had production capacities that surpassed domestic demand, and consequently drug smuggling from Germany to other countries was a major problem during the early Weimar years. As much was made clear in 1926 by the British representative to the Opium Advisory Committee, Sir Malcolm Delevingne (1868-1950): "Germany is very far from having clean hands in the matter of illicit traffic in drugs; but the use of forged labels on an extensive scale (many of them appear to emanate from Japanese sources) gives the German government and manufacturers a

---

465 "Medizinalrat Dr. Clauss to Minister of Welfare"(Düsseldorf, 6 December 1920) in GSa. PKb. I.HA Re76 VIII B Nr. 1246.

466 "Verordnung über den Verkehr mit Opium und anderen Betäubungsmitteln, 20 July 1920" *Reichsgesetzblatt* II, 1464.

467 "Gesetz zur Ausführung des internationalen Opiumabkommens vom 23. Januar 1912, 30 December 1920," *Reichsgesetzblatt* (1921), 2. See also "Bekanntmachung, betreffend das Internationalen Opiumabkommen vom 23. Januar 1912, 22 December 1920" *Reichsgesetzblatt* (1921), 6.

468 *Reichsgericht Entscheidungen Straftaten* (RGSt) vol. 60 (1926), I 184/26.

means of defense."[469] Proof that the German government actively helped drug manufacturers smuggle their wares was hard to come by. Enforcement of the drug laws, however, was unquestionably lax. The authority's inability to control drugs has been interpreted by some historians as evidence of the Weimar Republic's weak federal system of control, rather than proof of a lack of will in government.[470] Whatever the case might be, little serious debate took place in the Reichstag as Berlin formed its drug policies during the 1920s and 30s.[471]

When public demand for drug law reform did grow, in the mid-1920s, a major catalyst was the fear of soldiers returning home from war as addicts.[472] Two other key factors were the demand for penal code reform and the creation of a League of Nations-affiliated organization regulating international drug traffic. By 1928, five drug laws and ordinances had been passed in Germany. In a 1928 guidebook to the opium laws, toxicologist Louis Lewin and jurist Wenzel Goldbaum (1881-1960) noted that the unlawful use of drugs or the misuse of drug prescriptions carried a maximum punishment of three years in jail and a fine. Lewin and Goldbaum insisted, however, that drug addicts were sick persons, not criminals, and therefore deserved the protection of Article 51 of the penal code, which dealt with criminal accountability. Addicts, according to Lewin and Goldbaum, were not responsible for their actions while under the influence of drugs, and therefore deserved treatment instead of imprisonment. Judges in the Weimar era often agreed with this position,[473] but were unable to force treatment upon addicts and were known to set free criminals who had been deemed unfit to stand trial.

---

469 "Delevingne to Foreign Office, 10 May 1926," PRO FO 371/11711 quoted in Richard Davenport-Hines, *The Pursuit of Oblivion* (London: Phoenix Press, 2002), 218.

470 Friman, *NarcoDiplomacy*, 20-34.

471 For example, see the 49th sitting of the Reichstag on "Entwurf eines Gesetzes zur Ausführung des internationalen Opiumabkommens vom 23. Januar 1912" (A bill for a law to enforce the International Opium Treaty of 23 January 1912) on 17 December 1920 *Verhandlungen des Reichstages* (1920), Vol. 346, 1762B; or, 408th sitting of the Reichstag on "Entwurf eines Gesetzes zur Abänderung des Opiumgesetzes" (A bill for a law to amend the Opium Law) on 10 March 1924 *Verhandlungen des Reichstages* (1924), Vol. 361, 12697A.

472 Wissler, *Die Opiumfrage*, 139.

473 Lewin and Goldbaum, *Opiumgesetz*, 20-21; Holzer, *Die Geburt des Drogenpolitik aus dem Geist der Rassenhygiene*, 31-32.

Ambiguity also characterized Germany's participation in international efforts to control the drug trade. Berlin signed the International Convention Relating to Dangerous Drugs in February 1925, several months before Germany entered the League of Nations. But as it had with the Opium Convention of 1912, Berlin dragged its feet on ratification, taking four years before finally ratifying the convention. Great Britain, by comparison, implemented the necessary laws and ratified the treaty within a year of rendering its signature.

As mentioned above, some historians have since argued that the delay in ratification was caused by German industrialists bent on protecting their interests and keeping the administration in the dark about their dealings. While this may very well have been the case, there is no concrete evidence to support this theory. Germany ostensibly had nothing to fear from ratification, as the treaty had already gone into force in Europe's other major drug-producing countries – Britain, Switzerland, France and the Netherlands – by 1928. Furthermore, Germany's laws already nearly complied with all the requirements of the 1925 convention.[474] Germany's wary eye, however, was cast mainly at its primary industrial competitor, the United States. Washington, or rather its representative in Geneva: Stephen G. Porter (1869-1930), refused to sign the treaty, claiming that more stringent controls were necessary to thwart the illicit drug market.[475]

In 1929 Germany finally ratified the treaty, and sent Otto Anselmino (1873-1955), a professor of chemistry at the University of Berlin, as its representative to the Permanent Central Board. That December, Germany's two legislative bodies, the Reichstag and Reichsrat, passed a new unified German opium law, the *Opiumgesetz*. The law restricted the sale of specific drugs and their salts and alkaloids, including opium, cocaine and cannabis. The *Opiumgesetz*, which grouped the drugs together with little differentiation between them, contained no dramatic departures from existing law. Perhaps the only substantive change to the German system was the possibility of adding new drugs to the list, if scientific research proved they were as dangerous as the ones already listed.[476]

---

474 Wissler, *Die Opiumfrage*, 229.
475 McAllister, *Drug Diplomacy in the Twentieth Century*, 77.
476 "Gesetz über den Verkehr mit Betäubungsmitteln (Opiumgesetz), 10 December 1929" *Reichsgesetzblatt* I, 215. See Briesen, *Drogenkonsum und Drogenpolitik in Deutschland und den USA*, 107-110.

The Conference on the Limitation of Manufacturing of Narcotic Drugs, which was held in Geneva in June 1931, prompted the next step in the evolution of the drug control regime, and probably the most lasting change in German drug enforcement. According to the treaty signed in Geneva, all contracting parties were to submit estimates of their drug production for the following year to a newly created organization, the Drug Supervisory Body. Germany managed to protect its financial interests by creating a scheduled system; there were two degrees of enforcement, depending on the type of drug. The first governed drugs with no acceptable medical use, banning them altogether. The second allowed a regulated international trade in drugs, which had acceptable medicinal use, even if they contained opiates or were opiate derivatives. Finally, each contracting party was expected to create a law enforcement agency whose purpose was to deal with drug-related crimes.[477]

In June 1932, Interior Minister Wilhelm von Gayl (1879-1945) assured the newly appointed German chancellor, Franz von Papen (1879-1969), that he no longer expected real objection to the ratification of the 1931 treaty, and that a ratification proposal had been submitted to the Reichstag for deliberations.[478] That November, Papen informed the Interior Ministry and Ministry of Foreign Affairs that the government would not oppose ratification.[479] The Reichstag and the Reichsrat ratified the treaty on January 19, 1933, just days before the National Socialists took power and only two years since the treaty had been signed.

Three months into the job, Nazi Interior Minister Wilhelm Frick (1877-1946) sent a letter to Adolf Hitler urging a second amendment to the 1929 *Opiumgesetz*, citing the recent discovery of illegal traffic in benzylmorphine from Hamburg to Eastern Europe. Frick noted that he would order the police to treat Hamburg severely in order to demonstrate to the world that there was no connection between the German pharmaceutical industry and the illicit drug trade.[480] Frick was sensitive to international public opinion, and knew that benzylmorphine was explicitly banned in Chapter 1, Article 1, Group 1, Subgroup A of the 1931 Conference on the Limitation of Manufacturing of Narcotic Drugs. But drug

---

477 McAllister, *Drug Diplomacy in the Twentieth Century*, 96-102.
478 "Minister of Interior to the Reich Chancellor, 15 June 1932," BArch. R 43 II/736.
479 "Chancellery to the Ministry of Interior and Foreign Affairs, 29 November 1932," BArch. R 43 II/736.
480 "Frick to Hitler, 20 May 1933," BArch. R 43 II/736.

legislation moved no quicker in Nazi Germany than in the Weimar Republic, and it was not until the end of the year that the Interior Ministry passed the amendment. Benzylmorphine, meanwhile, was only added to the drug list the next year.

In a December 1933 letter to his fellow Cabinet members, Frick wrote that despite Germany's ratification of the treaty, Berlin had to promulgate laws corresponding to all of the agreement's articles in order to implement the treaty.[481] Two matters were likely on Frick's mind. The first was a sudden increase in drug smuggling cases in Germany, which peeked at 373 cases in 1934 but subsided to less than a third of that in the years to follow.[482] The second was the creation of a national drug police force, roughly equivalent to the Federal Bureau of Narcotics in the United States.

Frick's letter was indicative of Berlin's commitment to meet its obligations under the international drug control regime, a commitment that would hardly seem to square with Germany's withdrawal from the League of Nations in October 1933. Within weeks, Dr. Waldemar Kahler of the Interior Ministry informed the president of the Opium Commission that Germany was relinquishing its membership in the advisory body.[483] Germany also asked its representative to the Permanent Central Board, Otto Anselmino, to resign his position, which he did forthwith. On the surface Germany appeared to be isolating itself from the drug control regime, but nothing was further from the truth.[484]

Following Nazi Germany's withdrawal from the League of Nations and its affiliated bodies, the volume of drug-related correspondence between Berlin and the league only increased. The German consul general in Geneva represented his country's interests at the international body, and Kahler continued to correspond with the Permanent Central Board. The main change following Germany's withdrawal from the league was that Berlin was unable, at least on paper, to directly influence the board or the Opium Advisory Committee. Rather than a self-imposed act of isolation, however, the move was a way for Germany to accommodate the interna-

---

481 "Frick to the Cabinet, 28 December 1933," BArch. R 43 II/736.

482 Briesen, *Drogenkonsum und Drogenpolitik in Deutschland und den USA*, 112.

483 "Kahler an Praesidenten der Opiumkommission, 27 October 1933," Pol. Arch. AA. R 96839 quoted in Tilmann Holzer, *Globalisierte Drogenpolitik: Die protestantische Ethik und die Geschichte des Drogenverbotes* (Berlin, 2002), 150.

484 McAllister, *Drug Diplomacy in the Twentieth Century,* 111.

tional drug control regime without it impinging on Hitler's aggressive foreign policy.

Why did Germany forego the letter of the law but still observed its spirit? Perhaps Berlin hoped to avoid sanctions prescribed in the 1931 treaty, the imposition of which would have made it difficult to obtain raw materials for drugs from countries enforcing the treaty. However, finding a nation where drug enforcement was lacking was not particularly difficult during those years. Perhaps Germany saw no reason to further antagonize the world. Or perhaps Hitler simply favored a strong international drug control regime. Whatever the case may be, the Reich continued to report on legal and illegal drug traffic to Geneva and to the League of Nations, as dictated by the international treaties of 1925 and 1931.[485] In fact, Germany's records are among the only sources available today with comprehensive figures for smuggling cases prior to World War II.

When war did break out, in September 1939, the Permanent Central Board sent an inquiry to Germany asking whether Berlin intended to maintain contact with the League of Nations. That December, the matter was taken up by representatives of the Interior Ministry and the Ministry of Foreign Affairs, and it was agreed that the German government would do its utmost to adhere to the international opium conventions, albeit only those concerning illegal traffic of the drug and its derivatives. Germany, the Nazi officials decided, would continue recording the relevant statistics and calculations, but would cease submitting them to the Permanent Central Board and the Drug Supervisory Body. The German consul in Geneva relayed Berlin's decision to the League of Nations on February 28, 1940.

The consul in Geneva, not so incidentally, failed to mention that the Health Office had also stopped reporting on the import and export of narcotics, as required by the 1925 treaty. In a secret resolution, it was agreed by the Interior Ministry and Foreign Affairs Ministry to direct drug purchases via a third party, usually Spain or a neutral country in South America, in direct contravention of the 1925 treaty.[486] The move was an attempt to mask Germany's growing need for strategic raw materials. The

---

485 "Summary of the Stettin Conference, 10 October 1937," StA. München, Pol. Dir. 7582.

486 "Conferences between Min. Rat Dr. Imhoff of the Ministry of Interior and Reg. Rat Dr. Hoffmann of the Foreign Ministry 28 November 1939 and 11 December 1939," Pol. Arch. AA R 43.328.

size of the country's stockpiles of opium, morphine and cocaine was considered highly sensitive information, as the drugs were essential field medicine in the unfolding world war. Another such step was an agreement that by January the two ministries agreed to label drugs imported from South America as "*Arzeneimittel*" (medicine) rather than "*Betäubung-smittel*" (drug).[487]

Both illegitimate and legitimate drug traffic were an important strategic concern for wartime Germany. It needed raw opium to produce morphine and other opiates required to treat its wounded soldiers. Large amounts of drugs were bought abroad; opium was primarily procured from Turkey, Persia, Afghanistan and the Soviet Union. The Soviet Union, for example, sent two shipments after the outbreak of war totaling over 10 tons of raw opium, at a price of 20 Reichsmarks per kilogram of opium with 12 percent morphine content. The Afghan authorities delivered 3 tons of raw opium, containing 470 kilograms of morphine base, and claimed they could deliver another 4 to 5 tons of raw opium with 12 percent morphine content for the price of 24 Reichsmarks per kilogram. The drugs were to be delivered via the Soviet Union.

Persia sold Germany 6,083 chests (49.8 tons) of raw opium containing about six tons of morphine base, in accordance with an old contract. In 1940, Persia offered Germany 500 chests for $660 per chest, which turned out to be 60 percent more expensive than the previous deal. A deal was struck on June 16, and Germany bought 38.64 tons of raw opium for 84 pounds sterling per chest. Turkey, meanwhile, sold a thousand chests in February 1940. It had previously delivered two shipments, one with 267 chests (21.37 tons) of raw opium containing 2.74 tons of morphine base and one with 160 chests (12.8 tons) containing 1.63 tons of morphine base. When Yugoslavia was conquered, Germany confiscated 8 tons of raw opium, but 7 tons were sold to France for 24 Reichsmarks per kilogram, 10 Reichsmarks less than what Yugoslavia would have sold it for had it still been independent. Bulgaria, for its part, sold 12 tons of raw opium for 39 Reichsmarks per kilogram.[488] Preparation for war and the German withdrawal from the international drug control regime did not flood the world market with illicit drugs. On the contrary, the war and the

---

487 "Conference between Min. Rat Dr. Imhoff of the Ministry of Interior and Reg. Rat Dr. Hoffmann of the Foreign Ministry, 18 January 1940," Pol. Arch. AA R 43.328.

488 "Drug Consumption Report, (undated) 1941" Pol. Arch AA 43.327.

disruption to the shipping lanes proved to be the only successful remedy to the illicit drug trade.

International drug control was multi-faceted. As noted above, it primarily focused on curbing the international drug trade, but it was also directed internally. Among the many stipulations regulating scientifically approved drugs, and banning drugs deemed to have no medicinal value, each signatory power was expected to create an effective police force to enforce these laws.

On March 18, 1932, after signing the treaty of 1931 but before its ratification, Kahler convened a meeting at the Ministry of Interior where it was decided to create a drug unit for the Reich to comply with the convention.[489] The new unit was to expand the Prussian drug unit that had existed since 1925.[490] The Prussian unit's chief, Kriminalkommissar Thomas, was selected to head the new national drug police unit. In an amusing historical footnote, that July the American government officially congratulated Thomas on his appointment, presumably unaware that Thomas' rank, Kriminalkommissar, was the lowest pay grade for an officer in the German police – hardly a sign of Germany's determination to create a centralized drug unit.[491]

The creation of the Reich drug unit coincided with a wider Nazi effort at bureaucratic reform that centralized police authority in Berlin, with individual departments dealing with distinct offenses. Of the 11 new offices, the only one to have the word *Vergehen* or transgression in its name rather than *Verbrechen* or crime was the Reich Central Office for Combating Drug Transgression,[492] which was officially established on November 22, 1935.[493] The unit had 19 intelligence-gathering stations and

---

489 "Summary of Dr. Kahler's Conference, 18 March 1932," Pol. Arch AA R 43.43.289.

490 Kosmehl, *Der sicherheitspolizeiliche Einsatz bei der Bekämpfung der Betäubungsmittel,* BArch. RD 19/30; for the Geneva Conference of 1931 see above.

491 "United States to Germany, 29 July 1932," Pol. Arch. AA R 43.291; For Thomas' career, see BArch. SSO Thomas, Werner, 12.03.1895.

492 In German: *Reichszentrale zur Bekämpfung von Rauschgiftvergehen,* see Friedrich Wilhelm, *Die Polizei im NS-Staat* (Paderborn: Verlag Ferdinand Schöningh, 1997), 81-82.

493 "Announcement of the Minister of Interior Nr. 1935-III C II22 Nr. 513/34, 22 November 1935," *Reichsministerialblatt* 63:47 (29 November 1935), 840.

64 intelligence-gathering posts, with two more being added during the war.[494]

At the drug office's headquarters there were no more than a dozen policemen and administrators.[495] They were tasked with gathering information from various police stations, maintaining a card index of all known drug addicts and criminals, coordinating efforts against drug smuggling, including contact with foreign police forces, and ensuring enforcement of the 1929 opium law and 1930 prescription ordinance.[496] In practice, the head office did little more than extract information from the drug desks at existing police stations.

Such information was contained in the annual report from the Reich criminal police office for the years 1939-1940. The effectiveness of the intelligence gathering posts reflected the over all lack of zeal of the German government's attitude towards drug enforcement. In Berlin, just one case was investigated based on information from an intelligence-gathering station. In the rest of the Reich, 224 drug-related cases were investigated. Seventy-one of them involved the card index of known addicts and criminals, while 24 came about following interrogation following a crime. The most efficient police stations were Frankfurt am Main, with 40 cases obtained via intelligence, 10 using index cards and seven via interrogations; Hamburg, with 39, eight and eight; Munich, with eight, 40 and four; and Dresden, with 32 cases, five and one.[497]

The drug unit also conducted active field operations, with some degree of success. In October 1943, the intelligence-gathering post in Vienna reported on its efforts the previous year to control the drug stores in the Alpengau and Donaugau, in what is today upper Carinthia and lower Styria. But it noted that only 215 of the area's 713 stores had been examined, and that more pressing war issues precluded further investigation. The missive from Vienna was meant to encourage local police stations to

---

494 Holzer, *Die Geburt der Drogenpolitik aus dem Geist der Rassenhygiene*, 204; Kosmehl, *Der sicherheitspolizeiliche Einsatz bei der Bekämpfung der Betäubungsmittelsucht,* BArch. RD 19/30.

495 So deduced from a report in *Jahrbuch Amt V (Reichskriminalpolizeiamt) des Reichssicherheitshauptamtes SS 1939/1940*, 83-86, BArch. RD 19/29 1939/1949.

496 "Prussian criminal police announcement on the creation of *Rechszentrale zur Bekämpfung von Rauschgiftvergehen,* 1 March 1935," StA. München, Pol. Dir. 7582.

497 BArch. RD 19/29 1939/1940, *Jahrbuch Amt V (Reichskriminalpolizeiamt) des Reichssicherheitshauptamtes SS 1939/1940*, Anhang.

divert more resources to examining drug stores.[498] Similar calls were repeated in an April 1944 letter from the central drug office to the intelligence-gathering posts, in which an officer from Berlin urged police to conduct random checks of pharmacies. The missive, incidentally, went against the recommendation of the Interior Ministry's medical department that pharmacies be left alone unless there was suspicion of criminal activity.[499]

That there was a fair amount of suspicion among Nazi officials that pharmacists were indeed engaging in illegal practices can be gleaned from a 1937 directive issued by the Reich's top pharmacy official, ordering pharmacists to cooperate with the police:

> Order of the *Reichsapothekerführer* concerning cooperation with the criminal police: The justice authority notified me that a few pharmacists, due to their false understanding of their obligation to maintain confidentiality [...] did not hand the needed material on narcotics prescriptions to the criminal police. Every pharmacist is obliged to explain drug cases to the best of his ability. Therefore, I expect that in the future such incidents will not occur. I value immensely your collegial cooperation with the criminal police in this manner.

Six years later, a second, more stringent directive was issued to reinforce the 1937 order:

> Order about the cooperation with the criminal police: If the criminal police require the confidence of a pharmacist to combat narcotics misuse, it is self explanatory, that the pharmacist must keep the criminal police's secret. The pharmacist, who draws attention to the fact that the police is conducting an investigation, places himself in danger of a legal process.[500]

Control was tightened even further that December, when pharmacists were ordered to report all individuals buying drugs with prescriptions.[501] The need for repetition might indicate the lack of success in controlling illegal

---

498 Quotes from "Intelligence gathering post in Vienna to the *Reichszentrale zur Bekämpfung von Rauschgiftvergehen*, 16 October 1943" StA. München, Pol. Dir. 7582.

499 "*Reichszentrale zur Bekämpfung von Rauschgiftvergehen* to *Nachrichtensammelstelle*, 3 April 1944" StA. München, Pol. Dir. 7582.

500 Both quotes were taken from Police reproduction of "The *Reichsapothekerführer*'s orders to pharmacists, 1 June 1944" StA. München, Pol. Dir. 7582.

501 "Anordnung des RSHA—Reichszentrale zur Bekämpfung von Rauschgiftvergehen Tgb. Nr. 3473/43-B 3CT, 6 December 1943" StA. München, Pol. Dir. 7582.

drug flow from legitimate sources, such as prescriptions and pharmacists. Or it could have been due to concerns that, with World War II still raging, the authorities were worried about a new wave of addicted soldiers flooding the country. Whatever the cause, the authorities clearly believed that the weakest links in the German drug control system were pharmacists and physicians.

Physicians, for their part, were kept under an even more watchful eye by the authorities. In April 1937, the Reich Physicians Chamber ordered physicians to report every case in which they prescribed narcotics, with the information to be passed on to the criminal police.[502] The next year, the top health official in the Third Reich, Gerhard Wagner (1888-1939), issued a number of orders defining when physicians were allowed to prescribe narcotics.[503] And in February 1939, yet another directive required physicians to be personally familiar with a patient before prescribing drugs, a directive that was highlighted by Leonardo Conti after he took over from Wagner.[504] These directives were strictly enforced. Dr. Wilhelm Glasser of Bad Aibling, for example, was convicted in October 1941 of prescribing narcotics to a patient whom he had not seen. The presiding judge decreed that in so doing, Glasser had violated the procedures set down by the Prescription Ordinance.[505]

But for all the government's decrees, physicians and those close to them remained a problem for the authorities. From the 1920s on, most addicts brought into court were physicians and pharmacists, or their family members. For example, Charlotte Seebald, the daughter of a physician from Potsdam, was a typical defendant. Seebald received morphine for pain after undergoing an operation in 1937. Her consumption grew over time, but her father, who was administering the morphine, restricted her to three ampoules a day, each dose containing 0.02 grams of morphine. In August 1940 she began falsifying her father's prescriptions, changing the three ampoules a day to five. She went to several pharmacies to receive

---

502 "Summary of the Stettin Conference, 10 October 1937," StA. München, Pol. Dir. 7582.

503 Linz, "Behoerdliche Durchfuehrung des Opiumgesetzes: Ziele und Ergebinsse" in Gerhart Feuerstein (ed.), *Suchtgiftbekämpfung* (Berlin, 1944), 24-32.

504 "Richtlinien fuer die Anmeldung von Betaeubungsmitteln in der aerztlichen Praxis," official copy published in *Deutsches Reichsaerzteblatt* (February, 1939), 171.

505 StA. München, Pol. Dir. 7582.

her drugs. The pharmacists, who noticed the falsification, gave her the drugs anyway. In January 1941, Seebald was brought into court on prescription falsification charges, and two months later sent to the Brandenburg state sanitarium for rehabilitation.[506]

The German bureaucracy had several tiers. The criminal police was the only German agency dealing with drug control that had enforcement powers, but there were a number of other official or semi-official organizations that guided drug policy in the Third Reich. Prior to the outbreak of World War II, the most prominent among them was the Reich Study Group for Combating Drugs, which answered to the Interior Ministry's Committee for Public Health. The study group was intended to be an independent organization that would help the Interior Ministry create drug policy, but by the end of 1940 it had proved ineffectual. Among its more memorable achievements was the use of the term *"Rauschgiftsüchtiger,"* or "stupefying poison addict" as a catchall phrase to describe those who habitually used psychoactive substances.

According to the chief of the study group, Gerhart Feuerstein, its primary purpose was to propose efficient ways to combat the drug menace, as well as to raise public awareness of the dangers of nicotine and alcohol use. Beginning in 1938, patients released from sanatoria had to submit themselves to periodic medical examination by local members of the study group, who also held positions in local offices of the Reich Health Office.[507] In 1940, on the orders of Reich health leader Conti, the local branches were integrated into the study group as part of the Central District Posts for Combating Drugs.

The Reich Reporting Center for Combating Addiction, meanwhile, was created in December 1941 to regulate and keep the records of the various posts. Feuerstein was appointed the head of the organization, which was modeled after the Central Reporting Office for Opium Addiction established in East Prussia in 1937,[508] and managed to extend its authority to both the civilian population and the Wehrmacht.[509] The central district

---

506 "Landesgericht Beschluß: Charlotte Seebald," (Potsdam, 7 January 1941) Brandenburgisches Landeshauptarchiv Re12 B, Nr. 107.
507 "Summary of the Stettin Conference, 10 October 1937," StA. München, Pol. Dir. 7582.
508 Gerhart Feuerstein, "Ziel und Weg der Reichsmeldstelle fuer Suchtgiftbekämpfung" in *Suchtgiftbekämpfung*, ed. Gerhart Feuerstein, 7-15.
509 Ibid.

posts operated as local branches of the Reich reporting center in much the same way the criminal police's local stations answered to headquarters in Berlin. Two separate branches of the Reich bureaucracy, therefore, dealt with drug-related matters, one civilian and the other a part of the police.

The civilian branch was reformed several times, eventually coming under the joint authority of the Interior Ministry, Justice Ministry and Health Office. The Reich reporting center and its subsidiaries were instructed to examine the areas of medicine, health care and preventive action. The central district posts handled the paperwork coming in from physicians, who were required to file a report whenever prescribing narcotics to a patient for more than three weeks, a requirement first ordered locally in Berlin in 1937. Each post had a Working Group for Combating Addiction, an advisory committee that met biannually to assess the drug situation in the district and prepare comprehensive plans to clean it of addicts. The working groups were composed of physicians, dentists, veterinarians, chemists, officers, state attorneys, police officers and others.[510]

One such working group was established in the Munich-Upper Bavaria district in April 1942 on Conti's orders. Led by Dr. Harrfeldt, the working group included members of the regional physicians association, the chief state attorney, Kriminalkommissar Galster of the Munich criminal police, Ms. Sperling of the Munich-based *Deutsche Frauenwerk* women's organization, and Feuerstein representing the Reich Reporting Center for Combating Addiction. The chief purpose of the working group was to monitor physicians' compliance with the mandatory reporting of narcotic prescriptions, and to help bar from medical practice doctors suspected of drug addiction.[511]

Although the working groups did, to some extent, succeed in their limited mandates, they did little to reverse the increasing bureaucratization of Reich drug policy. Nazi Germany was as prolific in adding red tape as it was determined to be free of it, the working groups represented yet another example of the National Socialist proclivity for placing one new bureaucratic body on top of another in a chain of command that appeared clear only on paper. That bureaucratic inertia is perhaps the most noteworthy aspect of Reich drug policy speaks volumes, given the impunity

---

510 Ibid.
511 "The Formation of the Working Group for Combating Addiction in Bavaria, 1 April 1942," StA. München, Pol. Dir. 7582.

with which other arms of the Nazi bureaucracy murdered millions. Few if any of the drug laws and amendments promulgated in the Third Reich were infused with Nazi ideology. Racial policies had little impact on the drug laws, other than the influence of racial hygiene directives in Nazi penal code reform.

Continuity and singularity are the two words that come to mind when describing the German drug laws. From the Second Reich through the Weimar years and into the Third Reich, the German drug laws evolved in a linear path, despite foreign meddling and two revolutions. Germany retained its own unique laws that were meant to keep the public safe on the one hand, and regulate the drug traffic efficiently.

6. Treating a Biological Enemy

The pursuit of racial hygiene was a central tenet of Nazi ideology, and the determination to rid the *Volk* of those deemed biologically defective or anti-social pervaded both lawmaking and law enforcement in the Third Reich. The general omission of drug addicts from such categorization, therefore, is telling. The Nazis had no compunction about persecuting and murdering millions of people deemed to be defective, yet even the worst drug offenders suffered little for their crimes, at least by the lethal standards of the Third Reich.

Unlike nearly every other aspect of Reich policy, Nazi drug laws were generally devoid of racial and hygienic rhetoric. Even after the Third Reich began sending habitual criminals to concentration camps, drug addicts were spared. Indeed, save for a few confirmed cases, drug addicts were not maltreated, and in fact enjoyed a better life than they would have in the United States.

An examination of articles published during the Nazi era in the *Deutsches Ärzteblatt*, the official gazette of the Reich's Physician Chamber, revealed just one claiming a connection between drug use and race. Not a single article was written about addiction. When the head of the Health Office's Racial Hygiene and Criminal-Biological Research Department, Dr. Ritter, defined the Reich's views on biological defects and their criminal manifestations in 1941, drug crimes were not even mentioned once.[512]

That is not to say, of course, that there were not attempts by the Nazi leadership to have drug addiction categorized as an anti-social offense. Early in the war, a proposal on how to deal with "enemies of the community" was circulated within several Reich ministries.[513] Reinhard Heydrich

---

512 R. Ritter, "Die Aufgaben der Kriminalbiologie und der kriminalbiologischen Bevölkerungsforschung," *Kriminalistik* 15:4 (April 1941), 37-48.

513 Henry Friedlander, *The Origins of the Nazi Genocide: From Euthanasia to Final Solution* (Chapel Hill: North Carolina University Press, 1995), 154; Robert Gellately, *The Gestapo and German* Society (Oxford: Clarendon Press, 1992), 196; Jeremy Noakes, "Nazism and Eugenics: The Background to the Nazi Sterilization Law of 14 July 1933" in *Ideas into Politics: Aspects of European History, 1880-1950*, ed. Roger Bullen et al. (London: Croom Helm, 1984), 75-94.

(1904-1942), the head of the Reich Security Main Office, was the force behind the proposal, but when it was officially sent to Reich Chancellery secretary Hans-Heinrich Lammers (1879-1962) in June 1941; it came from Interior Minister Wilhelm Frick. The proposal codified the term "anti-social," and among those who would be subject to greatly expanded police powers were drug addicts. The bill, however, failed to pass the German cabinet.

A modified version of Heydrich's bill was resubmitted the following March, but it, too, was rejected, this time with particularly strong opposition from leading political figures. Those against it included Hans Frank (1900-1946), the governor-general of Poland and the Nazi Party's legal advisor; Konstantin von Neurath (1873-1956), a former foreign minister and governor of Bohemia; Johannes Popitz (1884-1945), the finance minister of Prussia; Otto Georg Thierack (1889-1946), the justice minister – and, most notably, Hermann Göring (1893-1946), the second-most powerful man in the Third Reich. Göring declared that the Allies would see the law as a sign of weakness, while Neurath was even more explicit, warning that a broadening of police powers would lead to public agitation.[514] Underlying their opposition to the proposal was opposition to the growing reach and power of Heydrich and his SS commander, Heinrich Himmler (1900-1945).

The Justice Ministry sent a third and final version of the proposal to the Reich Chancellery on February 1, 1943, by which time Heydrich had been assassinated. The Chancellery, however, did not respond to the proposal, nor forwarded it to another government body for consideration. Indeed, the proposal was forgotten almost as soon as it arrived – no surprise, perhaps, as it was received the same day as news that Field Marshall Friedrich Paulus had surrendered his army in Stalingrad.[515]

Disconnected from the Third Reich's racial policies, drug-related offenses remained in the realm of regular criminal law. Even there, such

---

514 "Schreiben des Reichs- und Preussischen Innenministers Dr. Wilhelm Frick an den Reichsminister ohne Geschäftsbereich und Chef der Reichskanzlei Dr. Hans Heinrich Lammers mit Entwurf eines Gesetzes über die Behandlung Gemeinschaftsfremder mit Begründung" (Berlin, 24 June 1941) in *'Gemeinschaftsfremde': Quellen zur Verfolgung von 'Asozialen', 1933-1945*, No. 114, ed. Wolfgang Ayass (Koblenz: Bundesarchiv, 1998).

515 "Entwurf des Ministerialrats im Reichsjustizministerium Otto Rietzsch für ein Gesetz über die Behandlung Asozialer" (Berlin, 1 February 1943) in *'Gemeinschaftsfremde'* No. 140.

offenses earned a far more lenient response from the authorities. Criminals operating under the influence of drugs were not considered criminally liable for their actions because of the diminished responsibility clause, the centuries old German legal concept that survived the Nazis' rise to power.

Possessing drugs unlawfully acquired through falsifying or stealing prescriptions was indeed prosecuted as a misdemeanor, but rarely to the full extent of the law. In 1934, the year with the highest number of drug convictions in the Third Reich, less than one-fifth of those convicted served a jail sentence of more than six months.[516] Instead of serving time in jail, offenders were often sent to a sanatorium for rehabilitation; in some cases, a fine sufficed.

The sanatoria in the Third Reich were hardly pleasant places. At some of these institutions, people were exterminated and children starved to death. But it is yet to be proven that drug addicts were ever purposefully sent to killing wards because of their addiction, and without question the treatment drug addicts received at such institutions was a far cry from the fate they would have suffered in prison, let alone in a concentration camp.

Drug addicts sent to treatment in a sanatorium were first given 24 hours to settle their affairs. Upon commitment they were sequestered in a closed ward, where they were forced to quit their habit cold turkey. After being clean for a week or two, they were released to the general population of the institution.[517] "The withdrawal process actually takes only five to ten days, but then follows a period of one to two months when the patient loses his habit," the Reich Central Office for Combating Drug Transgression explained in 1938. "During this time the body of the patient is still weak, inefficient and resistant to treatment. It is strengthened via a good diet [as well as] with physical and mental therapy."[518]

By law, incarceration in a sanatorium could be extended indefinitely, pending judgment by the physician in charge.[519] However, most sanatoria released their patients after a six-month treatment, if not earlier. The

---

516 62 out of 338 persons. See Holzer, *Die Geburt der Drogenpolitik aus dem Geist der Rassenhygiene*, 182.

517 "Summary of the Stettin Conference, 10 October 1937," StA. München, Pol. Dir. 7582.

518 "Information pamphlet of the *Reichszentrale zur Bekämpfung von Rauschgift-vergehen*, 1 July 1938 StA. München," Pol. Dir. 7582.

519 An exception was carved out for rehabilitation institutes (*"Entziehungsanstalt"*), where incarceration was limited to two years.

average weight of a patient increased between 15 to 20 kilograms when undergoing treatment.[520] The authorities boasted a success rate of nearly 75 percent,[521] but the veracity of the claim is impossible to verify, and is most likely false.

After release from a sanatorium, a patient was required to undergo periodical checkups coordinated by the local state attorney. If, during such checkups, a physician determined that there was a justified need to prescribe narcotics, special permission had to be obtained from the Health Office. The police had a name index of all patients released from sanatoria, and provided the information on demand to the local advisory posts of the Health Office that handled these cases. If a patient relapsed, the state attorney was to be informed, since that office had also the authority to return an addict to a sanatorium without trial. Regulations at the state attorney's office stipulated that tracking of a patient cease 15 years after the last visit to a sanitarium, though in practice tracking was stopped much earlier.

In most cases, depending on the judicial writ, German health insurance companies covered the hospitalization of drug addicts in sanatoria. The prices of the sanatoria were not particularly steep, and even when patients had to pay for their own hospitalization, it was affordable. The Eglfing-Haar sanatorium in Bavaria, for example, charged just 3 Reichsmarks a day for its rehabilitation program.[522] Given that state-assured health insurance companies recognized drug rehabilitation as coverable treatment, it is reasonable to conclude that the authorities acknowledged drug addiction to be a treatable disease, rather than a criminal behavior.

Eglfing-Haar's low daily fee for drug addicts stands in stark contrast to the more sinister policies carried out in other wards at the sanatorium. It was used as a collection point for the euthanasia program known as "T-4," after the program's headquarters at Tiergartenstraße 4 in Berlin. By the end of the first stage of the program in 1941, over 70,000 patients had been killed, and some more are believed to have been killed during the ensuing four years.[523] From the beginning of 1940, Eglfing-Haar had also

---

520 "Information pamphlet of the *Reichszentrale zur Bekämpfung von Rauschgift-vergehen*, 1 July 1938 StA. München," Pol. Dir. 7582.
521 Ibid.
522 StA. München, Staanwa. No. 17584.
523 Robert Proctor, *Racial Hygiene: Medicine under the Nazis* (Cambridge MA: Harvard University Press, 1988), 177.

a killing ward for "biologically deficient" children. Separated off from the rest of the institution, they were starved to death.[524] Drug addicts at Eglfing-Haar, however, suffered little of the horrific treatment meted out to others at the very same sanatorium.

Indeed, of the 70,000 victims of the T-4 program between 1939 and 1941, only eight are believed to have been drug addicts – and only one of the eight appeared to have been euthanized because of her drug addiction, but the exact details of her case are lost.[525] In light of the atrocities committed on a massive scale by the T-4 program, the relative insignificant number of drug addicts who may have suffered is telling. And yet, a closer look at some of these cases might shed a light on how addiction was viewed in the Third Reich, and explain the fine line between state sanctioned murder, murder for personal gain, and treatment.

Among the eight drug addicts killed through the T-4 program was pharmacist Wilhelm Ballast, who was committed to the Eichberg sanatorium for drug addiction in 1941. At Eichberg, the director of the children's ward, Dr. Walter Schmidt (1910-1970), employed Ballast as a pharmacist and relations between the two were friendly. "But since Ballast was able to obtain drugs," as a recent account put it, "his addiction continued, and he eventually contracted tuberculosis. Postwar investigators concluded that Schmidt killed him with an injection because 'his drug addiction had become inconvenient, and his behavior had become tiresome.'"[526] Ballast was killed because of his drug addiction, but less because it revealed a biological defect, and more because it had become an unwelcome nuisance to Schmidt.

Similar to Eglfing-Haar, Eichberg served as a transit point to the dreaded Hadamar sanatorium as part of the T-4's attempt to mask the euthanasia program from the German public. It was also the location of an experimental children euthanasia program. In 1941 several hundred children were killed under the supervision of Schmidt. In 1953, the Hessian minister-president reprieved Schmidt of his actions against children, but he was later convicted of murdering Ballast.[527] One crime – committed

---

524 Friedlander, *The Origins of Nazi Genocide*, 49-51; 167.
525 Holzer, *Die Geburt der Drogenpolitik aus dem Geist der Rassenhygiene*, 258-264.
526 Friedlander, *The Origins of Nazi Genocide*, 184-185.
527 Ibid., 108-109, 156-157.

against children – was pardoned; the other – committed against a drug addict – was not.

Another of the eight drug addicts killed through the T-4 program was the dentist Hermann Wirsing, who was sent to the hospital in Waldheim, Saxony. Unlike Ballast, Wirsing met his fate shortly after entering the sanatorium. He arrived on April 15, 1940, and was sent to his death the very next day.[528] The director of the Waldheim sanatorium reported Wirsing's case as follows:

> The dentist Hermannn Wirsing (born 16/8/83) was sent here from Dresden jail on 15/4/40 according to article 42b of the penal code; he was transferred out again the following day (on 16/4/40) with a collective transport of patients of the Charitable Patient Transport Corporation. He is a psychopath and a chronic morphine addict. His relatives have inquired a great many times by letter or telephone about his transfer and his present whereabouts.[529]

Although the director's report highlights Wirsing's morphine addiction, it is hardly conclusive that he was murdered because of his addiction. Indeed, it is far more likely that he was sent to his death because he had been deemed a psychopath.

As either a psychopath or a morphine addict, Wirsing would have been immune from criminal proceedings. And with either condition, he would have been a candidate for transfer to an asylum, in line with Nazi amendment to Article 42b of the penal code. Yet there is one point on which the two conditions diverge: There are numerous examples of mental patients and psychopaths killed by T-4, but barely any of morphine addicts, making it unlikely that Wirsing was killed because of his addiction. The Nazis cast a wide net to catch those who lived "lives unworthy of living," in an attempt to purify the race. The fate of those who were caught in the net was uncertain, regardless of the reason why they were in it.

Of the six other known instances of drug addicts killed through the T-4 program, little is known about five, save for the place of death, the Hadamar sanatorium.[530] The final victim, Frieda S., is the only victim of

---

528 Friedlander, *The Origins of the Nazi Genocide*, 173.
529 "Director of the Asylum Waldheim to the Minister of Interior of Saxony," (Waldheim, 2 August 1940), in *Nuremberg Trials*, doc. PS-624.
530 Rainer Scheer, "Die nach Paragraph 42 RStGB verurteilten Menschen in Hadamar," in Dorothe Roer and Dieter Henkek (eds.), *Psychiatrie im Faschismus: Die Anstalt Hadamar, 1933-1945* (Bonn: Psychiatrie-Verlag, 1986), 247.

T-4 confirmed to have been killed because of her drug addiction. Frieda S. was sent to Wittenau in 1937 for morphine addiction, and soon thereafter transferred to Wuhlgarten. She was released from the institution, but relapsed and was sent back to Wuhlgarten. From there, she was sent to her death.[531]

From the 1930s to 1945, there were no less than 683 cases against drug addicts in Berlin, out of which 392 were not prosecuted; 202 were sent to sanatoria; 20 were Jews who were either sent to sanatoria or concentration camps; five Aryans were sent to concentration camps, and the rest were foreign nationals who were either released or sent to sanatoria.[532] There are no typical cases of Aryans sent to concentration camps. Yet, the file on Paul Thormann allows a glimpse into the erratic ways of Nazi Germany as well as personal bad luck, and an unsupportive family. Thormann was a manual laborer from Berlin who led a normal life on paper: a war veteran, a husband and a father of two daughters. In 1926, he underwent a gall-stone removal operation. For his pain, doctors gave him morphine. By next year, it became clear that he developed a habit, which he tried to quit unsuccessfully.

In 1934, Thormann went to a private clinic for treatment, but without a lasting success. The following year, he was caught falsifying prescriptions and was forcibly sent to the Wittenau sanatorium in Berlin. He was released in 1937 under the supervision of the local health office. Every six months, professor Victor Müller-Heß (1883-1960) of the forensic and social medicine department at the university of Berlin checked him. Although traces of opiates were found in his urine in the four years that followed, the state attorney was satisfied with Thormann's claim of legitimate use of opiates, and decided against a commitment in a sanatorium, overruling Müller-Heß' recommendation.

On 16 February 1940, Thormann was sent to Wittenau after he was caught using aliases to obtain pantopon prescriptions. He stayed in the sanatorium until April 1941. Upon his release he was tested on a monthly basis. After failing five urine tests, the state attorney was convinced that a third commitment was necessary, and Thormann was sent to Wittenau in February 1942, where he stayed for two years.

---

531 Holzer, *Die Geburt der Drogenpolitik aus dem Geist der Rassenhygiene*, 262.
532 Crime Registry of the State Attorney of Berlin, USHMM, RG 14.070M. The registry mislabeled four cases erroneously marking them as victims of euthanasia, when in fact their files were simply lost.

Following a routine police inquiry in March 1943, the state attorney reopened Thormann's case, raising the possibility that his repeated offenses could be a sign of anti social behavior, rather than addiction. If the former were the case, medical treatment would prove useless and instead he should be sent to an 'improvement and education camp' (*Besserungs- und Erziehungslager.*) To determine the true character of the patient, the state attorney's office requested expert testimonies.

On 7 October 1943, the director of Wittenau had reported that unless other preventative measures are taken, Thormann could not be released from hospital, because he is not yet cured. Twenty days later, Müller-Heß had written a thorough psychological report on Thormann detailing his past problems with drugs. Müller-Heß emphasized that despite two spells in sanatoria, Thormann relapsed. Moreover, and perhaps more importantly, by occupying a hospital bed, he kept wounded soldiers from treatment. Therefore, Müller-Heß concluded that Thormann was indeed a psychopath who could not stop his craving. As a psychopath, Thorman did not require medical attention; instead he should be sent to an improvement and education camp so he could be isolated from the rest of the Volk. The length of stay in the camp had to be determined at a later date.

One of Thormann's daughters wrote a letter to the police in December 1943 in which she described her father as a man who had never worked an honest job in his life, stealing her mother's jewelry to satisfy his life of crime, which eventually culminated in their divorce in 1938. She also mentioned the fact that she could no longer pay for her father's treatments. For four months, the state attorney remained passive until another police inquiry was sent on 9 March 1944, asking whether a decision in this case was reached. A day later, the attorney signed an order to transfer Thormann to Sachsenhausen concentration camp with an indefinite release date. At this point, the paper trail ends. It is not known whether Thormann survived the war.[533]

Thormann's case betrays the distinction the authorities made between anti-social and psychopathic behavior, deemed incurable; and addiction, which required medical attention. Several factors were detrimental to his fate. The first was the criminal police's inquiries, while he was committed in a hospital. His long stay, and his daughter's testimony that he often

---

533 USHMM, RG 14.070M, reel 3074, fr. 1265-1334; reel 3075, fr. 1-185; reel 3076, fr. 1046-1349; reel 3077, fr. 1-169.

stole and never worked only helped creating his anti-social image; and in Nazi Germany, the fate of anti-socials was often incarceration in a concentration camp.

In Thormann's case, the concentration camp served as an *oubliette* for a man who simply took up space. As dreadful as the outcome might be, however, his case is an extreme exception to the rule. He, and the other four who were sent to concentration camps for addiction like him, represent less than one percent of the drug cases in Berlin. Instead, most drug addicts were treated with kid gloves with high survival rates in hospitals.

The Third Reich's soft approach to drug addiction is further evidenced by the treatment meted out to those of otherwise impeccable Aryan stock. Three examples offer a telling illustration of how addicts were viewed by, respectively, the Nazi leadership, party functionaries and local officials. The first involves the highest-ranking Nazi known to be a drug addict, Reichsmarschall Hermann Göring, the senior military officer in the Third Reich and Hitler's chosen successor. Göring was wounded in the failed Nazi coup in Munich in December 1923. After being smuggled out of Germany to the Austrian city of Innsbruck, he underwent an operation for which he was treated with morphine. He remained an addict ever since. In September 1925 he was hospitalized at the Langbro mental asylum in Sweden, where he ended up in the violent ward in a straightjacket after attacking a nurse for refusing to give him morphine. He was first released after three months, but soon relapsed and was voluntarily hospitalized. A few months later he was officially rehabilitated and released.[534]

After the Nazi takeover of power, Göring procured his record from Langbro and had it destroyed. But he could not entirely erase his past, as word of his addiction leaked out in the 1930s, including to members of the foreign diplomatic corps.[535] Over the course of the decade Göring underwent annual treatment by Hubert Kahle (1878-?), whose method of detoxification was to calm the nervous system by the administration of sleeping pills when withdrawal symptoms appeared. Göring underwent the treat-

---

534 Roger Manvell and Heinrich Fraenkel, *Herman Göring* (London: New English Library, 1962), 38, 42-43, 385; Blaine Taylor, "Hermann Goering and Josef Goebbels: Their Medical Casefiles (Part 1)," *Maryland State Medical Journal* 25:11 (1976), 35-47.

535 Manvell and Fraenkel, *Herman Göring*, 142.

ment either in Kahle's clinic in Cologne or at his mansion, where he later installed a sauna that was supposed to help him sweat out the drugs.[536]

Recent scholarship has called into question Göring's addiction, arguing that claims of his dependency on morphine are overblown:

> It has been widely rumored that [Göring] had become a drug addict. Such rumours were exaggerated. His addiction was not to narcotics but to the habit of taking pills. His physicians provided him with large numbers of harmless coloured pills, each containing a small quantity of paracodeine. The hundred pills consumed each day contained not much more than a number of aspirin tablets. The doctors who treated him after his capture at the end of the war found no difficulty in ridding him of the habit. He took pills at meetings and in interviews as other people might smoke.[537]

Whether the pills Göring consumed all day were indeed harmless, however, remains open to question. Paracodeine is unquestionably a narcotic, as it is a synthetic derivative of codeine – one of the many alkaloids found in opium. And despite attempts to suggest otherwise, Göring was quite dependent on the pills, which were first synthesized and marketed in Germany in 1911 as an analgesic and cough suppressant.

Colonel Burton Andrus, the American commandant of the Luxembourg interrogation center where Göring and other war criminals were held before being transferred to Nuremberg, reported that no less than 20,000 pills of paracodeine were found in Göring's suitcase. "He has been in the habit of taking 20 pills per dose, two doses a day,"[538] Andrus stated. Furthermore, Hitler's personal physician, Karl Brandt (1904-1948), informed his American captors that Göring consumed 20 times the normal daily dose of the drug.[539]

As for the assertion that the Reichsmarschall's doctors were easily able to cure him of his addiction, a closer examination of Göring's postwar incarceration paints a more nuanced picture. Douglas M. Kelley (1912-1958), the American psychiatrist attending Nazi war criminals during their stay first in the Luxembourg interrogation center known as "Ashcan" and afterward in Nuremberg, claimed to have rid Göring of his

---

536 Ibid., 143.

537 Richard Overy, *Goering* (London: Phoenix Press, 2000), 20.

538 Burton C. Andrus, *The Infamous of Nuremberg* (London: Frewin, 1969), 30, 48; Airey Neave, *Nuremberg: A Personal Record of the Trial of the Major Nazi War Criminals in 1945-6* (London: Hodder and Stoughton, 1978), 69; Gustave M. Gilbert, *Nuremberg Diary* (New York: Farrar, Straus, 1961 [1947]), 17.

539 Manvell and Fraenkel, *Herman Göring*, 315.

habit.[540] Göring's addiction, however, may have been more enduring than the American psychiatrist wished to admit. Given the breadth of Göring's crimes, Kelley had a near obligation to declare Göring healthy, a reflection of the American justice system and its requirement that the condemned must be of sound body and mind before being sentenced to death. If Göring had indeed been found to be a morphine junkie, it would have been far more difficult to paint him at the Nuremberg Trials as an arch-villain guilty of mass murder.

In fact, it is questionable whether Göring was cured at all. Gustave Gilbert (1911-1977), an American psychologist and interpreter who interviewed the Nazi leadership during the Nuremberg Trials, and Leon Goldensohn (1911-1961), Kelley's successor in Nuremberg, suspected that "although [Göring] has been deprived of drugs, his drug addiction is far from cured and he is still a basically weak character resorting to other means of frustration-evasion and ego-protecting."[541]

Göring's addiction was known to the party elite. Gilbert's notes from a talk with Göring in his cell on the evening of April 18, 1946 attest to the fact. While complaining to Gilbert about the direction in which the trial was heading, Göring claimed that had he known of the atrocities in the East, he would have confronted Hitler. In his notes, Gilbert added: "I still did not have the desire at this point to tell him what Ohlendorf[542] had said to this: that Göring had been written off as an effective 'moderating' influence, because of his drug addiction and corruption."[543] Confirmation that Göring's influence with Hitler was on the decline because of his addiction also comes from the testimony of Rudolf Semmler (1913-?), an aide to Joseph Goebbels (1897-1945). Semmler stated that he overheard Theodor Morell (1886-1946), Hitler's personal physician, tell Goebbels' wife that "Göring was becoming more and more a slave to the habit, and that even his doctors were powerless to stop him."[544]

Despite being an open secret, Göring's drug addiction did not prevent him from maintaining a position of enormous power. In fact, his fall from grace was far more likely due to his incompetence on the battlefield, and

---

540 Douglas M. Kelley, *22 Cells in Nuremberg* (New York: Greenberg, 1947), 57-58.
541 Gilbert, *Nuremberg Diary*, 326.
542 *SS-Gruppenführer* Otto Ohlendorf (1907-1951) was the commander of *Einsatzgruppe* D and the Inland SD.
543 Gilbert, *Nuremberg Diary*, 255.
544 Manvell & Fraenkel, *Herman Göring*, 260.

not, as Ohlendorf asserted, because of his drug habit. Hitler lost confidence in Göring because of a series of strategic losses, including the blunder at Dunkirk, defeat in the Battle of Britain and at Stalingrad, and the incessant air raids over Germany.[545]

As the second in command in the Third Reich and anointed successor to Hitler, Göring clearly enjoyed a phenomenal amount of power that provided protection from the fate suffered by ordinary German drug addicts. Yet the same soft approach to drug addiction is evident in examples of officials lower down the Nazi ladder. One such example is Enno Lolling (1888-1945), a former staff doctor in the Imperial Navy and a practicing physician in Neustrelitz, Mecklenburg.

Lolling's drug addiction was made clear in a letter from the physicians association in Mecklenburg to the chief physician of the SS, presumably in response to an inquiry into Lolling's character during a purge of SS members in 1936:[546]

> With reference to your query of 20 June 1936 we inform you that there is nothing objectionable against Herr Lolling MD, practicing physician at Neustrelitz-Strelitz [regarding his] professional, moral, collegial [behavior] or political worldview.
> Yet we wish to note that Herr Dr. L. was a morphine addict[547] and required repeated rehabilitation. We are obliged to report this to you without being able to produce documentation. Consequently, we are requesting from you to treat the matter with extreme discretion and perhaps, if you think it necessary, ask Herr Dr. L. directly whether he is an addict.[548]

The chief physician of the SS, taking up the suggestion to contact Lolling directly, sent the Mecklenburg doctor the following query: "I ask you for your word of honor as an SS man, whether you were a morphine addict or were addicted in any other way or [whether you] are [still addicted]. I await your honorable explanation by 30 July 1936."[549] On that date, Lolling replied: "I hereby hand over the insurance affidavit and declare on my word of honor as an SS [officer] that I have not taken morphine in any

545 Ian Kershaw, *Hitler, 1936-45: Nemesis* (London: Longman, 2000), 296, 535, 620-621, 644-645,.

546 Heinz Höhne, *The Order of the Death Heads* (London: Pan, 1969), 130.

547 In German: "*morphinsüchtig*"

548 "Physician Chamber Mecklenburg-Lübeck to Reichsführer SS-the Reich Physician of the SS, (Rostock, 21.7.36)," BArch. SSO Enno Lolling 19 July 1888.

549 "The Reich Physician of the SS to SS-Scharführer Dr. Lolling, (Berlin, 27 July 1936)," BArch. SSO Enno Lolling 19 July 1888.

form since 1932 and have been completely free ever since and suffered no aftereffects. Further addictions were and are not present."[550]

An addict's word of honor, no more, was enough to clear him from further investigation. Whether Lolling indeed remained clean is uncertain, particularly given that one of his colleagues later described him as a "heavy drinker."[551] What is clear is that Lolling's career was unaffected by his addiction. He became a physician in Dachau soon after his correspondence with the chief physician of the SS, and was later promoted to chief physician at Sachsenhausen. He eventually rose to become chief physician at the Concentration Camps Inspectorate, putting him in charge of all doctors and medical staff at all SS concentration camps.

Such soft treatment of drug addicts was hardly limited to SS members. In the Third Reich addiction was viewed as a disease like any other, and once it had been treated, the patient was usually declared healthy and allowed to resume work. The example of Dr. W. Horn of Bad Kissingen is illustrative. The authorities identified Horn as an opiate addict in 1942, when he was convicted in court of falsifying prescriptions. He was fined 500 Reichsmarks, likely no more than one-third of his monthly income, and then submitted to treatment in a privately-owned sanatorium in Bayreuth. Following treatment, Horn, like many addicts, relapsed. The local Health Office in Munich discovered that he had started taking opiates again, and informed the local police. An investigation revealed that had had written falsified prescriptions for his patients in order to supply himself with opiates.

Horn admitted his guilt to the police, and was subsequently convicted of breaking the Opium Law. The court fined the doctor 6,000 Reichsmarks and ordered him to pay for the costs of the trial, which amounted to 642.20 Reichsmarks. But beyond the financial penalty, Horn was neither hospitalized nor sent to jail.[552] And throughout the proceedings against him, Horn's medical license was never revoked. Indeed, he continued to practice as a physician well after the war's end.

The example of Dr. W. Horn is perhaps the most illustrative of the three, in that it points to an important influence on drug policy during the

---

550 "Dr. Enno Lolling to The Reich Physician of the SS, (Neustrelitz-Strelitz, 30 July 1936)," BArch. SSO Enno Lolling 19 July 1888.

551 Robert Jay Lifton, *The Nazi Doctors: Medical Killing and the Psychology of Genocide* (New York: Basic Books, 1986), 198.

552 StA. München, Staanwa. Nr. 17670.

Third Reich: addicts generally came from the higher classes of German society. Physicians in particular were known to be susceptible to drug addiction, given their easy access to drugs. Rather than antagonize the politically important medical community, successive German governments attempted to gain the cooperation of physicians and pharmacists in the effort to control drug use.[553] Widely acknowledged drug addiction among another politically important constituency, veterans of World War I, also contributed to the authorities' gloved approach to drug control.

But given the overriding Nazi preoccupation with racial purity, the single most plausible explanation for why drug addicts were generally spared in the Third Reich is that drug addiction was not considered to be hereditary. Being non-hereditary, it presented no danger to the master race, and the potential for a cure remained no matter how many times a patient relapsed.

Under a regime that went down in history as the most inhumane of all time, extremely few individuals have been deported to a concentration camp due to drug addiction, even those addicts who repeatedly violated the prescription laws. Furthermore, among the more than 350,000 victims of the Nazis' decade-long program of forced sterilization, not a single one is known to have been selected because of drug addiction.

Drug addiction itself was never considered a crime, nor was it grounds for forced treatment without a court order. Nor, for that matter, was drug use a known problem in German prisons, even those not operated by the iron-fisted SS. The law against habitual criminals did allow judges to order addicts into forced hospitalization, but the sentence was not meant, at least *de jure*, as a castigatory measure. And unlike with cases of severe alcoholism, physicians were not required to report cases of drug addiction to hereditary courts.[554]

While a multitude of factors shaped the Third Reich's atypically lenient handling of drug addicts, the underlying explanation surely lies in the long-held German view of drug addiction as a disease to which all are

---

553 A. Linz, "Behördliche Durchführung des Opiumgesetzes: Ziele und Ergebnisse" in Gerhart Feuerstein (ed.), *Suchtgiftbekämpfung* (Berlin, 1944), 24-32; "Summary of the Stettin Conference, 10 October 1937" StA. München, Pol. Dir. 7582; Erwin Kosmehl, *Der sicherheitspolizeiliche Einsatz bei der Bekämpfung der Betäubungsmittelsucht*, Barch. RD 19/30.

554 Andreas-Holger Maehle, *Doctors, Honour and the Law: Medical Ethics in Imperial Germany* (New York: Palgrave Macmillan, 2009), 47-68.

susceptible. For more than half a century, since Eduard Levinstein put his stamp on German drug treatment in the 1870s, it had been accepted wisdom that any individual who used drugs could fall prey to addiction, irrespective of class, state of mind or strength of will.

In contrast to the United States, where debate raged well into the 20th century over whether addiction was a crime or a disease, Germany had long since defined the parameters of drug addiction. It was not perceived to be criminal in nature, but rather a treatable mental disease, or a physical disease akin to influenza or tuberculosis. It was deemed to be both treatable and reversible, and most importantly, declared to be non-hereditary. Drug addiction, quite simply, was not viewed as a biological disease in need of eradication. In the cold calculus of the Third Reich, that was enough to spare drug addicts the horrific fate suffered by countless others.

Part II

7. Meat vs. Rice

After the Opium Wars, many poor Chinese emigrated in search of income. They left first for Southeast Asia, then on to Australia and the United States. Some went as free laborers, but most made the journey as indentured slaves, or coolies as they were colloquially known.[555] Where the Chinese went, opium soon followed.[556] Thus opium smoking became a bad habit by association with Chinese.[557] Even before coolies were brought across the Pacific in droves to build the transcontinental railroad and mine Californian gold in the 1860s and 1870s,[558] opium smoking and the Chinamen were associated with one another in America. Stories were told time and again of the decadent Oriental lying on a straw mat smoking his opium pipe, a caricature dating back to English Romanticism.[559]

"Liquor drinking is a new vice among the Chinese and though they have not attained a position that will compare with Anglo-Saxons, either in drinking or profanity, yet they have shown themselves to be apt scholars in drinking, as any one can see who will count the bottles disposed of at one of their funerals," an anonymous reader of the *New-York Daily Times*

---

555 William C. Hunter, *The 'Fan Kwae' at Canton* (Taipei: Ch'eng-wen Pub. Co, 1965 [1882]), 62.

556 Martin Booth, *Opium: A History* (New York: St. Martin's Press, 1998), 175-180.

557 John C. Burnham, *Bad Habits: Drinking, smoking, Taking Drugs, Gambling, Sexual Misbehavior, and Swearing in American History* (New York: New York University Press, 1993), 1-22.

558 See, for example, the treaty that allowed the immigration of Chinese to the United States and vice versa: "The Burlingame Treaty, 1868" in *The Search for Modern China: A Documentary Collection*, ed. Pei-kai Cheng, Michael Lestz and Jonathan Spence (New York: Norton, 1999), 163-164.

559 Gustave Doré and Blanchard Jerrold, *London, a Pilgrimage* (New York: B. Blom, 1970 [1872]), 147-148; Terry Parssinen, *Secret Passions, Secret Remedies: Narcotic Drugs in British Society, 1820-1930* (Philadelphia: Institute for the Study of Human Issues, 1983), 61; Meyer Howard Abrams, *The Milk of Paradise: The Effect of Opium Visions on the Works of De Quincey, Crabbe, Francis Thompson and Coleridge* (Cambridge, MA: Harvard University Press, 1934); Alethea Hayter, *Opium and the Romantic Imagination* (London: Faber, 1968), 13, 331-341; Marcus Boon, *The Road of Excess: A History of Writers on Drugs* (Cambridge MA: Harvard University Press, 2002).

wrote in a letter to the editor in 1852. "But if they come short in liquor drinking, they make up the deficiency in the free use of opium."[560]

Stories also migrated north from Panama, where legions of Chinese laborers worked on the Panama railroad during the 1850s. "Last Sunday great numbers of these Chinese came into town, and in every street might be seen some of them with partially filled bottles of bad liquors, slung by a handkerchief to a pole they carried on their shoulders, gazing at the women who were passing to and from church, or leering at them with their big, half-drunken moose-eyes, while others were buying or piteously begging for opium at the bar-rooms and apothecaries' shops," read one 1854 report in the *New-York Daily Times*.[561] Panama was depicted as a depraved and unwholesome environment where alcohol, opium and leering heathen Chinese sinfully mixed. It was that reputation which preceded the wave of Chinese immigrants that began reaching American shores in the mid-1850s.

In 1853, there were but a handful of Chinese in San Francisco. By 1855, 3,000-4,000 Chinese had already settled in the city, and their numbers continued to swell, driven by increasing demand for cheap labor. Exact population estimates are somewhat difficult to ascertain, as the figures reported at the time often varied by political bent. One anti-Chinese politician declared that 75,000 Chinese settled in San Francisco alone, while an official federal census put the number of Chinese in the entire United States at 105,448 in 1876.[562]

As the number of Chinese working in the mines and on the railroads of California, Oregon and Washington rose, anti-Oriental movements sprang up among white laborers, spreading hatred and fear of the coolie. Anti-Chinese sentiments were prevalent even before the economic depression of 1873, as a result of the growth of the mining economy in the West in the late 1860s. It was believed that once the cheap Chinese laborers were free from mining and railroad construction, they would spread across the

---

560 "Gov. Bigler and the Chinamen," *New-York Daily Times* (21 June 1852), 2.
561 "From the Isthmus," *New-York Daily Times* (27 April 1854), 2.
562 Robert McClellan, *The Heathen Chinee: A Study of American Attitudes toward China, 1890 - 1905* (Columbus OH: Ohio State University Press, 1971), 5. Another estimate established that there were 104,731 Chinese in the United States in 1876. See H. H. Kane, *Opium-Smoking in America and China: A Study of Its Prevalence, and Effects, Immediate and Remote, on Individual and the Nation* (New York, 1882), 17-18.

country and take over the labor force like locust. Legislation targeting Chinese immigrants was abundant in California, including, among other measures, a special tax imposed on the "Mongolian race."[563]

The Panic of 1873 left the United States with the gold standard, deflation and a six-year stretch of high unemployment.[564] Labor unions, which had enjoyed a period of growth after the Civil War, crumbled as membership declined, and many laborers had trouble finding year-round employment. As jobs became scarcer but more profitable, Chinese coolies presented a clear threat to the white American worker.[565] As it were, white workers already feared competition from freed black slaves, even though the newly emancipated black workers were heavily concentrated in the former Confederate states.

A range of trade unions, even those with a socialist bent, voiced criticism of Chinese workers. Methods ranged from calling for a boycott of Chinese-made cigars in 1874 and other Chinese products in the early 1880s, to expelling the coolie by force out of white men's professions in 1885.[566]

The Chinese menace seemed so clear and present a danger that even those with no interaction whatsoever with Chinese workers still felt the need to guard against the yellow peril. An 1887 report from the Colorado Bureau of Labor tells of a miner from Lake County who expressed his desire for the imposition of laws against coolies, lest they take away his job – even though not a single Chinese person lived in Lake County five years before or after the statement was made.[567]

Self proclaimed drug experts, aided by a rabble-rousing press, played a major role in linking opium and Orientals. Harry Hubbell Kane (1854-?), a

---

563 "An Act to Protect Free White Labor against Competition with Chinese Coolie labor, and to Discourage the Immigration of the Chinese into the State of California," (26 April 1862) at: http://www.druglibrary.org/schaffer/History/1870/anticoolieact.htm.

564 Kathleen Auerhahn, "The Split Labor Market and the Origins of Antidrug Legislation in the United States" *Law & Social Inquiry* 24:2 (1999), 417.

565 Philip S. Foner, *History of the Labor Movement in the United States: From Colonial Times to the Foundation of the American Federation of Labor*, Vol. 1, (New York: International Publishers, 1975), 439-440.

566 Auerhahn, "The Split Labor Market and the Origins of Antidrug Legislation in the United States," 419.

567 McClellan, *The Heathen Chinese*, 8-10; Herbert Hill, "Anti-Oriental Agitation and the rise of Working-Class Racism," *Society* 10:2 (1973), 43-54.

prolific expert and a proprietor of a clinic treating habitués in New York, spent much of the 1880s and 1890s associating the Chinese with opium imports into the United States. Kane claimed that the smoking of opium had been virtually unknown in America before the arrival of the Chinese, and that the habit threatened to spread faster and with less excuse than medicinal opium.[568]

Alonzo Calkins (1804–1878), another American drug expert, reported as early as 1867 that there were about 60,000 Chinese coolies along America's Pacific coast, most of them adult males. In that same year, nearly 23 tons of smoking opium was imported to cater the growing American market, at an estimated value of $374,000. And those figures, Calkins warned, undercounted the real amount, as they did not take into account illegal smuggling.

While estimating the smuggled opium entering the United States, Calkins betrayed his own biases:

> An addition to the custom-house entries of ten per-cent, to be credited to smuggling, would be a good deal within the mark unquestionably; for every month about there is a fresh immigration of Coolies into San Francisco, who invent all sorts of ingenious contrivances to get within the gate of their El Dorado, without challenge from scrutinizing tide-waiters.[569]

In rather archaic terms, Calkins made clear that the opium appetite had prompted illegal smuggling into the United States in the 1860s, just as it had prompted illegal smuggling into China two decades earlier. Reports of smuggling soon reached the American public. Calkins, Kane and other drug experts were aided in their campaign by a sympathetic press, which

---

568 Diana Ahmad, *The Opium Debate and Chinese Exclusion Laws in the Nineteenth-Century American West* (Reno: University of Nevada Press, 2007), 15, citing H. H. Kane, "Opium Smoking - A New Form of the Opium Habit amongst Americans *Gaillard's Medical Journal*, vol. 32/2 (Feb. 1882), 103. Kane pointed out that Chinese had indeed brought opium smoking with them to the New World, but by the time of his study in 1882, the vice was taken up by Whites. His conclusions, though might sound racist to a modern ear, were certainly not for a contemporary and should be considered as progressive.

569 Alonzo Calkins, *Opium and the Opium Appetite: With Notices of Alcoholic Beverages, Cannabis Indica, Tobacco and Coca, and Tea and Coffee, in their Hygienic Aspects and Pathologic Relations* (Philadelphia, 1871), 38. For an attempt to determine the amount of smuggled opium by the tabulation of the number of users, see Kane, *Opium-Smoking in America and China*, 19-20. The calculation resulted in 7,999 pounds of opium or less being smuggled in 1880. The veracity of this report remains debatable.

drew the public's attention to the issues of race, opium and illegal smuggling.

"The Custom-house authorities at San Francisco discovered a very ingenious Chinese trick, which led to the seizure of another lot of smuggled opium," *The New York Times* reported in 1864, under the headline "A Chinese Trick." It read: "Among the cargo of the bark *Ceres* were 400 tubs, invoiced as eggs, value stated at $1 each. The eggs were coated with a peculiar kind of varnish to preserve them. One of the officers, in examining the eggs, scraped off a little varnish and disclosed a metallic case, egg-shaped, filled with opium. Each metallic egg is worth $300. So far as the examination had proceeded, five hundred have been found."[570]

Chinese immigrants and their opium pipes were considered to be a threat to the law of the land. Import tariffs had been imposed on opium as far back as 1842; but the drug was permitted into the country. In order to restore law and order and eradicate the drug smuggling once and for all, many Californians argued, America had to get rid of those who had brought opium to America's shores in the first place.[571] Drugs were not yet an evil to be reckoned with, but the Chinese coolies most certainly were.

In the 1870s America reckoned with its growing Chinese population by enacting a range of laws against the immigrant laborers. Whether it was a desire to ban opium that led to anti-Chinese legislation being passed in America, or whether it was a general antagonism toward Chinese immigrants that led to the condemnation of the drug habit with which they were inextricably linked, the belief at the time was that by eliminating immigration from China, America could eliminate the opium trade.[572]

In March 1875, Congress passed the Page Act, which, by requiring that immigration into the United States be free and voluntary, legally closed America's doors to Chinese coolies and prostitutes. Eight months later, the City of San Francisco enacted the Opium Den Ordinance, making it a misdemeanor to be a proprietor or a patron of an opium den.

The Page Act led to a substantial decrease in the number of Chinese women who were brought into America for sex, while the Opium Den

---

570 "A Chinese Trick," *New York Times* (20 July 1864), 2.
571 Charles E. Terry and Mildred Pellens, *The Opium Problem* (New York, 1928), 745-747.
572 Ahmad, *The Opium Debate and Chinese Exclusion Laws in the Nineteenth-Century American West*, 74-76.

Ordinance criminalized the use and provision of the drug. The legal crackdown on opium smoking and prostitution – the two activities that brought solace to the lone, male Chinese worker – had one goal in mind: to drive the Chinese out of the United States.[573]

The association of opium with sex was hardly an American construction. In 15th- and 16th-century China, opium was used as an aphrodisiac and luxury commodity for the rulers of the empire. Over time, opium use in China evolved. With the introduction of the practice of smoking opium, consumption of the drug spread across the empire. The emperor himself switched from eating opium to smoking it, and the practice percolated down the social strata. By the end of the 19th century, opium smoking had reached the lowly coolie, whose existence was no better than that of a beast of burden.[574]

Despite the continual evolution of the use of the drug, across centuries, countries and classes, sex remained ever-present alongside opium consumption. The association in America of opium with sex for hire, therefore, was but a natural extension. Chinese laborers, who had come seeking a better life across the Pacific, brought with them their practices for solace. For the San Franciscan looking down at Chinatown from his balcony, it looked as if one sin was following the next, brought by the Chinese: gambling, opium and prostitution, all sinfully mixed in together. And far more pernicious, in the eyes of Americans, was the undeniable fact that opium smoking and promiscuous sex were not staying in the confines of Chinatown. Opium dens began to host, in addition to the heathen coolies, white males and females.[575] Opium smoking, a practice alien to proper American society, threatened to spread from low to high and from old to young. It was only a matter of time before public hysteria broke out.

In 1881, the San Jose Mercury shrilly warned that the "impending evil, that, transplanted here, if not rooted out, would before the dawn of another century, decimate our youth, emasculate the coming generation, if not

---

573   Ibid., 4, 51-54. See also "Page Act of 1875" at: http://w3.uchastings.edu/wingate/pageact.htm (Last access: 20.12.2015).
574   Yangwen Zheng, *The Social Life of Opium in China* (Cambridge: Cambridge University Press, 2005), 11-12, 183-184. Kane, who experimented with opium smoking, reported that his sexual desires were heightened while under the influence. See Kane, *Opium Smoking in America and China*, 52.
575   McClellan, *The Heathen Chinee*, 38.

completely destroy the white population of our coast."[576] The twin enemies of Chinese immigrants and sexual promiscuity had been identified. A panic was in the making.

Although the Chinese had long tied opium with sex, in America the connection was laden with racial overtones. Testimony given in 1878 to the California Senate left little doubt about the authorities' underlying concern: "San Francisco police claimed they had 'found white women and Chinamen side by side under the effects of this drug – a humiliating sight to anyone with anything left of manhood.'"[577] The degradation caused by smoking opium was leading to an even greater fear: interracial sex.

Through the late 1870s, the debate continued to rage about the degree to which opium smoking was endemic among America's Chinese. According to testimony given at a federal hearing into the issue, the Joint Committee of Congress to Investigate Chinese Immigration, which was convened in San Francisco in 1877, only one out of 20 Chinese smoked opium, and just one in 100 was a confirmed habitué. Yet at the very same hearing, a San Francisco policeman claimed that no less than 99 percent of Chinamen in California smoked opium on a regular basis. More moderate estimates elsewhere generally ranged from 15 percent to 40 percent.[578] In all probability, there was a spike in the consumption of opium among Chinese in America from 1870 to 1880, reaching roughly 10 percent of the population.[579]

An accurate estimate of the number of Chinese opium addicts in America, however, was hardly needed to convince the public of the growing threat. By the early 1880s, the drumbeats had grown inexorably

---

576 Quoted in Auerhahn, "The Split Labor Market and the Origins of Antidrug Legislation in the United States," 420.

577 Steven B. Duke and Albert C. Gross, *America's Longest War: Rethinking our Tragic Crusade Against Drugs* (New York: Putnam's Sons, 1993), 90-91, quoting "Chinese Immigration, Its Social, Moral and Political Effects," *Testimony of the San Francisco Police Department recorded in California State Senate Committee* (Sacramento, 1878), 152.

578 David T. Courtwright, *Dark Paradise: A History of Addiction in America* (Cambridge MA: Harvard University Press, 2001), 68; McClellan, *The Heathen Chinee*, 38-39. Sensing a moral crusade involving women in lewd positions, medical authorities began to ask whether the numbers were true, never receiving a definite answer. See "Is it True?" *Medical News* 41:1 (1 July 1882), 12.

579 John Helmer, *Drugs and Minority Oppression* (New York: Seabury Press, 1975), 28.

louder for the authorities to tackle the menace from the Chinese and their opium. In 1881, following the example set by the City of San Francisco, California passed a state law restricting the public sale of opium. Yet, in an opium case heard by the California Supreme Court six years later, the presiding judge made clear the intent of the law: "The object of the police power is to protect rights from the assaults of others, not to banish sin from the world or make men moral."[580]

In hindsight, San Francisco police were more lenient in practice than on paper. As long as an opium den only served Chinese, the police generally refrained from taking action.[581] The growing racial antagonism toward all things Chinese was tempered by the demand for menial labor, which, shunned by many white Americans, was filled in large part by Chinese immigrants. Despite the increasingly morality-tinged crusade against the Chinese heathen, there were still those who attempted to inject a measure of perspective into the debate. As one American politician put it bluntly, in a notable juxtaposition with Americans' propensity to drink and the domestic violence it helped to engender, "some of them smoke opium, but the opium-smoker does not beat his wife."[582]

In the 19th century, opium smoking, sinful as the habit was, was not yet the target of the authorities. Rather, it was the Chinese. As the Supreme Court made clear, America could not abide the threat of the heathen Chinese assaulting upstanding American citizens, and therefore the Chinese vice had to be contained. A year after California passed its opium law, the United States Congress enacted the Seclusion Act, which barred Chinese immigrants from entering the United States.[583] More federal laws followed in 1888 and in 1892. Criminal syndicates responded by smuggling both opium and Chinese laborers into the United States, often

---

580 Dale Gieringer, "125th Anniversary of the First U.S. Anti-Drug Law: San Francisco's Opium Den Ordinance (Nov. 15, 1875)," (November, 2000) at: http://www.drugsense.org/dpfca/opiumlaw.html (Last access: 20.12.2012).

581 Jesse B. Cook (former chief of police), "San Francisco's Old Chinatown," *San Francisco Police and Peace Officers' Journal* (1931) at: http://www.sfmuseum.org/hist9/cook.html (Last access: 20.12.2015).

582 Quoted in McClellan, *The Heathen Chinee*, 119. America's attitude towards the Chinese remained ambiguous, as they were tolerated in some communities, and shunned from others, resulting in an inconsistent attitude towards them. See ibid., 120-129, 249-254.

583 "The Exclusion act, 6 May 1882" at: http://www.ourdocuments.gov/doc.php?doc=47&page=transcript (Last access: 20.12.2015).

offering laborers a reduced fares in exchange for their agreeing to smuggle opium on their persons.[584]

In 1886, the Federal District Court of Oregon upheld the incarceration of a Chinese man who had been jailed by a state court on an opium-related charge. The ruling affirmed that the drug, although used as a medicine by whites, was in fact a poison when used recreationally, and as such could not be considered legitimate property. "Smoking opium is not our vice, and therefore it may be that this legislation proceeds more from a desire to vex and annoy the Heathen Chinese in this respect, than to protect the people from the evil habit," the ruling acknowledged. "But the motives of legislators cannot be the subject of judicial investigation for the purpose of affecting the validity of their acts."[585]

Aside from upholding the state court's position, Matthew Deady (1824-1893), the first judge of the federal district, made his nativist opinion known: opium smoking was not a white man's problem, and its prohibition was intended to keep the Chinese away from America. Deady did not perceive the evil opium habit itself to be of much concern to whites.

The federal Seclusion Act achieved its aims, and the number of Chinese entering the United States declined. However, the number of opium smokers continued to increase. In fact, smoking spread throughout the United States, from the West eastward. The amount of opium entering the country increased from 315,121 pounds (143 tons) in 1870 to 533,510 pounds (242 tons) in 1880,[586] reaching an average of 924,908 pounds (420 tons) a year in the 1890s. During that timeframe, the number of Chinese decreased by nearly one-quarter, from an estimated 110,000 in 1882 to 103,620 in 1890 to 85,341 in 1900.[587] Clearly, white smokers had taken to the habit and replaced the heathen Chinese as consumers of the drug.

In 1882, Wallis Nash (1837-1926), an English lawyer of some notoriety who was to become one of the founders of Oregon State University,

---

584 Jeffrey S. McIllwain, *Organizing Crime in Chinatown: Race and Racketeering in New York City, 1890-1910* (Jefferson NC: McFarland & Co. 2004), 60-61.

585 Quoted in Richard J. Bonnie and Charles H. Whitebread II, "The Forbidden Fruit and the Tree of Knowledge: An Inquiry into the Legal History of American Marijuana Prohibition," *Virginia Law Review* 56:6 (1970), 996-998.

586 H. H. Kane, *Drugs that Enslave: The Opium, Morphine, Chloral and Hashisch Habits* (Philadelphia, 1881), 6; idem, *Opium Smoking in America and China*, 16.

587 Ahmad, *The Opium Debate and Chinese Exclusion Laws in the Nineteenth-Century American West*, 77.

described how drunkenness and opium smoking were punishable in his town of residence, Corvallis, Oregon. There, offenders could be seen cleaning the muddy streets shackled to a ball and chain. And yet, he presciently observed, "It is strange to find that opium-smoking in these dens is not altogether confined to the Chinese, but some degraded white men are occasionally captured by the marshal in a raid on a China house. Such as not only punished, but scouted, and still they repeat the offense, proving the hold the practice gains when once yielded to."[588]

Opium smoking, according to contemporary accounts, spread like a disease, and climbed the social ladder.[589] Harry Hubbell Kane identified the first white opium smoker in California in 1868. He then allegedly taught others to smoke the drug, spreading the diseased vice across the country's Western frontier.[590] Like wildfire, opium smoking spread from the Chinese to the underworld, from the underworld to the poor, from the poor to the middle class, and from the middle class to the wealthy.

Laws against dens were enacted, but opium continued to be smoked by white men and women. Notably, despite the increasing consumption by white Americans, the press and popular opinion continued to portray the Chinese as the source of the vice.[591] The press was not alone in this bias. As late as the 1920s and 30s, local police departments made sure to mention the status of Chinese opium smokers in their reports to federal agencies.[592]

Local government attempts to control opium smoking failed, and in some cases made the problem even worse. Such was case in San Francisco, where an 1875 ordinance against opium dens unintentionally helped broaden the drug's appeal. Whereas clerks, schoolboys and the less risqué parts of society were inclined to avoid Chinatown and its vile dens, the 1875 ordinance pushed whites who sought out the drug to smoke else-

---

588 Wallis Nash, *Two Years in Oregon* (New York, 1882), 208.
589 Helmer, *Drugs and Minority Oppression*, 30-31; Kane, *Opium-Smoking in America and China*, 72-73.
590 Courtwright, *Dark Paradise*, 69-70; Kane, *Opium-Smoking in America and China*, 1.
591 Ahmad, *The Opium Debate and Chinese Exclusion Laws in the Nineteenth-Century American West*, 70-99.
592 See for example, "Captain Frank Kleren (Detective Division, Bureau of Police, Philadelphia) to Levi G. Nutt (Chief of Narcotic Division), 1 February 1929," NARA RG 170 Acc# 170-73-1, box 40, file 120-5, folder #3.

where, leading to the establishment of more respectable places to acquire the habit.[593]

Thomas D. Crothers (1842-1918), a leading expert on drugs and a temperance advocate, noted in 1902 that the number of smokers in New York City alone had reached over 5,000, spreading up the social order from the squalid dens of the lower classes to the palatial clubs of the upper classes.[594] As opium smoking spread both high and low, it was clear that a crisis was in the making. Observers noted that unlike morphine users, who at the time were known to take their drugs in solitude, opium smokers sought out company. Dens served as gathering places for social outsiders, and offered the expertise of experienced smokers who could prepare and "cook" opium, a difficult task for the inexperienced or initiated.[595]

The opium epidemic, which brought together high and low society, was also linked with another social disease: syphilis. After all, Kane noted, "female smokers, if not already lost in point of virtue, soon become so."[596] Women and men smoking opium congregated with one another in close quarters and squalid conditions, and frequently engaged in promiscuous and interracial sex. Physicians warned that opium would transmit syphilis from the den to the home, bringing the scourge to respectable society. There were even reports of syphilis being contracted from the mouth-pieces of opium pipes, as smokers often shared their pipes with others.[597] In this regard, opium shared a place with alcohol, since by the turn of the century liquor was also being blamed for the spread of syphilis. By some estimates, no less than 70 percent of men under the age of 25 contracted syphilis while being drunk.[598]

In what turned into a perennial source of stories and scoops, journalistic fervor continued to fuel the opium panic. Sex and opium were bundled

---

593 *San Francisco Chronicle* (25 July 1881), quoted in Ibid., 14; Nayan Shah, *Contagious Divides: Epidemics and Race in San Francisco's Chinatown* (Berkeley: University of California Press, 2001), 96.

594 Thomas D. Crothers, *Morphinism and Narcomanias from other Drugs, their Etiology, Treatment and Medicolegal Relations* (Philadelphia, 1902), 208, 215-216.

595 Courtwright, *Dark Paradise*, 69-73; Kane, *Opium-Smoking in America and China*, 70-71.

596 Ibid., 81.

597 Shah, *Contagious Divides*, 90-97.

598 James H. Timberlake, *Prohibition and the Progressive Movement, 1900-1925* (Cambridge MA: Harvard University Press, 1963), 58.

together by outraged newspapermen, who were intent on both warning against the seductive nature of opium and on selling more copies. Californian newspapers, for instance, published a series of articles in the early 1880s on the vile effects of opium on married couples and the seduction of Chinese opium-den proprietors. One such article ran in June 1882 in the *Los Angeles Times*. The report told of a married woman who was ready to elope with a "disreputable scalawag named Billy Somerset," but repented after passing through the law courts. The husband was naive enough to accept his wife back, but soon found out that she had fallen back to her old habit of meeting her lover in his apartment. Upon hearing about this indecency, the husband stormed the apartment with a friend, only to find that "there was evidence not only of a most heinous crime, but there was also an opium-smoking outfit, the fire all lighted and the deadly pipes, showing that they had but just been dropped by the guilty pair [...]. The two gentlemen left the apartment to the degraded pair, allowing them to enjoy each other's society and the soothing, delusive and death-dealing drug in peace. No legal measures are contemplated, we understand; but here the paths of husband and wife diverge, each traveling that road which inclination may direct."[599]

Yet it was economic fears that most fueled anti-Chinese sentiment at the turn of the century. In 1902, in preparation for the renewal of the Chinese Seclusion Act, American Federation of Labor leader Samuel Gompers (1850-1924) published a pamphlet titled "Meat versus Rice." In the pamphlet he warned that Chinese laborers endangered American workers by forcing wages down. Not only did Chinese coolies settle for lower wages,[600] Gompers argued in an echo of Republican Senator James Blaine of Maine (1830-1893), they also economically elbowed out their white counterparts because their diet consisted primarily of rice, whereas Americans ate more costly beef.[601]

Gompers warned that Chinese immigrants to the United States were foreign in nature and could not assimilate into the developing American

---

599 "The Denouement," *Los Angeles Times* (28 June 1882).

600 Samuel Gompers, "Meat vs. Rice: Some Reasons for Chinese Exclusion: American Manhood against Asiatic Coolieism" (Washington DC, 1902) at U.S. Senate, 57th Congress, 1st sess., doc. 137.

601 James G. Blaine, "Chinese Immigration" Speech U.S. Senate, (14 February 1879), in *James G. Blaine, a Sketch of his Life*, ed. Charles W. Balestier (New York, 1884), 122-123.

culture. In addition, they were hurting Americans' economic prospects as well, he argued, noting that Chinese syndicates had taken over European and American trade. As an example, he cited the dissolution of Russell & Co., whose business was taken over by Chinese corporations. The exact nature of Russell & Co.'s business – the opium trade – was naturally omitted from Gomper's tract.[602]

Others in the American trade-union movement went even farther, claiming that the smoking of opium – at the time considered to be a stimulant – gave the Chinese a leg up in the job market. Opium, the argument went, enabled the coolies to work more than the average white laborer.[603]

According to Gompers, himself a Dutch-Jewish immigrant from England, immigrant Chinese laborers posed more than just an economic and moral danger, real as they were. The debased Chinamen and their habits also posed a health hazard. As evidence, he pointed to an 1885 report to San Francisco's Board of Supervisors regarding the city's opium dens: "Without exception, the smell of these establishments was so repugnant as to assault four out of the five human senses." Opium dens were not only places of degradation and moral promiscuity, but also dirty insalubrious locales that broke multiple municipal health codes.[604]

The 1885 report was neither the first nor the last to note the stench emanating from the opium dens. By the 1890s, tourists who wished to "visit the Orient" with a short excursion to the local Chinatown often reported on the foul odors of the Chinese lairs, as well as the "human bundles [laying] on shelves, overcome by poppy fumes."[605]

Gompers claimed at the turn of the century that on a walk through the streets of San Francisco's Chinatown, one would meet "a number of what were once men and women, but are now but mental and physical wrecks of humanity."[606] Gomper's description of these gaunt and emaciated shells presented the opium fiends as barely human, with little control over their faculties and desires. "Who and what are these beings, and why are they

---

602 Gompers, "Meat vs. Rice," 9.
603 Auerhahn, "The Split Labor Market and the Origins of Antidrug Legislation in the United States," 419. David F. Musto, *The American Disease* (Oxford: Oxford University Press, 1999), 5-6, 43.
604 Gompers, "Meat vs. Rice," 21-22.
605 McClellan, *The Heathen Chinee*, 32-33.
606 Gompers, "Meat vs. Rice," 28.

seen only in San Francisco, one of nature's most favored cities?" he asked rhetorically, before answering:

> Some time in the past these poor miserable and degraded wrecks were the beloved children of fond parents, who perhaps [built] upon their bright prospects, but are now hopelessly lost to them forever. They have become what is known in the parlance of the street as 'dope heads,' opium fiends in the ordinary language. In some manner, by some wily method they have been induced by the Chinese to use the drug. Time was when little girls no older than 12 years were found in Chinese laundries under the influence of opium. What other crimes were committed in those dark and fetid places when these little innocent victims of the Chinamen's wiles were under the influence of the drug are almost too horrible to imagine. The police have largely broken up these laundry opium joints, but there are hundreds, aye thousands of our American boys and girls, who have acquired this deathly habit and are doomed, hopelessly doomed, beyond a shadow of redemption. Better death a hundred times, than to have become a victim of this worst of all oriental opium habit.[607]

Gompers touched on three themes that would remain a mainstay in the American discourse on drug control. The first was the fallen potential of the drug fiend, as if the addict would have had a marvelous life if only he or she had not touched the drug. In the second, the foreigner tempted the innocent young American and degraded him – and more insidiously, her – to a life not worth living. Third, boys and girls were the target of drugs; thus, a ban on drugs was justified for the sake of protecting the youth from bad habits, even in a free society.

Although San Francisco was considered the beachhead of Chinese immigrants to America, California was hardly the only state concerned about opium's powers of seduction among whites. Other western states, from Oregon in the north to Wyoming in the East, enacted laws against opium smoking and opium dens. Laws against the sale of opium and opium dens were enacted in Nevada in 1877, in North Dakota and South Dakota in 1879, in Utah in 1880, in California and Montana in 1881, in Wyoming in 1882, in Arizona in 1883, in Idaho and New Mexico in 1887, and in Washington in 1890.

Anti-opium laws also crossed the Mississippi, with Pennsylvania passing its legislation in 1883, Ohio in 1885, Maryland in 1886, Wisconsin in 1891, Georgia in 1895 and New York in 1897. By 1914, no less than 29 states had passed laws governing the sale of opium and

---

607 Ibid., 29.

restricting opium dens. Only six states, however, prohibited possession of the drug altogether, with Oregon pioneering such laws.[608]

The federal government took steps against opium as well. In 1884 a bill banning the smoking of opium in ports was proposed by a California congressman, but failed to pass. In 1887, the American-Chinese Commercial Treaty of 1880 was enacted into law, codifying restrictions on the ability of Americans to import opium into China, and more importantly for those who feared opium smoking, restricting the Chinese from importing opium into America.[609] This legislative move, however, was meant to add teeth to the 1880 treaty, since unruly American traders continued to hoist the United States flag on opium freighters in 1884 and 1885 off the Chinese coast.[610]

In 1886 and again in 1888, bills were introduced to ban opium smoking in the District of Columbia, but they both failed to pass because of the excessive powers they would have given law enforcement.[611] In 1883, the federal government increased the tariff on smoking opium in addition to the general tariff on opium, but in a spark of pragmatism reduced the tax in 1897 to control excessive smuggling.[612] This policy barely lasted a decade, and in 1909 Congress banned the importation of smoking opium into the United States, limiting the importation of opium for medicinal use only to specific ports.[613]

The *Los Angeles Times* gleefully announced in August of that year that the importation ban was "the death sentence of Chinatown," reporting that dozens of Chinamen "are dying monthly because forced to abstain from the 'dream pipe.'"[614] Prices shot up, and the price of smoking opium went from roughly $12 a pound to more than $70.[615]

---

608 Bonnie and Whitebread, "The Forbidden Fruit and the Tree of Knowledge," 985-986.
609 Courtwright, *Dark Paradise*, 78-79.
610 Hosea Ballou Morse, *The Trade and Administration of the Chinese Empire* (Taipei: Ch'eng-wen Pub. Co, 1966 [1907]), 341.
611 Courtwright, *Dark Paradise*, 78-79.
612 McIlwain, *Organizing Crime in Chinatown*, 63.
613 "Smoking Opium Exclusion Act," (9 February 1909), entering force on April 1; Courtwright, *Dark Paradise*, 104-105; Musto, *The American Disease* 27-28.
614 "Without Opium, Chinamen Die," *Los Angeles Times* (17 August 1909), quoted in Dale Gieringer, "The Opium Seclusion Act of 1909," *CounterPunch*

The law proved difficult to enforce, as smugglers found ways to circumvent it by keeping the tax stamp paid for legal opium imported before the law entered into force on April 1, 1909, and attaching the stamp to the smuggled goods. Up against the claim that the opium was purchased and imported before the law took effect, state law enforcement could not win convictions in court. Other drug peddlers simply changed their wares, selling morphine and heroin instead of opium. In an attempt to stop the smuggling of opium, Congress passed an amendment to the importation ban in January 1914 that outlawed the importation of smoking opium altogether. This time, Congress instated on the same day a prohibitive tax of 300 dollars per pound on poppy crops that were destined to find their way to the market as smoking opium.[616]

Congress, for constitutional reasons, could not meddle with state affairs, and therefore was restricted to regulating foreign trade and imposing taxes. Yet its legislative stance fit the perceived drug menace like a glove – after all, it was foreigners who had brought opium to America in the first place, and it was foreign trade that continued to feed the growing number of addicts in the country.

Close America's doors to Chinese immigration, many members of Congress believed at the turn of the century, and the scourge of opium would disappear along with the unwanted coolies. When the vile drug outlasted America's welcome of Chinese laborers, Congress dug in its heels and extended the argument to the foreign opium trade.[617]

Domestic consumption, the government made clear, was not the real problem, but rather seduction from abroad. This nativist perception of the drug problem resulted in a nativist solution: Stop the foreign element – be it the Chinese themselves, or those who trade with them – and thereby stop the opium problem. For much of the 20th century, this essentially nativist sentiment would serve as a recurring theme in American drug

---

(6-8 February 2009) at: http://www.counterpunch.org/gieringer02062009.html (Last access: 20.12.2015).

615 McIllwain, *Organizing Crime in Chinatown*, 63.

616 Courtwright, *Dark Paradise*, 225n.88.

617 Douglas C. Kinder, "Shutting the Evil: Nativism and Narcotics Control in the United States" in *Drug Control Policy: Essays in Historical and Comparative Perspective*, ed. William O. Walker III (University Park: Pennsylvania State University Press, 1992), 117-142.

policy, focusing the country's attention more on controlling the drug trade than on treating those ensnared by its wares.

8. The Birth of a Panic

During the late 19th and early 20th century, opium was rarely sold in an unadulterated form in the West. It was usually available as a tincture, or as an alcohol-based solution called laudanum.[618] Opium smoking began as an anomaly in America, as it was brought over by the Chinese for the sole purpose of relaxation and indulgence. Opium itself, however, was not entirely foreign, having been eaten by Americans as far back as the early Republic, if not earlier.

William Rosser Cobbe (?-1907), a journalist and recovered addict, drew a strong distinction between the two forms of taking opium, arguing that the opium smoker was different from the eater because the former sought out the addiction. Opium eaters, unlike smokers, succumbed to their disease mostly out of ignorance, or medical malpractice. Thus, Cobbe reasoned, the habitué who sought out addiction for pleasure had something inherently wrong with him or her.

In the minds of many Americans at the time, addiction resembled slavery, as evidenced in the title of Harry H. Kane's 1881 book, "Drugs that Enslave." The United States, built on the premise of a free society, could not tolerate those individuals who wished to enslave themselves by choice.[619]

Though America's anti-opium ire was overwhelmingly directed against the Chinese, they were hardly alone in being blamed for the spread of opium. In 1891, Cyrus Hamlin (1811-1900), an American missionary to Turkey who would later become the president of Middlebury College in Vermont, railed against the British Empire for supplying the Chinese with opium:

> We, as Americans, have a closer relation to this question than that of sympathy with the wrongs and sufferings of the Chinese. The curse has trav-

---

618 Virginia Berridge, *Opium and the People: Opiate Use and Drug Control Policy in Nineteenth and Early Twentieth Century England* (London: Free Association Books, 1999), 21-37.

619 On freedom and addiction, see Mariana Valverde, *Diseases of the Will: Alcohol and the Dilemmas of Freedom* (Cambridge: Cambridge University Press, 1998), 32-33.

eled across the Pacific to San Francisco and many other cities. Whenever the Chinese go, they have their 'joints' for smoking opium.... [Opium] enters unawares. It blinds its victim, paralyzes his will, and makes him a vessel fitted for destruction, before he knows his danger.... The Englishman counsels government 'not to make war again upon the strong and lasting feeling of mankind.' What China demands is, that England shall not force upon her a commerce that is destructive to her very life. And what every Christian and every patriot must demand of our government is, that swift penalties shall be visited upon those who are offering the insidious temptation to the seekers of pleasure in our own cities.[620]

The British Empire was also held responsible for introducing countless Americans to stories about opium dens and decadence, as described in the many pictures, books and journals by British authors that found their way across the Atlantic. Thomas de Quincey (1785-1859) and other Englishmen who wrote in the early 19th century about their opium-induced oriental fantasies were well known in America.[621]

By the end of the century, Victorian authors were regaling readers, many of them American, with tales of the decadent nature of the drug and the criminals who dealt with them.[622] Sir Arthur Conan Doyle (1859-1930) made famous the character of Sherlock Holmes, who was both a morphine and cocaine user himself and an investigator of decadent opium smokers in their dens.[623] Oscar Wilde (1854-1900), whose popularity in the United States far exceeded his problematic relations with his government and readers at home, wrote about the cleansing effects of the decadent opium dens. He even dared to suggest that the upper crust of

---

620 Cyrus Hamlin, "The Anti-Opium Resolution in Parliament," *Our Day* 8:45 (September, 1891), 153-160. It is interesting to note that the *Woman's Temperance Publishing Association* financed this journal.

621 A few famous examples: Thomas de Quincey, *Confessions of an English Opium-Eater* (London, 1997 [1821-1822]); Samuel Taylor Coleridge, "Kubla Khan or, a Vision in a Dream, a Fragment," (1816); Lord (George Gordon) Byron, "Don Juan" (1824), 4/19.

622 Julian North, "The Opium-Eater as a Criminal in Victorian Writing," in *Writing and Victorianism*, ed. J. Barrie Bullen (London: Longman, 1997), 120-136; Terry Parssinen, *Secret Passions, Secret Remedies: Narcotic Drugs in British Society, 1820-1930* (Philadelphia: Institute for the Studies of Human Issues, 1983), 61.

623 Arthur Conan Doyle, "The Man with the Twisted Lip," in *The Illustrated Sherlock Holmes Treasury* (New York, 1984 [1891]), 70-84. See also Berridge, *Opium and the People*, 223-224. Sherlock Holmes' use of cocaine was used and known in America, often repeated in anti-cocaine literature. See "The Cocaine Fiend," (undated) *Drug Pamphlets*, Library of Congress, CLC RM 41.

society might enjoy the vice, by having Lord Henry Wotton smoke opium-tinted cigarettes in *The Picture of Dorian Gray*.[624]

Novelist Sax Rohmer's (1883-1959) answer to Doyle's Sherlock Holmes, Sir Denys Nayland Smith, was known across America for hunting the insidious criminal mastermind Dr. Fu Manchu in one opium den after another.[625] By the 20th century, parents had been instilled with a fear that their children would be lured into experimenting with drugs and turn into drug fiends, just by reading Oscar Wilde and other decadent literature.[626]

British novelists were not the only writers bringing opium to the attention of Americans in the early 20th century. Countless "true accounts of the dope underworld," inevitably featuring seedy Chinese opium dens, were published by journalists during the 1920s.[627] Newspapers featured them so often that readers came to expect such drug stories. Their veracity, however, was not always clear.

The popularity of drugs in the 19th and 20th centuries followed a pattern. Whenever a new drug was discovered and banned, users flocked to a new one. As the Massachusetts State Board of Health argued in 1872, people turned to opium when alcohol was unavailable, as evidenced by the fact that wherever the temperance movement was strong, the opium trade flourished.[628] The prohibition of alcohol in Iowa in 1886 exerted pressure on pharmacists to provide users with alternative intoxicants, presumably in the form of opium and tonics.[629] High taxes and importation bans, in

---

624 Oscar Wilde, *The Picture of Dorian Gray* (London, 1992 [1891]), 6, 112, 213, 216-217.

625 Sax Rohmer [Arthur Henry Sarsfield Ward], *The Insidious Dr. Fu-Manchu* (London, 1913). The book, and its sequel, *The Return of Dr. Fu-Manchu* (1916) were serialized by the *Collier's Magazine* in the United States.

626 Susan L. Speaker, "'The Struggle of Mankind Against its Deadliest Foe' Themes of Counter-Subversion in Anti-Narcotic Campaigns, 1920-1940" in *Journal of Social History* 34:3 (2001), 591-610; Boon, *The Road of Excess*, 54-55.

627 See, for example, Fred V. Williams, *The Hop-Heads: Personal Experiences Among the Users of 'Dope' in the San Francisco Underworld* (San Francisco, 1920), 91-98, 112-117.

628 F. E. Oliver, "The Use and Abuse of Opium," *Massachusetts State Board of Health, Third Annual Report*, (Boston, 1872), 162-177.

629 Committee of Fifty, *The Liquor Problem: A Summary of Investigations Conducted, 1893-1903* (New York, 1970 [1905]), 64-65. Hamilton Wright, a driving engine behind the Federal drug law, denied the charge before Congress in 1910 that prohibition caused drug use, or a ban on drugs would induce drinking.

turn, made smoking opium expensive in the first two decades of the 20th century, forcing many users to turn to morphine to sooth their addictions. Morphine turned from the 19th-century drug of middle-aged white women into the drug of young, lower-class men.[630]

By the end of the 19th century, morphine had also become known as a poison. In 1891 in New York City, Helen Potts was poisoned with morphine by her husband, a medical student who was also married to another woman. He was executed for murder shortly afterward. The next year, another morphine murder was committed by a physician wishing to get rid of his wife. The doctor used atropine and morphine in an effort to mask the poisoning, and appeared to have gotten away with the crime until an investigative reporter revealed the truth and the doctor was sent to the execution chamber.[631]

While physicians fought to keep morphine in the medicine cabinet as a powerful analgesic, the association of the drug with crime and addiction led them to seek out alternatives in synthetics or semi-synthetics. Some progress was made in their research, notably the production of desomorphine in 1932, but overall no wonder drug was discovered. With every new analgesic physicians rejoiced anew, believing they had found a non-addictive substance to replace morphine, only to discover soon afterward that the new drug was also addictive.[632]

A few years after morphine replaced opium as the street drug, it, too, became prohibitively expensive. Cost and legal limitations drove addicts

---

He used Kansas as an example: a dry state since 1881, which had no drug problem. See "Importation and Use of Opium," *Hearing before the Committee on Ways and Means of the House of Representatives*, 61st Congress, 3rd Session, (14 December 1910 and 11 January 1911), 93. Wright's source remains unknown and his claim is suspect of ulterior political motives. Furthermore, Kansas despite its strict dry constitution *de jure* was notoriously wet, with illegal bars found in every city. Following the logic of this argument, there was no reason to use drugs because alcohol was readily available. See Richard F. Hamm, *Shaping the 18*[th] *Amendment: Temperance Reform, Legal Culture, and the Polity, 1800-1920* (Chapel Hill: University of North Carolina Press, 1995), 1-2; Paul Johnson, *A History of the American People* (New York: Harper Collins, 1997), 697.

630 Courtwright, *Dark Paradise*, 99-100.

631 Patrick M. Wall, "The Annals of Manhattan Crime," *New York Magazine* 21:45 (1988), 43-46.

632 Caroline Jean Acker, *Creating the American Junkie: Addiction Research in the Classic Era of Narcotic Control* (Baltimore: Johns Hopkins University Press, 2002), 62-97.

to seek out other, more readily available drugs. Importation bans enacted in 1909, 1914 and 1922 reduced the supply of opium and morphine into the American market, and into the void stepped a German import, heroin.[633]

In 1924, Congress set its sights on heroin, which had become increasingly popular thanks to its potency. By that time nearly all physicians and drug experts had concluded that the drug caused crime, and therefore ought to be targeted by federal drug laws, particularly given that heroin was not believed to possess any redeeming medical qualities.[634] In one measure against heroin, the surgeon general of the United States Army ordered in 1923 that the military's stockpiles of the drug be incinerated..[635]

Mass produced by the German company Bayer since 1898, heroin became popular among American addicts because, as *The New Republic* magazine reported in 1916:

> It was cheap, it demanded neither layout nor hypodermic syringe, and could be taken for a long time without disturbing the health. It stopped the craving without diminishing working capacity to a degree which would prevent the earning of money to buy the drug, and last, but not least, as it is sniffed through the nose on a 'quill,' the addict could take it without much fear of being interfered with [...]. The majority of the present takers are boys and young men whose easy scalability has been developed in the gangs who later flock together in leisure hours at the dance halls, the movies and at that form of entertainment which they all seem to like best, vaudeville [...]. Some examined by the Binet-Simon test show mental defects, but the majorities are not materially defective in intellectual qualities.[636]

On the streets of New York, morphine was being sold for as high as $80 an ounce,[637] and demand for the drug kept prices high across the country. In 1935, the street price of morphine in Chicago reached $90 to $100 an ounce. Heroin, meanwhile, was only $38 to $40 an ounce.[638] Small wonder that many addicts turned to the cheaper and more powerful drug.

The New Republic reporter maintained that young men succumbed to the heroin habit "ignorantly and innocently," as if the American public,

633 Courtwright, *Dark Paradise*, 98-109.
634 Ibid., 242n.131.
635 Arnold S. Trebach, *The Heroin Solution* (New Haven: Yale University Press, 1982), 46-52.]
636 Pearce Bailey, "The Heroin Habit," *New Republic* 6:77 (1916), 314-316.
637 Terry and Pellens, *The Opium Problem*, 485.
638 Courtwright, *Dark Paradise*, 242n. 131.

especially young men who lived in the vicinity of older habitués, did not know what addiction was. Yet another panic appeared to be in the making, with the press again warning the public against a drug that corrupted the youth.

The magazine stressed that physicians were not to be blamed for heroin addiction, as was the case with morphine, because heroin was rarely used in remedies and cures. The claim, however, was not entirely true. When heroin first appeared on the market, it was hailed as a panacea, a non-addictive opiate produced by modern science.[639] Addiction to heroin was soon identified, but even then not fully understood. As late as 1913, in fact, a prominent specialist on addiction proclaimed, "codeine and heroin can be used for longer period without formation of addiction than any of the other preparations of opium."[640] The products of modern science were deemed safer than the smoked drugs of the orient.

With doctors still debating the use of heroin, journalists looking for a bogeyman instead turned their pens on that old standby, the insidious lower-class criminals who introduced the drug to the young:

> Oftentimes one old addict will corrupt at one sitting ten or twenty boys. A common story is of a group of boys being together at a dance, or a show, at some outdoor gathering in the summer. One of the number produces a 'deck' or 'package' of heroin and tells the others that the taking of it is wonderfully enjoyable.... From all these considerations, which are drawn from the class of boys who have gone to the public schools, it would seem that heroin taking is closely allied with the factors which make inebriety in some form inevitable in the poorer classes in large cities. Boys and young men seem to want something that promises to make life gayer and more enjoyable, and the particular 'fillip' they hit upon depends on their personal temperament and their surroundings.[641]

---

639 For the clinical uses of heroin by Bayer chemists, see: Theobald Floret, "Klinische Versuche über die Wirkung und Anwendung des Heroins" in *Therapeutische Monatshefte* (1898), vol. 12/9, 512; *idem*, "Weiteres über Heroin" in *Therapeutische Monatshefte* 13:6 (1899), 327-329; Dreser, "Pharmakologische über einige Morphinderivate [sic]" in *Therapeutische Monatshefte* 12:9 (1898), 509-511. See also David F. Musto, ed. *One Hundred Years of Heroin* (Westport, CN: Auburn House, 2002), xiv-xvi; Courtwright, *Dark Paradise*, 89-93; Terry and Pellens, *The Opium Problem*, 76-85.

640 George E. Pettey, *The Narcotic Drug Diseases and Allies Ailments: Pathology, Pathogenesis, and Treatment* (Philadelphia, 1913), 3-4.

641 Bailey, "The Heroin Habit," 314-316.

Boys, not women or girls, as had been the case during the mid-19th century, were the prime candidates to succumb to the heroin habit.[642] Rear Admiral Richmond P. Hobson (1870-1937), an ardent prohibitionist revered for his heroics in the Spanish-American war, led the charge in spreading the warning: Heroin caused crime. "Heroin addiction can be likened to contagion," he declared in a radio broadcast in 1928. "Most of the daylight robberies, daring holdups, cruel murders and similar crimes of violence are now known to be committed chiefly by drug addicts."[643]

Newspaper and magazines echoed the shrill warnings issued by Hobson and other like-minded public figures:

> Once the habit is acquired, the addict will not try to work without 'dope.' He will, as he expresses it, 'do almost anything to get the 'dust.'' It is at this point particularly that heroin habituation becomes an important incentive to crime. Among the frequent misdemeanors charged against the heroin boys besides those directly concerned with the use or possession of the drug, are stealing and destruction of property.[644]

Such misdeeds, and the drug that caused them, were an urban plague, according to contemporary press accounts. "The heroin habit is essentially a matter of city life, as in rural communities it does not exist as it does in New York," reported *The New Republic*. "For example, the records of State Hospital at Trenton, New Jersey, which recruits from a rural community, show that of the drug addicts who have gone there for treatment since the passage of the Harrison law, not one has been a taker of heroin and not one had acquired the habit through social usage."[645]

Heroin had become the new bogeyman. As had been the case with opium decades before, a drug panic was spreading across America. Heroin was taking over the streets, stronger and cheaper than any drug previously known to man. The press depicted defenseless children falling victim to its easy high, turning them into drug fiends who would do anything, including criminal behavior, to get their next fix. This incurable urban disease was being fed by a steady influx of young men, who flocked to America's cities in search of gainful employment, only to be corrupted irreparably by the vile drug.

---

642 Terry and Pellens, *The Opium Problem*, 484.
643 Richmond Hobson, "Mankind's Greatest Affliction and Gravest Menace," (1928), reproduced in *Drugs in America*, ed. Musto, 271-275.
644 Bailey, "The Heroin Habit," 314-316.
645 Ibid.

The panic stretched from coast to coast, from San Francisco to New York City. The press regularly featured stories of white men and women congregating in secluded apartments, where fiends injected their "c" or "m," sometimes freebasing the drug. These addicts were shells of their former selves, all bearing, in the words of one journalist, the "branding marks of the drugs to which they were slaves – the uncanny brightness of their eyes, the deathly pallor of their skins, the swift, jerking movements of their shoulders, arms and legs."[646]

In the press, the addicts were all criminals; the men resorted to thievery and begging while the women dabbled in prostitution. Some were doctors, entertainers and professionals who had fallen, their potential left unfulfilled because of the dope. While under the influence, the users were paranoid and potentially violent. Many were found scratching their skin with nails and needles to fight off the hallucination of bugs eating their flesh,[647] a common occurrence among heavy cocaine users first identified by Viennese neurologist Heinrich Obersteiner (1847-1922) in 1886.[648]

The stories of how users succumbed to addiction followed a standard plotline, one marked by tropes of crime, destitution and strife. A familiar version had a man introducing a woman to opium smoking. She soon discovers that her vice has turned into a habit. After the police crack down on opium, she turns to heroin, and from heroin to cocaine, morphine and whatever else is available. The life of crime and easy money soon follow, all to feed the craving. But the real threat of addiction was the lack of cure.

The sad soul at the center of every such story inevitably wanted to quit, to go straight, but could not. They were slaves to their addiction. The progressive press assigned blame on everyone: doctors, policemen, jailors, all of whom clearly knew nothing about addiction. Hospitals cost money and the law only sent addicts to prison. The police maltreated the dope fiends, on the beat or in jail, oppressing addicts, taunting and demanding bribes from them. Corruption spread everywhere, from government on down to little girls forced to carry drugs for local peddlers.[649]

A panic was also in the making with cocaine, and as with opium it had a pronounced racial undertone. In place of the Chinese coolies and their

---

646 Williams, *The Hop-Heads*, 17.
647 Ibid., 1-17, 50, 63, 71-72.
648 Heinrich Obersteiner, "Ueber Intoxicationspsychosen," *Wiener medizinische Presse* 24:4 (1886), 116.
649 Williams, *The Hop-Heads*, 18-29, 39-40, 47-48, 59, 81-81.

insidious opium dens the cocaine panic centered on blacks in America. White Americans feared that the slave of old would turn violently on his former master, making a stimulant like cocaine a real threat.

Predominantly black laborers on the waterfront in New Orleans used cocaine to ease their hard labor.[650] Cocaine use then spread upriver on the Mississippi, and from there east and west to mine workers and farmhands. Employers, upon learning of the stimulating effects of the drug, distributed it to their workers, who in turn came to expect it.[651] Unlike their experience with morphine, heroin and other manufactured drugs, physicians quickly came to understand that cocaine was addictive.[652] By the turn of the century, the country's leading experts were already tracking the spread of the drug. "The cocaine habit is said to have already invaded some northern cities, though in none of them is it as general a vice as among the Negroes of the South," the *Journal of the American Medical Association* reported in 1901.[653]

In 1903, *The New York Tribune* reported that many black saloons in Atlanta were going out of business because patrons preferred to sniff cocaine rather than drink hard liquor. A quarter or half-dollar's worth of cocaine could last a full week, and was even available in the agreeably drinkable Coca-Cola.[654] *The New York Times*, meanwhile, reported that the Southern habit "had fixed itself to an alarming degree on Negroes. The curse of cocaine, in fact, is said to be as great if not a greater menace to the peace of that section of the country than the liquor habit."[655] The popularity of cocaine in the United States could not be denied. According to some estimates, the United States imported no less than 600 to 1,000

---

650 Joseph F. Spillane, *Cocaine: From Medical Marvel to Modern Menace in the United States, 1884-1920* (Baltimore: Johns Hopkins University Press, 2000), 91.
651 Ibid., 92-93.
652 Ibid., 25-42.
653 "The Cocaine Habit," *Journal of the American Medical Association* 36:5 (1901), 330.
654 Colonel J. W. Watson quoted in "Cocaine Sniffing," *New York Tribune* (21 June 1903), 11. The Georgia legislature debated the fate of the drink available to the public and the Coca-Cola Company decided to withdraw cocaine from its drink the same year. See Spillane, *Cocaine*, 136.
655 "Cocaine Forbidden in the U.S. Mails," *New York Times* (17 July 1908). Southern politicians, who subscribed to dry politics and feared blacks from procuring their cocaine by mail, demanded the ban on the alcohol and cocaine traffic by mail.

tons of cocaine annually from South America by the beginning of the 20th century.[656]

At the turn of the century, cocaine and morphine were available in nearly every pharmacy, and could even be received by mail-order cata- logue. The shipment of cocaine was so rampant that in July 1908 the Post Office Department, which concerned itself with moral problems at the time, issued a ban on delivering the drug by mail, invoking the same regu- lations forbidding the delivery of alcohol from wet to dry states, or pornography.

Cocaine, as a stimulant leading to an increase in workers' productivity, ought to have expected a bright future in the harsh capitalistic environ- ment of late 19th-century America. This was all the more so given that the country had a long tradition of self-medication and tonics to increase a person's energy. And yet as quickly as cocaine entered the American market in the mid-1880s, it faded out in rapid fashion thirty years later.

The price of the drug plummeted to roughly $2 an ounce, making it newly affordable to the poor, and to criminals.[657] Reports from Southern states claimed that the drug induced violence among blacks. As one Geor- gian politician told the *New York Tribune* in 1903: "I am convinced that if some stringent law is not enacted and enforced against its use the habit will grow and extend to such proportions that great injury will result. In fact, great injury has already resulted, for I am satisfied that many of the horrible crimes committed in the Southern states by the colored people can be traced directly to the cocaine habit."[658]

Blacks, cocaine and crime were bundled together for public consump- tion, just as Chinese laborers, opium and prostitution had been earlier; and, corruption of the youth, as before, became a cause for concern. "The use of cocaine is not confined to negroes of the South, by any manner of means," warned the Georgian politician, "The young white men have taken up the habit, and its effect could be seen on their faces."[659]

---

656 Paul Gootenberg, "Between Coca and Cocaine: A Century or More of U.S.-Peru- vian Drug Paradoxes, 1860-1980," *Hispanic American Historical Review* 83:1 (2003), 121-122.

657 David T. Courtwright, "The Rise and Fall and Rise of Cocaine in the United States," in *Consuming Habits: Drugs in History and Anthropology*, ed. Jordan Goodman, Paul E. Lovejoy and Andrew Sherratt (London: Routledge, 1995), 209.

658 Watson quoted in "Cocaine Sniffing," 11.

659 Ibid.

Fear of the conjugal mixing of the races, also as before, helped drive the drug panic. Dr. Christopher Koch of Pennsylvania claimed in 1914 that "most of the attacks upon white women of the South are a direct result of the cocaine-crazed Negro brain."[660] Four years earlier, Koch testified before the U.S. House of Representatives that between 45 percent and 48 percent of all criminals were dope fiends. The doctor recounted to the congressional members of the Committee on Ways and Means colorful stories of "Chinks" forcing their white concubines to do all the housework while they smoke opium. He claimed that cocaine was essentially an American vice, one primarily adopted by blacks but also increasingly by white boys.[661]

Cocaine, like opium, was believed to promote sexual promiscuity. But unlike the sedative effects of opium, cocaine's stimulating effects were blamed for promoting rape, violence and deadly accuracy in shooting.[662] According to the police chief of Atlanta, cocaine was responsible for no less than 70 percent of all crimes committed in the city.[663] He also claimed that a black man under the influence of cocaine could forget his rightful, docile place in society, and commit the unthinkable: raping a white woman. Once again, interracial sex had become the true danger to America. The danger was not in the form of seduction, as had been the case with opium and the Chinese coolies, but rather in the form of violence.

The police departments readied their arms. It has even been suggested that one of the reasons why policemen switched from .32 to .38 caliber guns was to deal with the cocaine-crazed Southern black man.[664] That the

---

660 Christopher Koch, *Literary Digest* (28 March 1914), quoted in Musto, *The American Disease*, 305n.15.

661 "Importation and Use of Opium," *Hearings before the Committee on Ways and Means of the House of Representatives*, 61st Congress, 3rd Session (14 December 1910, 11 January 1911), 71; Timothy A. Hickman, *The Secret Leprosy of Modern Days: Narcotic Addiction and Cultural Crisis in the United States, 1870-1920* (Amherst: University of Massachusettes Press, 2007), 109-111. A similar voice was heard in the same hearing that debated the ill-fated Foster Anti-Narcotic Bill by Hamilton Wright. See David F. Musto, "The History of Legislative Control over Opium, Cocaine and their Derivatives," at http://www.druglibrary.net/schaff er/History/ophs.htm, n. 32. (Last access, 22.1.2016).

662 Williams, "Negro Cocaine 'Fiends' Are a New Southern Menace."; Hickman, *The Secret Leprosy of Modern Days*, 77-78.

663 Musto, *The American Disease*, 304n.15.

664 Ibid., 7.

facts did not necessarily support the idea of a craze was, at least in much of the press, conveniently ignored. In a survey conducted in a Georgia asylum in 1914, a total of two of the 2,100 blacks who had been admitted were found to be cocaine users. The surveyor concluded that blacks were too poor to buy the drug.[665]

Though racial attitudes strongly colored the cocaine panic, blacks were not the only part of the population to be blamed for the spread of the drug. Even before the black cocaine scare, stories appeared in the press about increasing cocaine addiction among doctors. An 1886 article in *The New York Times*, "Work of an Awful Habit," told the story of a Chicago physician named Charles H. Bradley: "Once a brilliant physician, he experimented with cocaine and became a slave to it [within two years, thus ruining] himself and his family by the use of cocaine."[666] Bradley's notoriety derived from his research into cocaine. After first experimenting with the drug on animals, he then practiced on himself and then eventually his wife. Enslavement to the drug turned into economic ruin, as the doctor neglected his duties and his medical practice collapsed. He was sent to a mental asylum for half a year, after which he was declared cured. Soon thereafter, however, his cocaine habit turned into an opiate habit. He was eventually arrested for acquiring syringes from fellow doctors under false pretenses, namely seeking the opium that came with the syringe cases.[667]

Numerous newspaper articles recounting how doctors had had their lives ruined by addiction soon followed. In 1886, Dr. Morehouse of New York City was sent to Bellevue Hospital in a state of near-dementia induced by cocaine. His descent into drug addiction landed him on the front page of *The New York Times*.[668] The cocaine-induced madness of Dr. C. N. Moore, a native of Erie, Pennsylvania, got him on the cover in 1887.[669] Dr. John Le Grand Schaffer was profiled after losing his sanity due to the overuse of morphine and cocaine,[670] while Dr. F. M. Hamlin of

---

665 Ibid., 8.
666 "Work of an Awful Habit; the Sad Story of Dr. Charles H. Bradley" *New York Times* (30 November 1887), 3. See also "Cocaine's Destructive Work" *New York Times* (24 January 1887), 2.
667 Ibid., 2.
668 "Charged against Cocaine" *New York Times* (23 August 1886), 1.
669 "A Physician's Sad Plight; Driven mad by the use of Cocaine to Allay Pain" *New York Times* (16 January 1887), 1.
670 "Crazed by Drugs" *New York Times* (8 March 1887), 8.

Auburn, New York, was featured after the drugs sent him to a mental asylum in Utica in 1888.[671]

With white doctors and poor blacks seemingly succumbing in droves to cocaine addiction, the warnings in the press grew sharper, with strong echoes of the warnings against opium in years past. "The boy slaves of dope ceased to be human beings," asserted an investigative reporter in 1920 "They become creeping, crawling things without the power of connected speech or thought. They wallowed in the filth and refuse under the sidewalks, suffering the dread illusions to which the slaves of cocaine are heir."[672]

The burgeoning movie industry soon followed with a series of films about dealers who seduced young innocent white boys – and more insidiously, white girls – to take drugs. "The Cocaine Fiends," a film released in 1935, opened with the following words:

> Among the many evils against which society struggles, one of the most vicious is the traffic in dope. In every community where the menace developes [sic] all the forces which society can mobilize, including social agencies, doctors, law enforcement officials and government band together to stamp it out… Without such activity the dope evil would run rampant. Yet it has long been recognized that one other powerful force is necessary before the struggle can be completely successful. That force is an aroused and educated public awareness. It is in the hope of aiding in developing such awareness that this picture has been produced. What happens to Jane Bradford may happen to anyone. There will always be 'Jane Bradfords' until you, Mr. Citizen, co-operate with the forces now fighting the dope evil to forever stamp it out in our land.[673]

Even without viewing the film, one can imagine the horrible cocaine-induced fate that befell the character of Jane Bradford. At the time "The Cocaine Fiends" was being shown in cinemas across America, a third drug panic was in the making, this time with marijuana. The flower of the cannabis plant was associated with Mexican laborers, who brought their "reefer" with them across the border, as well as with blacks from the West Indies who settled along the Gulf Coast. As with cocaine and opium before it, marijuana became dirty by racial association, this time with Mexicans as the bogeymen. After all, there is a reason why American

---

671 "Used Morphine and Cocaine" *New York Times* (24 March 1888), 3.
672 Williams, *The Hop-Heads*, 70.
673 William A. O'Connor (dir.), "Cocaine Fiends," (1935).

English adopted the Spanish 'marijuana' for the buds of the cannabis plant.

Despite the growing public outcry against the drug, Congress was slow to enact laws against it, passing federal legislation banning marijuana only in 1937. State and local governments, however, took steps earlier. Laws against marijuana existed as early as 1914 in Louisiana, Maine and Massachusetts. That same year municipal legislation curbing the drug also began to be passed, such as a 1914 ordinance in El Paso, Texas.[674] It was not long for Washington to remain uninvolved in the unfolding debate over marijuana.

Sensing the public fear of the drug, the chief of the newly founded Federal Bureau of Narcotics, Harry J. Anslinger, joined together with Courtney Ryley Cooper (1886-1940), a popular true crime author, to publicly rail against marijuana. At first, Anslinger was hesitant to commit the Federal government against marijuana, believing that controlling the weed was best left to the states. Yet demand and political pressure, as well as the opportunity to expand his own Bureau changed his mind. He and Cooper described the drug as an assassin of youth, citing cases of suicides, murders, robberies and deeds of maniacal insanity.

Marijuana, they warned, was smoked not only by drug fiends, but also by "all-American girls" who simply wanted to try something different, and thus ending up puffing "homemade" cigarettes with a "real kick." Sensationally written, with the sole purpose of frightening readers, Anslinger and Cooper listed the dangers of marijuana, perhaps most pernicious of which was its unpredictability. "No one knows, when one places a marijuana cigarette to his lips, whether he will become a philosopher, a joyous reveler in a musical heaven, a mad insensate, a calm philosopher, or a murderer," they cautioned.[675]

The drug was unpredictable, but how it was distributed was clear to all, at least according to Anslinger and Cooper. Like opium and cocaine before it, those peddling marijuana preyed on America's innocent youth, spreading the drug through society by targeting its most impressionable members. "That youth has been selected by the peddlers of this poison as

---

674 Richard J. Bonnie and Charles H. Whitebread II, *The Marijuana Conviction: A History of Marijuana Prohibition in the United States* (New York: Lindesmith Center, 1999), 32-52, 354.

675 Harry J. Anslinger and Courtney R. Cooper, "Marijuana: Assassin of Youth," in *American Magazine* 124:1 (July, 1937), 18-19, 150-153.

an especially fertile field makes it a problem of serious concern to every man and woman in America," Anslinger and Cooper explained. "[And] therein lies much of the cruelty of marijuana, especially in its attack upon youth. The young, immature brain is a thing of impulses, upon which the 'unknown quantity' of the drug acts as an almost overpowering stimulant."[676]

The drug was allegedly available under every stone and behind every corner; it could be obtained from the janitor in school, at the local dance hall, or from countless street peddlers. The poisonous drug was ensnaring America's youth, with one puff threatening to lead them on a downward spiral that eventually led to murder or death.[677]

In promising devastation for anyone who lit up a marijuana joint, Anslinger and Cooper were hardly alone. Doomsday warnings abounded, with perhaps the most enduring among them coming at the end of "Reefer Madness," a film produced in 1936 for a Christian anti-drug organization and espoused by the Bureau of Narcotics. "The next tragedy may be that of your daughter's, or your son's, or yours, or yours," the school headmaster warns at the conclusion of the film, before turning to the camera and addressing the audience directly: "... or yours!"[678]

During the 1930s and 40s pamphlets on the dangers of marijuana circulated around America, stirring public sentiment against the drug in an attempt to rally support for the Marijuana Tax Act. The stories they recounted were truly horrific, if of questionable accuracy, as in the following example:

> A Young boy who has become addicted to smoking Marihuana cigarettes, in a fit of frenzy, because, as he stated while still under the Marihuana influence, a number of people were trying to cut off his arms and legs, seized an axe and killed his father, mother, two brothers and a sister, wiping out the entire family except himself.
> A man under the influence of Marihuana actually decapitated his best friend; and then, coming out of the effects of the drug, was as horrified as anyone over what he had done.[679]

---

676 Ibid.
677 Ibid.
678 Louis Gasnier (dir), "Reefer Madness," (1936).
679 "Marihuana, Killer Drug," (undated, was archived on 18 April 1940 and probably published before August 1937), *Drug Pamphlets*, Library of Congress, CLC RM 41.

Anslinger favored such stories, often stressing, as in a speech delivered in March 1937, that the users of "'cannabin,' the active narcotic principle of cannabis sativa... are said to develop a delirium rage after its administration during which they are temporarily, at least, irresponsible and liable to commit violent crimes."[680] Anslinger's claims were dubious, to say the least. To begin with, the Israeli scientist Raphael Mechoulam (1930-) discovered the active principle of cannabis only in 1964 – nearly 30 years after Anslinger's cannabin. And already during Anslinger's time such arguments were being rejected. A report submitted to New York City mayor Fiorello La Guardia (1882-1947) in 1944 refuted claims that cannabis caused violence or crime.[681] But it was already too late; by then cannabis had been virtually outlawed.

All drugs were labeled as bad, and with active encouragement from the press and politicians, the American public grew accustomed to loathing drug users. A telling example is a letter sent in late 1934 by one Paul A. Learneel of Los Angeles to J. Edgar Hoover (1895-1972), director of the then-Bureau of Investigation.

> A prison sentence is a joke for addicts. They get caught up on their sleep or kick out of a habit, after which [they] are prepared for future peddling, now, if a death sentence faced such, those rats and murderers, I predict all foreigners would coat-tail it out of our country and all users would take the cure and make fair citizens again.[682]

The matter was forwarded to the Federal Bureau of Narcotics, which in turn courteously replied to Learneel and then summarily filed the letter without any serious consideration.[683] The government received numerous such letters, which had no impact on policymaking but nonetheless repre-

---

680 Harry J. Anslinger, "Marihuana," A speech delivered for the *Women's National Exposition of Arts and Industry* (New York City, 30 March 1937), NARA, RG 170, Acc #170-73-1, box 44, file 0145, gen. Folder #1.

681 Mayor's Committee on Marihuana, *The Marijuana Problem in the City of New York* (1944), known as the *La Guardia Committee Report on Marihuana* at: http://www.druglibrary.org/schaffer/library/studies/lag/lagmenu.htm.

682 Paul A. Learneel to J. E. Hoover (Director of the Federal Bureau of Investigations), (12 December 1934), NARA RG 170, Acc# 170-73-1 box 44 file 0135-5 folder 1926-1949.

683 Will S. Wood (Acting Commissioner of Narcotics) to Paul. A. Learneel, (16 January 1935), NARA RG 170, Acc# 170-73-1 box 44 file 0135-5 folder 1926-1949.

sented the degree to which Americans' attitude toward drugs had hardened.

By the time of Learneel's letter, anti-drug sentiments were widespread, pushed along in large part by the fourth and final drug panic to hit America in the early 20th century: patent medicines and physician's malpractice. In the latter part of the 19th century, tonics and other home-made remedies were popular in the United States. Often containing psychoactive substances, they were available to all on the open market. The 1897 Sears, Roebuck & Co. catalogue, whose wares were available for shipment to every corner of America, had among its many offers a product labeled "Peruvian Wine of Coca." Manufactured by the same innovator of Coca-Cola, to "sustain and refresh both body and brain," it was available for just $10 a dozen.[684] Vin Mariani, a French wine laced with cocaine sold between 1884 and 1913, boasted a long list of famous customers, among them King Alfonso XIII of Spain, Jean-Martin Charcot, Thomas Alva Edison, Pope Leo XIII and President William McKinley.[685] And in the catalogue of New York wholesaler Charles N. Crittenton, no less than 19 different brands of coca wine were available for sale to the public.[686]

The mail-order catalogues went out of their way to meet customers' requests. A solicitation in the 1902 Sears catalogue makes clear just how easy it was to acquire drugs in America at the turn of the century: "If you will send your doctor's prescription or any other prescription to us, you can rest assured it will be given professional care."[687]

If it was not Sears and other such businesses that facilitated the spike in drug sales, then it was the doctors themselves who set the patients on the path to addiction. It was no coincidence that white women, who frequented physicians more than men and were prescribed tonics to treat their ailments, comprised the bulk of the addicted population at the turn of

---

684 *Sears, Roebuck & Co. Catalogue*, (1897); Joseph F. Spillane, *Cocaine: From Medical Marvel to Modern Menace in the United States, 1884-1920* (Baltimore: Johns Hopkins University Press, 2000), 75.

685 "The Mariani Album: 1884-1913," in *The Coca Leaf and Cocaine Papers*, ed. George Andrews and David Solomon (New York: Harcourt Brace Jovanovich, 1975), 243-246.

686 Spillane, *Cocaine*, 79.

687 *Sears, Roebuck & Co. Catalogue*, (1902).

the century.[688] Bluntly put, doctors got many of their patients hooked on drugs.

"America's earliest narcotic addiction problems were iatrogenic in nature," notes modern addiction expert William L. White. "They were spawned by the isolation of morphine and codeine, the introduction of the hypodermic syringe, the widespread distribution of opiate drugs by physicians, and the aggressive marketing of opiate-laced medicines (such as Dr. McMunn's Elixir of Opium [sic] and Mrs. Winslow's Soothing Syrup) by a multimillion-dollar patent medicine industry whose sales grew from $3.5 million in 1859 to $74.5 million in 1903. Narcotic addiction arose in a nineteenth-century America that had few nonnarcotic alternatives for the management of acute and chronic disease or trauma."[689]

Patients could not trust their cures, whether prescribed by their doctors or ordered from a catalogue. There were bottled home-cures for addiction, promoted by the same patent medicine industry that also sold opium and alcohol remedies. "These medicinal specifics that claimed to cure narcotic addiction – products with such names as Denarco, Opacura, and Antidote, almost all containing high dosages of morphine – provided little more than disguised drug maintenance."[690]

The story of Mrs. E. W. Morse of Windsor, Vermont, offers a telling example of addiction spreading through those most trusted by patients. As recounted by *Our Day*, a journal published by the Woman's Temperance Publishing Association, Morse fell victim to opium for 13 years after being treated for an illness by her physician husband. "The disease manifests itself in various forms – the most pronounced effects upon the intellectual faculties are dullness of observation, impaired judgment, loss of memory," Morse warned, after recovering from her long addiction, "The will is weakened. The opium habit undermines the moral nature. It dulls the senses of right and wrong. Duties and responsibilities are regarded lightly under its influence and reluctantly attended to." To overcome the opium disease, Morse underwent seven months of treatment under the care of a physician from Winchendon, Massachusetts. The doctor gradually reduced her doses of opium, and together with "good nourishment"

---

688 Musto, *The American Disease*, 2-3; Courtwright, *Dark Paradise*, 42-52.
689 William L. White, "Trick or Treat? A Century of American Response to Heroin Addiction" in *One Hundred Years of Heroin*, ed. David F. Musto (Westport, Conn., 2002), 131-147.
690 Ibid.

and "suitable tonics," succeeded in turning the woman away from the ghastly habit.[691]

Morse's story bore three of the hallmarks of drug literature at the turn of the century. It featured a recovered habitué who has beaten the vile drug and is on a crusade to show the light to others who have fallen victim. The habitué is a physician's spouse who became addicted to a drug after treatment. And the recovery included treatment with unidentified tonics that in all likelihood contained opium.

Until the 20th century opium remained a staple in American medicine, especially in northern states, well after European doctors had adapted morphine into their practice. It was primarily dispensed as a cure in serums and tinctures such as laudanum, and was often taken without medical supervision. When typhus made its way down the East Coast a decade before the Civil War, local Southern physicians began treating the fever with a myriad of remedies. Some resorted to measures like bloodletting and purging, but others turned instead to nursing, opium and quinine.

For much of the 19th century, quinine, tincture of opium, paregoric (camphorated opium) and castor oil were the drugs most commonly found in Southern pharmacies. For all the spread of opium and its derivatives, however, whiskey remained the most popular panacea. A cure-all for nearly every disease, its popularity was due, if not to availability, then certainly to its low price. Whereas opium retailed for 50 cents to $1 per ounce, whiskey sold at 40-50 cents a gallon.[692] Well into the 20th century, in fact, physicians used alcohol – rather than morphine or even opium – to treat ailments.

That American doctors viewed alcohol as a universal panacea for so long is a testament to the limited medical education available in the country in the mid-19th century. Many physicians, in fact, had no formal medical education; most attained their training as apprentices, not in universities. With no government licensing system, the relative few who held medical degrees often received them from diploma mills.[693]

---

691 E. W. Morse, "What are the most effective methods of cure of the Opium Habit?" *Our Day* 9:55 (July, 1892), 530-533.
692 John Duffy, "Medical Practices in the Ante Bellum South," *The Journal of Southern History* 25:1 (1959), 62-65.
693 Richard H. Shryock, *Medical Licensing in America, 1650-1965* (Baltimore: Johns Hopkins University Press, 1967), 53; John S. Haller, *American Medicine in Transition* (Urbana: University of Illinois Press, 1981), 201 - 203.

In 1877, Illinois was the only state in the nation to require that doctors register their diplomas with the Board of Health for approval. The requirement was tellingly opposed by many older physicians, who claimed that it amounted to state interference in medicine.[694] Even the doctors who studied at respected medical schools rarely had access to modern instruments and books. The result was that the average American physician lagged far behind his German counterpart. High educational standards for doctors were first set in Prussia in the early 19th century, and by mid-century had been adopted in other German principalities.[695]

In America, by contrast, the professionalization of medicine was far longer in coming. It was not until the reform of American medical schools that followed the publication of the Flexner report in 1910 that American doctors attained a consistent standard in the practice of medicine.[696] Yet even into the mid-20th century, professionalism came slow to some parts of the country. Well into the 1940s, older doctors in some Southern states were known to freely dispense drugs to known addicts.[697]

The poor quality of medical education in the United States was heavily blamed for the spread of addiction in the country. Jansen B. Mattison, a leading expert on addiction at the time, was among those who testified that physicians and their malpractice were the cause of America's growing addiction problem. The solution, Mattison argued, was to curb physicians' propensity to dispense drugs.[698]

William Rosser Cobbe, a journalist and recovered addict, was even more strident in his condemnation of doctors: "Understanding, as they undoubtedly must, the weakness of humanity, it is incomprehensible that physicians should resort to opium with such frequency and use it so recklessly."[699] For most of the 19th century, physicians in America relied on

---

694 Shryock, *Medical Licensing in America*, 201 - 203.
695 Ibid., 13, 43-44.
696 Stephen J. Kunitz, "Professionalism and Social Control in the Progressive Era: The Case of the Flexner Report," *Social Problems* 22:1 (1974), 16-27.
697 David Courtwright, Herman Joseph and Don Des Jarlais, *Addicts Who Survived: An Oral History of Narcotic Use in America, 1923-1965* (Knoxville: University of Tennessee Press, 1989), 254.
698 J. B. Mattison, "The Responsibility of the Profession in the Production of Opium Inebriety," *Medical and Surgical Reporter* 38 (1878), 101-104. See Charles W. Earle, "The Opium Habit," *Chicago Medical Review* 2 (1880), 442-446.
699 William Rosser Cobbe, *Doctor Judas: A Portrayal of the Opium Habit* (Chicago, 1895), 171.

literary examples, rather than medical ones, to describe the habitué. Alonzo Calkins relied on Coleridge's poems and Quincey's "Confessions,"[700] while Harry Kane turned to Charles Dickens in the "Mystery of Edwin Drood."[701] Doctors would eventually develop a more scientific basis for discussing addiction and its etiology, but it would not be until the early 20th century.[702]

Indeed, the issue of drug addiction itself played a key role in the professionalization of medicine in the United States. The American Medical Association asserted its monopoly over the medical profession in part by insisting that only professional physicians be allowed to prescribe medicine and drugs, including opiates.[703]

The public increasingly clamored for more professionalism from doctors, as well as more accountability from drug manufacturers.[704] With the Socialist and progressive press aflame with stories of patent medicine and processed food poisoning the American stomach in 1906,[705] President Theodore Roosevelt signed into law the Pure Foods and Drugs Act. The law, which required that the ingredients in patent medicines be clearly listed, was primarily aimed at curbing the rampant mislabeling of patent medicines that brought unsuspecting users closer to drugs than they had imagined.[706]

---

700 Calkins, *Opium and the Opium Appetite*, 84, 91-93.
701 Kane, *Opium-smoking in American and China*, 46-50.
702 Gordon Coonfield, "Mapping Addiction," (Ph.D. dissertation, Michigan Technological University, 2003), 19.
703 Timothy Alton Hickman, "The Double Meaning of Addiction: Habitual Narcotic Use and the Logic of Professionalizing Medical Authority in the United States, 1900-1920," in *Altering American Consciousness: The History of Alcohol and Drug Use in the United States, 1800-2000*, ed. Sarah W. Tracy and Caroline Jean Acker (Amherst: University of Massachusetts Press, 2004), 189
704 Terry and Pellens, *The Opium Problem*, 74-76.
705 See for example, Upton Sinclair, *The Jungle* (1906); Samuel Hopkins Adams, "The Great American Fraud," *Collier's* (7 October 1905) at http://www.museumo fquackery.com/ephemera/oct7-01.htm (Last access: 22.1.2016).
706 After the Supreme Court decided in 1911 that the Pure Foods and Drugs Act referred only to the ingredients of medicine and not their therapeutic value, Adams published a series of articles in the *Collier's*: "Fraud Medicines Own Up," (20 January 1912), "Tricks of the Trade," (17 February 1912), "The Law, the Label and the Liars," (13 April 1912), and "Fraud Above the Law," (11 May 1912). Public uproar led politicians to amend the law.

In 1883, Mattison, echoing the works of Eduard Levinstein in Germany, dropped yet another bombshell: many physicians themselves suffered from addiction, to the point of being the leading professional group to be addicted, comprising in some cities thirty to forty percent of the addicted population. He cited their ignorance regarding the effects of drugs as the primary reason for their addiction, but also mentioned stress and curiosity, yet discounted proximity and easy access to the drugs.[707]

Three decades later it became common knowledge among doctors that addicted physicians tended to treat their patients and families with drugs, explaining why wives of addicted doctors were addicts too.[708] The stories of cocaine-crazed doctors that appeared in the press in the years to follow, therefore, should be read in light of Mattison's warnings.[709] Addicted doctors were seen as a menace to society; a fact that resonates to this day.

According to the annual report of the Wisconsin State Board of Medical Examiners of 1948, of the four licenses revoked that year, three were for narcotic violations. Twelve physicians were investigated in conjunction with the Federal Bureau of Narcotics, of whom two voluntarily entered a state institution, two were committed to a state institution, one was committed to a federal institution, three were making effort to rehabilitate themselves and four were still under surveillance. As for alcoholics, only one was investigated and his case was pending.[710]

The birth of the panic was clear at hand. Drugs, whether opium, cocaine or marijuana, went hand in hand with public uproars. They were associ-

---

707 J. B. Mattison, "Opium Addiction Among Medical Men," *Medical Record*, vol. 23 (1883), 621-623 reproduced in *Yesterday's Addicts: American Society and Drug Abuse, 1865-1920*, ed. H. Wayne Morgan (Norman: University of Oklahoma Press, 1974), 62-66; idem, "Morphinism in Medical Men," *Journal of the American Medical Association*, 186:5 (1894), 186-188. An earlier version of this idea was delivered in a talk before the *American Association for the Cure of Inebriates* in 1878, see idem, "The Responsibility of the Profession in the Production of Opium Inebriety," 101-104. Mattison's claim was supported by various articles he published. For example, J. B. Mattison, "Triple Narcotic Addiction: Opium, Alcohol, Cocaine," *Times and Register* 21:22 (1890), 504.
708 Courtwright, *Dark Paradise*, 49, 211n. 114.
709 J. B. Mattison, "The Dangers of Cocaine," *Medical News*, vol. 50/16 (1887), 446. Mattison sent this article to the editors of *Medical News* to alert them that, contrary to what they have published in a previous issue, the malefic effects of cocaine were known and recorded.
710 *Annual Report: Wisconsin State Board of Medical Examiners* (1 July 1948), *Arch. Div. Wisc. Hist. Soc.*, series 1616, box 2, folder 4.

ated with all that was wrong with 19th and early 20th century America: promiscuous sex, interracial relations, crime and uncontrollable Chinese, Blacks and Mexicans. Exacerbating public fears, patent medicines and poor medical education were blamed for spreading drug use, as Americans began to describe the phenomenon in a medical term: a drug epidemic.

The two key actors harping on public opinion played with the common American's fears. The press had a field day, while selling more copies, instilled the fear of the spread of an incurable disease or a violent former slave running amok with cocaine in his blood. And doctors, upon realizing their own fault in spreading the disease, tried to exonerate themselves by insisting on a monopoly over dispensing drug prescriptions. The question is, therefore, not why politicians acted against drugs; but rather, why did it take them so long.

9. Moral Diseases

Racial prejudice was unquestionably a major catalyst for the change in America's attitude toward drugs, but it was hardly the sole reason Americans learned to loathe them. Toward the turn of the 19th century, addiction increasingly became accepted as a disease that caused men and women to lose their free will.[711] The pernicious disease was perceived not just as a physical and mental ailment, but as a moral evil as well, leading to widespread belief that drugs were, simply put, bad. The result was a hybrid best described as a moral disease.

Alcohol and inebriates troubled physicians well before drugs and drug addicts. In a survey conducted by the Massachusetts State Board of Health in 1870, 97 of 164 physicians responded that alcohol was "very destructive to life and health" or "injurious in a greater or less degree."[712] Contemporary doctors suggested that help, rather than chastisement, could relieve the suffering of drunkards, resulting in a compassionate understanding of alcoholics, if only for a brief period of time. The softening of attitudes even found its way into legislation and health care, with some states building special asylums for inebriates, a departure from the standard practice of condemning alcoholics to the madhouse.[713]

---

711 On whether addiction was a new or an old concept touched by physicians, rather than men of the cloth, see Harry G. Levine, "The Discovery of Addiction: Changing Conceptions of Habitual Drunkenness in America," *Journal of Studies on Alcohol* 39:1 (1978), 143-174; Roy Porter, "The Drinking Man's Disease: The 'Pre-History' of Alcoholism in Georgian Britain," *British Journal of Addiction* 80:4 (1985), 385-396; Jessica Warner, "Before there was 'Alcoholism': Lessons from the Medieval Experience with Alcohol," *Contemporary Drug Problems* 19:3 (1992), 409-428; Peter Ferentzy, "From Sin to Disease: Differences and Similarities between Past and Current Conceptions of Chronic Drunkenness," *Contemporary Drug Problems* 28:3 (2001), 363-390.

712 Robert Druit, "Drunkenness as Modified by Race; with an analysis of the Report on Drunkenness in Various Parts of the World, issued by the Massachusetts State Board of Health," *Medical Times and Gazette* 1 (1871), 420-423.

713 Arnold Jaffe, *Addiction Reform in the Progressive Age: Scientific and Social Responses to Drug Dependence in the United States, 1870-1930* (New York: Arno Press, 1981 [1976]), 16-17; Mariana Valverde, *Diseases of the Will:*

The majority of doctors in America, however, continued to believe that the disease was a vice requiring only willpower to overcome. With public debate on the issue still raging, the American Medical Association's section on Public Hygiene and State Medicine convened in June 1876 in Philadelphia to once and for all settle on a definition of drunkenness. Neither those believing inebriety to be a disease nor those convinced of drunkards' moral depravity were able to win the day, and in the end, alcoholism was declared to be both a disease and a vice – a moral disease. The medical association went on to proclaim that specialized institutions had to be erected to treat the morally sick.[714] The physicians' call to action was apiece with long-held views on the drinking disease in America. From Benjamin Rush's essays in the late 18th century onward, discussion of alcohol in the country was heavily steeped in moral condemnation, as those who wished to prove the existence of the disease were also those who wished to reform humans into better, more responsible beings.[715]

The mystery that challenged contemporary doctors was as simple to articulate, as it was difficult to decipher: Why did some succumb to the disease, while others did not? For some, drunkenness, and certainly habitual drunkenness, was merely a vice, a temptation that god had presented before man to test his will and virtue.[716] This religious explana-

---

Alcohol and the Dilemmas of Freedom (Cambridge: Cambridge University Press, 1998), 2, 51-67.

714 Tracy, Alcoholism in America, 26. Thomas D. Crothers, in his somewhat inaccurate history on the history of the disease theory of alcoholism, explains the tension. See idem, The Disease of Inebriety from Alcohol, Opium and Other Narcotic Drugs, its Etiology, Pathology, Treatment and Medico-Legal Relations (New York, 1893), 20-21. A slightly more elaborate account is found in idem, Inebriety: A Clinical Treatise on the Etiology, Symptomology, Neurosis, Psychosis and Treatment and the Medico-Legal Relations (Cincinnati, 1911), 24-28.

715 Benjamin Rush, Sermons to the Rich and Studious, on Temperance and Exercise (London, 1772); idem, An Inquiry into the Effects of the Spirituous Liquors upon the Human Body, and their Influence upon the Happiness of Society (Edinburgh, 1791 [1784]); idem, Essays, Literary, Moral & Philosophical (Philadelphia, 1798 [1796]), 258.

716 The religious explanation of temptation can be traced back to pre-Christian Greece, where the civilized Greeks had to resist temptation from drinking like Barbarians, and therefore becoming like them. See James Davidson, Courtesans and Fishcakes: The Consuming Passions of Classical Athens (New York: St. Martin's Press, 1998), 139-144. On Christianity, whether Catholic or Protestant, see Beverly Ann Tlusty, Bacchus and Civic Order: The Culture of Drink in Early

tion might have been enough for priests and pious doctors, but was not enough for secular physicians who sought to heal their patients using science rather than prayer. If the drink was not solely a sin, then something must be either wrong with the drinker, or with the drink itself.

If one assumed that the drinker was at fault, one could claim that the individual constitution or mental capacities of the inebriate were too weak. If, however, the drink were at fault, then alcohol itself must be poisonous, and if it were drank enough, anyone would succumb to the disease. Some said alcohol, and later drugs, was intrinsically poisonous and that it attacked the nervous system and the organs. Others argued that an individual's constitution or dosage would determine the pace of poisoning.[717]

The second question confounding doctors at the time was even more elemental: Why did people drink? In addition to moral weakness, physicians debated social causes for the disease. In the America of the second half of the 19th century, modern civilization greeted the flood of new urban dwellers. Americans migrated in droves from the countryside to cities, where they encountered an industrial, fast-paced and tense life.

The influential French psychiatrist Bénédict-Augustin Morel claimed in 1857 that modernity ultimately resulted in speed, noise and vice, from sexual promiscuity to obsessive drinking. "Mental degeneracy," as Morel labeled it, was hereditary and was caused by an external disturbance to the nervous system. Civilizations' sensory overload proved to be so powerful as to pass the ailments down the generations, he argued, with each generation suffering more than its forebears, eventually resulting in extinction. The causes of degeneration were, first and foremost, hereditary, but could also be contracted by intoxication from opium or alcohol, malnutrition, nervous disorders or poor hygiene. Degeneration was a mental process that could be identified by distinct physical markings. Morel dubbed it "stigmata," perhaps echoing a religious bent.[718]

Modern Germany (Charlottesville: University of Virginia Press, 2001), 70-76, 82-84; Valverde, *Diseases of the Will*, 14-15; Hasso Spode, *Die Macht der Trunkenheit: Kultur- und Sozialgeschichte des Alkohols in Deutschland* (Opladen: Leske & Budrich, 1993), 117.

717   Edward L. Youmans, *Alcohol and the Constitution of Man* (New York, 1853), 71-74.

718   Richard F. Wetzell, *Inventing the Criminal: A History of German Criminology, 1880-1945* (Chapel Hill: University of North Carolina Press, 2000), 46-47; Marcus Aurin, "Chasing the Dragon: The Cultural Metamorphosis of Opium in the United States, 1825-1935," *Medical Anthropology Quarterly* 14:3 (2000),

Neurasthenia, popularized by American psychiatrist George M. Beard (1839-1883) in 1869, was yet another disease caused by the modernization of society. It caused a weakening of the nerves, and was triggered by the appearance of the telegraph, sewing machine and other industrial devices in the West. Neurasthenia, like Morel's degeneracy, was both physical and hereditary, but did not necessarily condemn the sufferer to eternal hell. The neurasthenic was not insane, but merely ill. The disease was simply an unfortunate byproduct of modernity; one that society would eventually learn to overcome through advances in science and medicine. [719]

Americans, who were more dynamic and open to the wonders of modernity than their European brethren, succeeded in convincing themselves that they were more susceptible to neurasthenia, and consequently, to the drinking disease and drug addiction.[720] The more nervous a person was, the greater his or her susceptibility to stimulants and narcotics.[721] Thus, according to Beard, women, who by nature were more delicate and nervous than men, were more susceptible to be addicted to stimulants and opium, a notion that was repeated by numerous contemporary physicians.[722]

Neurasthenia, the precursor to what is now known as chronic fatigue syndrome, became accepted wisdom in the United States and even gained acceptance in France and Germany. The concept of neurasthenia, in fact,

---

419-420; Charles E. Rosenberg, *No Other Gods: On Science and American Social Thought* (Baltimore: Johns Hopkins University Press, 1976), 43-44.

719 German physicians used the term *Nervenschwäche*, or nervous weakness to describe similar symptoms to neurasthenia before Beard coined the term. See *Journal of Mental Science* (*British Journal of Psychiatry*) 33:144 (1888), 602-603.

720 Leslie E. Keeley, *The Morphine Eater; or, From Bondage to Freedom* (Dwight, Ill., 1881), 20, 44-47 and Edward Thwing, "American Life as Related to Inebriety," *Quarterly Journal of Inebriety* 10 (1888), 43-50, both reproduced in H. Wayne Morgan, *Yesterday's Addicts: American Society and Drug Abuse, 1865-1929* (Norman: University of Oklahoma Press, 1974), 92-100; Jaffe, *Addiction Reform in the Progressive Age*, 19; Rosenberg, *No Other Gods*, 98-108.

721 Timothy A. Hickman, "'Mania Americana': Narcotic Addiction and Modernity in the United States, 1870-1920," *Journal of American History* 90:4 (2004), 1269-1295.

722 George M. Beard, *Stimulants and Narcotics: Medically, Philosophically, and Morally Considered* (New York, 1871), 138-139; Stephen R. Kandall, *Substance and Shadow: Women and Addiction in the United States* (Cambridge MA: Harvard University Press, 1999), 28-30.

was essential to the development of Americans' understanding of the drinking disease.[723] In his 1871 book "Stimulants and Narcotics," Beard drew a distinction between the two types of substances. Stimulants, he argued, were those agents that "correct, economize, or intensify the forces of the system," while "narcotics are those agents which produce greater or less degree of paralysis of some portion of the nervous system."[724] Any drug could be either a narcotic or a stimulant, depending on dosage; smaller doses led to stimulation, while larger amounts led to a dampening of the senses.

Since amounts differed from one organism to the other, and from one race to another, Beard divided drugs into three categories: substances that contained alcohol; substances that were drunk, injected, smoked, snuffed or chewed, such as tobacco, coffee, cocoa, chicory and opium; and combustible substances, such as chloroform.[725] The primacy of alcohol was clear, as it received a category of its own, though it arguably could have fit into either of the other categories.

Beard believed that chronic alcoholism was "a degeneracy of the brain, resulting from long excess in alcoholic liquors." Dipsomania, methomania or oinomania were specific types of monomania, a disease of the brain caused by excessive drinking that manifested itself in the inability to stop drinking. Opiomania was effectively the same disease, other than being caused by opium rather than alcohol.[726] Beard's followers pointed toward inebriety as an example of neurasthenia, bearing many of the markings of the disease. Beard himself, however, preferred the term "intemperance,"[727] dubbing it first a disease and then a vice:

> Intemperance from disease is the form which is most frequently found among the intellectual and cultivated; intemperance from a bad organization is the form which is most frequently found among the ignorant and degraded, and among the so-called criminal classes; and yet both forms appear in all grades of life. Some men are born to intemperance, just as the sparks are prone to fly upward. Crime of all kinds is to a certain extent organic, and many of our

---

723 Jaffe, *Addiction Reform in the Progressive Age*, 19; Rosenberg, *No Other Gods*, 108; Jan Ellen Goldstein, *Console and Classify: The French Psychiatric Profession in the Nineteenth Century* (Chicago: University of Chicago Press, 2001), 335-336.

724 Beard, *Stimulants and Narcotics*, 5-6.

725 Ibid., 6-7.

726 Ibid., 61, 64.

727 Ibid., 63.

criminals are often subjected to their own evil organizations, even more than to the laws.[728]

Beard's work on intemperance was rife with contradictions between vice and disease, and social and racial biases certainly influenced his work. But while his peers discarded his theory on stimulants and narcotics relatively quickly, Beard managed to set the parameters of medical debate on addiction in America, particularly regarding heredity, for decades to come.

In a study conducted in 1888 at the Inebriates' Home in Fort Hamilton, New York, for example, no less than 265 of the 600 individuals examined showed inebriate ancestry, primarily patrilineal. Another 38 cases at the Inebriates' Home showed other insane ancestry.[729] The study was taken as firm evidence that inebriety was degenerative and hereditary, and several medical authorities went on to add that it attacked the nerves of the brains and the spinal cord.[730]

Widespread acceptance for such theories, however, would be longer in coming, and were held back by well-entrenched views on individual responsibility. The Association of Medical Superintendents of American Institutions for the Insane asserted in 1875 that drunkards disrupted the regular workings of their institutions, which were dedicated to more severely ill patients. The association's official journal even called into question the very notion of the "inebriate disease," pointing as evidence to the low cure rate. There could be, the association argued, "only two possibly interpretations for these apparent contradictions: either the diseased were being released uncured, or the disease was drunkenness and the cure was simply sobering up."[731]

Other doctors refused, on moral grounds, to acknowledge drunkenness or addiction as a disease. "It is becoming altogether too customary in these days to speak of vices as disease, and to excuse the men and women for the performance of indulgence of certain acts which not only ruin themselves and families but brings burden on the community," Charles W. Earle wrote in 1880. "I propose to fight this pernicious doctrine as long as is necessary." Yet even Earle, moral convictions notwithstanding,

---

728   Ibid., 70-72.
729   Lewis D. Mason, "The Etiology of Dipsomania and Heredity of 'Alcoholic Inebriety'" *Quarterly Journal of Inebriety* (1888), reported in *The American Journal of Psychology* 2:3 (1889), 500.
730   Jaffe, *Addiction Reform in the Progressive Age*, 30-31.
731   Ibid., 28-29.

conceded that the continual consumption of drugs would eventually turn into a disease, and that physicians were overly administering drugs to their patients.[732] Old views retained their hold on many physicians, but a slight ideological shift was underway.

On November 29, 1870, preachers, doctors and asylum directors from the Northeast and Midwest founded the American Association for the Cure of Inebriates. From its inception, the association was dedicated to the belief that inebriety could be cured by medical means. Doctors, rather than law enforcement, were to be entrusted with treating drunkenness.[733] The founders of the association aimed to change the manner in which the public saw drunkenness, turning it from a vice to a disease.[734]

The American Association for the Cure of Inebriates was based on the work of Joseph Edward Turner, who insisted as early as 1846 that inebriety was a disease, and a curable one at that.[735] The organization quickly grew, and succeeded in persuading both private and public institutions to invest in treatment. By 1878, 32 facilities were either open or soon to open. In 1888, the organization changed its name to the American Association for the Study and Cure of Inebriates, and in 1904 it merged with the American Medical Temperance Association, perhaps hinting at the political and moral stance these physicians ended up regarding prohibition.

Science led to prohibition, or so claimed its proponents. Mary Weeks Burnett, a registered nurse who presided over the Frances E. Willard National Temperance Hospital in Chicago, advocated the total prohibition of alcohol, save for medicinal uses. As early as 1889, she argued that without liquor, the neurotic cases caused by alcohol would not exist.[736]

---

732 Charles W. Earle, "The Opium Habit," *Chicago Medical Review* 2 (1880), 442-446.

733 Jaffe, *Addiction Reform in the Progressive Age*, 21-22; William L. White, "Trick or Treat? A Century of American Response to Heroin Addiction" in *One Hundred Years of Heroin*, David F. Musto (Westport CN: Auburn House, 2002), 131-147.

734 Tracy, *Alcoholism in America*, 1-2.

735 Crothers, *The Disease of Inebriety from Alcohol*, 22-23.

736 "Prohibition and Inebriety," *Journal of Mental Science* (*British Journal of Psychiatry*), 5:149 (1889), 121-122. The hospital was opened in 1886, but was incorporated a few years later. See Martha M. Allen, *Alcohol-A Dangerous and Unnecessary Medicine, How and Why: What medical Writers Say* (New York, 1900), 41-47.

Her logic may have been straight, but impractical. Physicians were unable to convince the public to stop drinking until they were able to take advantage of the propaganda machine wielded by the temperance movement.

The alliance at the turn of the century made for rather odd bedfellows. Members of the Association for the Study and Cure of Inebriates often ridiculed as unscientific and overly moralizing the work of the Woman's Christian Temperance Union, unquestionably one of the main engines driving Prohibition.[737] And yet in the first years of the 20th century, the president of the inebriates association sat on the scientific temperance advisory board of the temperance union.

The cooperation between the two organizations was portrayed more as a pragmatic political move than a shift in the medical understanding of the disease.[738] But it proved to be its undoing. By the beginning of World War I, the Association for the Study and Cure of Inebriates was barely active, and the hospitals it had helped found had nearly emptied of patients. Prohibition spelled the end of the Association; with alcohol banned, its *raison d'être* no longer held.[739]

From its earliest years, internal rifts tore the Association. An ideological struggle between moralistic reformers and their more scientifically minded brethren unfolded at the organization's annual meetings in the late 1870s. In 1876 the association's moralist members repeated calls heard at the American Medical Association's meeting in the same year to distinguish between the vice and the disease, but the Association for the Study and Cure of Inebriates ultimately decided against committing itself to a moralistic view of addiction. The association later argued that while drunkenness may have originated in sin, its end result – inebriety – was a disease of the nervous system, and should be treated as such.[740] Thomas D. Crothers, the editor of the association's journal, later celebrated the anti-moralistic stand, arguing that "the decline of the moralizing influence

---

737 "Alcoholism," *Medical News* 59:4 (1891), 109. The argument in this article is that in the same manner that opium and morphine are not banned from medical practices, even though they can potentially cause a disease, so should alcohol not be taken away from the medicine cabinet.

738 Tracy, *Alcoholism in America*, 78-84.

739 Jaffe, *Addiction Reform in the Progressive Age*, 27, 35, 43-44. For a similar development in Britain, see Virginia Berridge, "Morbid Cravings: The Emergence of Addiction," *British Journal of Addiction* 80 (1985), 233-243.

740 Jaffe, *Addiction Reform in the Progressive Age,* 28

eventually led to greater scientific respect for, and interest in, the new association."[741]

Moral issues aside, the reformist bloc in the association demanded that inebriety, as an involuntary disease, ought to be treated by doctors, rather than imprisoned, as was custom in the late 19th and early 20th centuries. They believed that inebriety was both a mental disorder and a physical disease; consequently, the diseased bore less responsibility for their actions than the average man. In other words, reformers argued that inebriates who committed crimes should bear limited to no criminal responsibility for their actions; and, treatment under the capable care of physicians, rather than incarceration under unprofessional prison wardens, was the proper way to deal with the disease.[742] The American reformers wished, in essence, to imitate the German law governing criminal responsibility and drunkenness. Their efforts, however, would not come to pass.

The American public had – and still has – little patience for drunkards. After all, drunkenness and drug use inspired stupor, loose morals, poor fiscal responsibility and an uncanny inability to pay debts – all of which were vices, not diseases. Americans and their politicians were not in the habit of rewarding vice by incarceration in a hospital, and preferred that treatment be provided in prison. In late 19th century America, unlike in Germany at the time, individuals were held responsible for their own fate, and if they transgressed they were expected to bear the punishment. This was even true for a while with the insane and those who today might be considered unfit to stand trial.[743]

Crothers, for example, believed in the coercive confinement of inebriates in hospitals. "Sanitary science teaches clearly that no one had a right to destroy himself and peril the health and comfort of others," he declared in an October 1893 lecture to the American Public Health Association. "The inebriate is a criminal pauper and madman, whose conduct forfeits all rights to personal liberty, and who is practically an outlaw to his own and all other interests. The only remedy is legal control and quarantining in hospitals; not as criminals, but as diseased and helpless."[744]

---

741 Quoted in Ibid., 23.
742 Ibid., 49.
743 Jaffe, *Addiction Reform in the Progressive Age*, 56.
744 Quoted in Ibid., 53. See also, Crothers, *The Disease of Inebriety from Alcohol*, 28, 117, 146-152. On the irregular treatment of drunkenness in the Criminal courts in England, see George H. Savage, "Drunkenness in Relation to Criminal

Crothers was among the most ardent proponents of defining inebriety as a disease, and has since been hailed by historians as one of the more humane doctors to treat inebriates and addicts in the 19th century. Yet even he treated the victim of the medical disease as a social villain.[745] His views of inebriates, one could argue, differed less from those of his less humane contemporaries than what has been previously suggested. His proposed method of dealing with drunkards – criminal paupers and madmen in his words – differed primarily in the place of treatment. Instead of prison, he and his colleagues advocated for sending society's drunkards to the hospital.[746]

A more critical interpretation of Crothers' advocacy is that the disease concept of addiction was nothing more than an attempt to usurp the powers of incarceration from policemen, shifting the right to persecute, prosecute and incarcerate the drunkards from lawyers and prison guards to doctors and their nurses.

Although he claimed otherwise, Crothers viewed drunkards through a moralistic lens. Perhaps his lens was not as shaded as the ones worn by his more moralistic colleagues, but it was moralistic nonetheless, in stark contrast to most German physicians of the time, whose more objective and scientific approach sent them on a path to sterilize severe alcoholics.

In Crothers and physicians of his stripe, one finds a classic example of professional hypocrisy. Doctors insisted on calling alcoholism a disease, claiming that they had not condemned their patients, for they were sick and not fallen souls. Yet they continued to treat them as if they were fallen souls who indulged in a vice: the perfect social villains. One could argue that it was so because doctors started viewing diseases as an unnatural aberration in the human organism, and any aberration was an evil to be smitten, rather than a natural phenomenon to be dealt with.[747] It seems reasonable to suspect, however, that the American Public Health Association's attitude toward drunkenness was at least in part shaped by the general moralistic attitude toward drunkenness in America.

Civilization and modernity, the culprits in Beard's neurasthenia, were not the sole cause of inebriates. Blame for the rise in drunkards was also

---

Responsibility," *Journal of Mental Science* (*British Journal of Psychiatry*) 32:137 (1886), 23-30.
745 Jaffe, *Addiction Reform in the Progressive Age*, 54.
746 Ibid., 51-52.
747 Grob, *The Deadly Truth*.

assigned to the Civil War that tore the United States apart in the early 1860s. As one physician explained in 1876, wars induced the alcohol disease on those whose nerves were too weak to handle the constant excitement of four years of industrialized warfare;[748] nor where physicians the only ones to view the war as a cause for inebriety. The deputy governor of the eastern branch of the Soldiers' Homes, the sanitaria that housed disabled war veterans, said in 1878:

> Drunkenness is the chief source of disorder; but even that is periodic, following hard upon pay-day. Seven years' experience has taught me to look with charity upon the failings of these poor men, or wrecks of men, rather; and I can not help thinking, when my patience is most tried by the deceit and ingratitude of the bad ones – I say, I can not help asking, how much are they to blame? When I know they were initiated into the army upon whiskey; had whiskey forced into them, as a *prophylactic*, before they were wounded, or taken sick, and finally had whiskey poured into them, in hospital, either as a stimulant, to quiet pain, or as a sedative, to keep them quiet otherwise.[749]

Sixty percent of those who were dishonorably discharged from the Soldiers' Homes were inebriates. Furthermore, it was believed that "a large percentage of the mortality by violence, crime or exposure" was due to the bad habit of drinking.[750] Blaming the Civil War for causing the drinking disease was but a mere echo of complaints raised as early as Napoleon's invasion of Russia in 1812.[751]

As the debate raged in the 1880s and 1890s over whether war, modernity or some other societal ill caused inebriety, various definitions for the disease took turns in the limelight. Crothers wrote in 1893 that drunkenness could be divided into two main categories, inebriety and dipsomania.[752] Inebriety was suffered by accidental or incidental inebriates, emotional inebriates, solitary inebriates, and pauper inebriates. Inebriety, therefore, had a strong connection to crime, poverty and prostitution, resulting from brain and nerve degeneration. Dipsomania, on the other

---

748 Tracy, *Alcoholism in America*, 63-64.
749 "The Soldiers' Home at Dayton, Ohio," *National Repository* 3 (1878), 202-203.
750 Ibid.
751 C. von Brühl-Cramer, *Ueber die Trunksucht und eine rationelle Heilmethode derselben* (Berlin, 1819), 10-11.
752 On the meaning of the various terms to describe the drinking disease in America, see Tracy, *Alcoholism in America*, 25-62. Over time, the American medical establishment abandoned the term inebriety and began to espouse the more medical sounding dipsomania and alcoholism.

hand, was a form of neurosis that ebbed and flowed within the body, occasionally attacking it like epilepsy, hysteria or paranoia.[753]

Dipsomania manifested itself in three ways: acute, periodic and chronic. The periodic form of dipsomania is notable for being induced by physical injury. Those suffering from this type of dipsomania possessed no morals, Crothers argued, nor could they be blamed for their state as they became ill through no fault of their own. Such patients "show this perversion, or rather, absence of morals, in almost all their dealings with their friends and relations, and it is on this account that the disease is such a scourge to the friends and relatives," he declared. "The patient will give the most solemn promises not to take any stimulant, but the backs of those whom he has made the promise are no sooner turned than he violates it, either by obtaining the liquor himself or not refusing the first or any temptation that is set before him."[754]

Chronic dipsomaniacs, by far the most common, were people who drank constantly, resulting in lazy and base individuals. Their lack of morals resembled that of the periodic dipsomaniac, who often suffered from complications of the disease, such as delirium tremens and diseases of the liver.[755] According to Crothers, heredity did not play a major role in inebriety and dipsomania, but rather signified a tendency toward the disease. Even if the progeny of alcoholics did not suffer from the drinking disease, he concluded, they were almost always feeble and degenerate.[756]

Leslie E. Keeley (1836-1900), perhaps the doctor most responsible for convincing the American public that habitual drunkenness was a disease,[757] was skeptical about whether inebriety was indeed hereditary. Keeley believed inebriety was an illness like any other, and was suspicious

---

753 Crothers, *The Disease of Inebriety from Alcohol*, 27-28. Crothers definition of dipsomania is a modification of the thesis of his friend Joseph Parish, who believed that alcohol inebriety was first, and foremost, a hereditary neurosis, not to be confused with the vice of drunkenness that often led to crime. Parish claimed that the difference between the vice and the disease was in the physical longing to alcohol. See Joseph Parish, *Alcoholic Inebriety from a Medical Standpoint* (Philadelphia, 1883), 11-39.

754 Crothers, *The Disease of Inebriety from Alcohol*, 29-33.

755 Ibid., 35-38.

756 Ibid., 152-160.

757 Tracy, *Alcoholism in America*, 84-91. For the favorable reception of Keeley and the idea that dipsomania was a disease, see "Dipsomania a Disease," *Chicago Daily Tribune* (11 October 1891), 12.

of uncertain general causes for it. "People do not inherit disease," he wrote. "They inherit a weak resistance and 'catch' the disease. Inebriety, in relation to heredity, reaches back no further than the cradle and the nursery." He claimed that the same was true for all forms of inebriety – irrespective of whether it was caused by alcohol, opium or any other drug.[758] Alcohol was a poison that penetrated the nerve cells, modified them and created a perpetual need that culminated in addiction. Since the strength of nerves varied from one person to another, depending on both nature and nurture, Keeley could explain why some people were more susceptible to the disease than others.

If indeed inebriety was a disease like any other, a treatment was also possible, and Keeley let America know that he held the patent for a cure.[759] The "Keeley Cure," a comfortable regimen in an institute where shots of "gold bichloride" were given to patients, promised a near 100 percent success rate in curing all forms of inebriety.

At the height of the Keeley cure in 1896, no less than 118 institutes were treating an estimated 500,000 inebriates. The commercial success of the cure was undeniable, but physicians, particularly members of the American Medical Association and the American Association for the Study and Cure of Inebriates, remained unconvinced. Indeed, they dismissed Keeley and the widespread advertising of his cure as quackery.[760]

Compared to many physicians in the United States at the time, however, Keeley was hardly an uneducated amateur. He attained his medical degree from Rush Medical College in Chicago and served as a physician for the Union army during the Civil War. He seemed to have deviated from the American Medical Association norm in advertising his cures, but as regards the cure itself he was not much different from his peers, both those with and without medical degrees. Perhaps envious of his success, physicians accused Keeley of misleading the public and promising success rates that were not achievable. He probably believed in his cure, and some

---

758 Leslie E. Keeley, *The Non-Heredity of Inebriety* (Chicago, 1896), 196.

759 Morgan, *Drugs in America*, 75-83. See also Courtwright, *Dark Paradise*, 250-251 n55.

760 Lakehurst Sanitarium (Oakville, Ontario), *A Popular Treatise on Drunkenness and Opium Habit and their Successful Treatment with the Double Chloride of Gold-The Only Cure* (Toronto, c. 1890-1900), at: http://www.archive.org/details/ alberta_01294 (Last access: 22.1.2016).

patients were pleased with it, especially since the cure required attending physicians to give their patients more attention than they normally would.[761] Whether he was a quack or not, even Keeley's many detractors acknowledged that he was instrumental in convincing countless Americans that inebriety was indeed a disease, and a curable one too.[762]

Other for-profit addiction centers operated franchises throughout the country. Two such centers were the Neal Institute and the Gatlin Institute, which catered to alcoholics and drug addicts who could afford the treatment. Some institutes, such as the Keeley, gave discounts to addicts of limited means. Specialists also ran private institutions dedicated to the treatment of drug addiction, including the De Quincey Home, operated by Harry H. Kane in New York City; the Brooklyn Home for Habitués, operated by Jansen B. Mattison in Brooklyn; and the Walnut Lodge Hospital, operated by Thomas D. Crothers in Hartford, Connecticut.

Crothers proclaimed that asylums like his would help wipe away the "tramp problem" that went hand in hand with alcohol.[763] The link between alcohol and pauperism had, by the end of the 19th century, been firmly established. The Committee of Fifty, a body of lawyers, scholars and industrialists that studied the alcohol question over the course of the 1890s, concluded in 1899 that 25 percent of paupers in America, whether born in the New World or not, owed their financial state either directly or indirectly to liquor. In almshouses, matters were even worse, with no less than 37 percent of paupers finding their way there because of the drink.[764]

In addition to the asylums run by Crothers and others, there were also institutions run by religious and temperance organizations, as well as county- and state-owned hospitals. In 1857, the New York Senate and Assembly passed an act calling for the establishment of the New York State Inebriate Asylum, the first hospital in the world dedicated to treating the drinking disease. The asylum, which opened in 1864, was the product of a public-private partnership. Since government support was not enough,

---

761 Tracy, *Alcoholism in America*, 87-91.
762 Ibid., 91.
763 Jim Baumohl, "Inebriate Institutions in North America, 1840-1920," *British Journal of Addiction* 85 (1990), 1187-1204.
764 James H. Timberlake, *Prohibition and the Progressive Movement, 1900-1925* (Cambridge MA: Harvard University Press, 1963), 57; John Koren (an investigation made for the Committee of Fifty under the direction of Henry W. Farnam), *Economic Aspects of the Liquor Problem* (Boston, 1899), 21-29; Committee of Fifty, *The Liquor Problem*, 108-120.

Joseph Edward Turner, the secretary of the asylum's board of trustees, turned to temperance activists and churches for help in raising the money required to complete the project.[765]

In the decades to come, several other states followed suit. In 1893, the State Hospital for Dipsomaniacs and Inebriates opened its doors in Foxborough, Massachusetts.[766] And 1904 and 1908, respectively, Iowa and Minnesota opened similar, albeit smaller, institutions. By 1919, however, such hospitals had all been closed down. Progressive proposals for treating inebriates ran up against the wall of government budget constraints.[767] The State of California voted for an asylum in 1889, but just four years later voted against it, before ground had ever been broken. By the mid-20th century, all that was left of the state hospitals were colonies for inebriates. Built between 1910 and 1925, they were occasionally paid for by public welfare, but more often than not were connected with county jails.[768] Drunkards of that time, especially those without means, were destined for jail, not the hospital.

By the 1930s and 1940s, most American physicians were extremely hesitant to declare the drinking disease to be hereditary in nature. An article published in 1942 in both the *Tennessee State Medical Journal* and the *Military Surgeon*, "Alcoholism: Some 'Causes' and Treatment," is representative of common medical wisdom in America at the time. Alcoholism might be hereditary, the author conceded, but "there is no unassailable positive evidence (yet) that alcoholism is hereditary (strictly speaking) or that it directly injures the stock of a family, or that it influences longevity favorably or unfavorably to any marked degree."[769]

The term alcoholism itself had, by that time, already entered the standard medical lexicon in the United States. As defined by a textbook widely read in American medical schools: "Alcoholism denotes the state of the body following the ingestion of relatively large amounts of ethyl

---

765 J. Edward Turner, "An Appeal," *Ceremonies, Etc., New York State Inebriate Asylum, Binghamton, New York* (New York, 1859), 157-169.
766 Tracy, *Alcoholism in America.*
767 For the case in Iowa, see Ibid., 196-225.
768 Baumohl, "Inebriate Institutions in North America, 1840-1920," 1198.
769 Merrill Moore, "Alcoholism: Some 'Causes' and Treatment" in *The Military Surgeon* 90:5 (May, 1942), 481-496.

alcohol. The sequelae of alcoholism depend on whether it is acute or chronic."[770]

Acute alcoholism was the poisoning of the central nervous system, which caused a temporary "disorder of the faculties so as to render him unable to execute the occupation in which he was engaged at the time, thereby causing danger to himself or to others."[771] Dipsomania was a special form of acute alcoholism, "associated with emotional difficulties. At times this tendency is inherited. With an uncontrollable urge the subject goes 'on a spree.' Between attacks he is rather quiet and often subdued, and exhibits no craving for alcohol."[772]

Chronic alcoholism was markedly different from acute alcoholism and dipsomania in that it indicated a substantive development of acute intoxication. Some drinkers never degenerated into chronic use, but others developed an addiction that affected both mind and body. Those succumbing to chronic alcoholism usually suffered from a weak nervous system, and were defined as having "inferior personalities." Only psychiatrists could treat those suffering from such a condition, even though chronic alcoholism was thought to have also physical manifestation in the form of *delirium tremens*.[773]

Alcohol itself was no longer perceived to be a threat; instead, specific individuals suffered from it, and had to be treated accordingly. It was, according to some historians, a historic shift in medical thinking about addiction, away from a "temperance paradigm" and toward an "alcoholism paradigm."[774]

One of the treatments of alcoholism was the use of amphetamine sulfate (Benzedrine), a drug that was used to treat obesity of neurotic origin, relaxing the gastrointestinal tract and postencephalitic Parkinson's disease.[775] The press, ever on the lookout for a cure to the disease, hailed

---

770 Soma Weiss, "Alcoholism" in *A Textbook of Medicine by American Authors*, ed. Russel L. Cecil and Foster Kennedy, 3rd ed., (Philadelphia, 1938), 556.
771 Ibid.
772 Ibid., 557.
773 Ibid., 558-559.
774 Ron Roizen, "The American Discovery of Alcoholism, 1933-1939," (PhD. dissertation, University of California-Berkeley, 1991).
775 Wilfred Bloomberg (Boston City Hospital, Dept. of Neurology), "Treatment of Chronic Alcoholism with Amphetamine (Benzedrine) Sulfate" in *New England Journal of Medicine* 220:4, (26 January 1939), 129-135.

benzedrine as the new panacea for alcoholism.[776] The use of benzedrine to treat alcoholism was apiece with a long tradition of treating addiction by substituting one drug for another – treating the drinking disease with morphine, morphinism with cocaine or ether, and heroin with methadone. Sometimes it was claimed that the new drug was a cure, while at other times it was merely argued that it was a better substitute for the addict.[777]

Whether drunkards ought to be held criminally liable remained a source of debate in both America and Europe in the late 19th century. But no legislation was ever passed freeing drunkards from standing trial in the United States. Alcoholism and crime, in fact, remained inextricably linked by both professionals and the public alike.

In 1902, the Committee of Fifteen (not to be confused with the Committee of Fifty), a New York City-based private research group that lobbied for a ban on prostitution and gambling, declared that alcohol and prostitution were related, since prostitutes prowled saloons soliciting drunken men.[778] The Committee of Fifty reported three years earlier that intemperance was responsible in some degree for no less than 50 percent of all crimes. Convicts in the Eastern Penitentiary of Philadelphia, perhaps in an attempt to downplay personal criminal culpability for their crimes, claimed that 70 percent of crimes committed in Pennsylvania were caused by alcohol.[779]

Three decades later, two physicians at Boston City Hospital set out to determine once and for all if a correlation existed between alcoholism and criminality. Between 1936 and 1939, they surveyed some 2,500 prisoners in Massachusetts state prisons. Among the 1,637 men studied, 66.3 percent were found to be suffering from alcoholism. Among the 928 women, the figure was 49.4 percent. The researchers shied away from declaring a causal link between crime and alcoholism, but noted that most criminals were alcoholics. Although they found no racial links to alco-

---

776 "Drug Held Cure for Alcoholism," *New York Times*, (28 December 1938), 17.

777 Richard Davenport-Hines, *The Pursuit of Oblivion: A Social History of Drugs* (London: Phoenix Press, 2001), 110-111. Mike Jay, *Emperor of Dreams* (London: Daedalus, 2000). Coca cola, for example, was first sold as a cure for neurasthenia and the morphine habit. See Mark Pendergrast, *For God, Country and Coca-Cola: The Unauthorized History of the Great American Soft Drink and the Company that Makes it* (New York: Basic Books, 1993), 32.

778 Timberlake, *Prohibition and the Progressive Movement, 1900-1925*, 58.

779 Ibid., 57-58; Koren, *Economic Aspects of the Liquor Problem*, 30-31; Committee of Fifty, *The Liquor Problem*, 121-125.

holism, they did manage to trace a hereditary cause, but stopped short of calling alcoholism a purely hereditary disease.

"Glueck expressed a belief as long ago as 1918 that the criminal act was the resultant between a particular constituted personality and a particular environment," the two doctors, M. Geneva Gray and Merrill Moore, wrote in 1941. "He believed that not all criminal persons were predestined to commit crimes. In addition, there probably is an imponderable factor which we can not [sic] uniformly evaluate. The fact that so many alcoholic men and women who are sentenced to penal institutions come from environments which are shaped unfavorably by the alcoholism of their parents, marital partners and other relatives *suggests that the frustration caused by an alcoholic environment elicits aggressive drives which manifest themselves in the socially inacceptable* [sic] *form of behavior* which we call crime."[780]

Gray and Moore relied on an unquantifiable factor, social environment, rather than heredity to explain the link between alcohol and criminals. According to them, frustration at a lack of success in life drove people to alcohol and crime. The environment was not only responsible for alcoholism, but also sex offenses, drug use, psychoses and suicides. In broad terms, alcoholics were not considered to be intrinsically criminal, but rather tended to commit crimes only under the influence of the learned habit of alcohol.

The Boston researchers acknowledged, however, that alcoholism was a form of anti-social behavior. The answer to the alcohol problem, therefore, had to be societal, rather than biological or heredity-based. They suggested treatment rather than punishment for alcoholics, and advocated for "hereditary counseling" in the education system and better social conditions.[781] What exactly constituted hereditary counseling is difficult to ascertain, but judging from the negation of the biological aspect of alcoholism, one can assume that such counseling had very little to do with genetics, but rather with a change in the social environment of the drinker aimed at ensuring that his offspring would not succumb to the drink.

---

780 M. Geneva Gray and Merrill Moore, "The Incidence and Significance of Alcoholism in the History of Criminals," *The American Journal of Psychiatry* 98:3 (November 1941), 347-353.

781 Gray and Moore, "The Incidence and Significance of Alcoholism in the History of Criminals," 347-353.

The temperance movement achieved its greatest success with the passage of the 18th Amendment shortly after the end of World War I. One of the strongest weapons employed by the advocates of prohibition was that drinking, in the words of historian Andrew Sinclair, "was more than a crime against God. It was a crime against society, self, and race. According to them, the findings of medicine and science proved absolutely that alcohol turned even the moderate drinker into the bad citizen, who infected his innocent children with the diseases of liquor."[782]

Science and medicine were used to persuade the public that prohibition was the only way to stop the drinking disease. Until the turn of the century, poverty, crime and vice had all been deemed personal individual failures. The prohibitionists adhering to the Progressive credo, by contrast, argued that in addition to saving the life of the individual, the environment in which alcoholic individuals wallowed also had to be saved. The government, in the form of the Volstead Act of 1919, had to intervene to rid America of alcohol-generated crime and vice.[783]

Within a decade, prohibition came and went – but the notion that society was responsible for the alcoholic remained. His environment had to be changed for him to break free from the disease. As Progressives turned into New Dealers after the Great Depression, the physical, biological or hereditary origins of alcoholism – all aspects that targeted the alcoholic as an individual – all but disappeared in American medical thought. It was, perhaps, a reflection of the social reform advocated by the new deal for Americans. Society, not its individual members, had to be treated and reformed.

Optimism regarding the ability of modern medicine to cure all ailments was abundant during the Progressive Era. Science, impersonal and objective, was to teach humanity how to create a better society. Unlike Keeley's turn-of-the-century gold bichloride cure, smacking as it did of that era's suspect mail-order patent medicines, physicians of the 1930s were insistent on proving their work through scientific rigor.[784]

For a cure to work, the new logic went, it had to be scientific. And scientific rigor was exactly what Charles B. Towns (1862-1947) claimed to have bottled in his cure against addiction. His cure consisted of one part

---

782 Andrew Sinclair, *Prohibition: The Era of Excess* (Boston: Little, Brown, 1962), 66.

783 Timberlake, *Prohibition and the Progressive Movement, 1900-1925*, 60.

784 Hickman, *The Secret Leprosy of Modern Days*, 64-66, 112-113.

fluid extract of prickly ash bark; one part fluid extract of hyoscyamus, which contains scopolamine and hyoscamine; and two parts of 15 percent tincture of belladonna, the active ingredient of which is atropine. In addition, strychnine was sometimes given to purify the stomach of the patient, a customary practice at the time.

An unknown individual sold this cure to Towns, who was a successful insurance salesman from Georgia that came to New York for a new challenge in life. To establish the legitimacy of his cure, Towns sought out the endorsement of Alexander Lambert (?-1939), at one point the chairman of the American Medical Association. After a brief trial, Lambert embraced the cure. The endorsement opened for Towns countless doors, including those of government, since Lambert happened to be the personal physician of President Theodore Roosevelt. Towns claimed that his cure had an extremely high success rate of getting addicts off drugs – 70 percent to 90 percent – figures he derived from the fact that only 10 percent came back for the cure a second time.[785]

During the first years that the federal government enacted laws against drugs, beginning in 1914 and continuing through the early 1920s, Lambert and the government believed that a cure for addiction was at hand. An attempt to ban drugs and the addicts was not inhumane, it was reasoned, since alternatives were believed to exist for those who were forced to give up their drugs cold turkey. As for those addicts who refused the cure, or who were not cured, they were viewed as having something wrong with them. As it turned out, however, Towns' cure was as flawed as his logic, with a success rate of about 4 percent. After the 1920s, the search for a cure was virtually abandoned, as the idea that a physical affliction caused addiction was forsaken in the United States. The Progressives were no longer so optimistic.[786]

Alcoholism served as a precursor to drug addiction, as physicians often confused the effects of drugs with alcohol, explaining the effects of one substance by describing the other.[787] The American psychiatrist, Stewart Paton (1856-1942) recounted the general symptoms caused by continual

785 Musto, *The American Disease*, 80-82, 87-90.
786 Ibid.
787 See for example: Richard von Krafft-Ebing, *Textbook on Insanity* (Philadelphia, 1904) quoted in Charles E. Terry & Mildred Pellens, *The Opium Problem* (New York, 1928), 184; F. Chotzen, "Zur Kenntnis der Psychosen der Morphiumabstinentz," *Allgemeine Zeitschrift fuer Psychiatrie und psychisch-gerichtliche*

use of morphine, from a mild case of hysteria to untrustworthiness and the lack of a sense of duty. "The whole character [of the addict]," he summarized, "deteriorates and the defects are in many respect similar to those belonging to certain stages in alcoholism although they are altogether different from others."[788] Edward H. Williams (1844-1930), an ardent temperance supporter called both alcohol and other drugs, including tobacco: "substances with narcotic effects."[789]

Before the 1880s, alcohol was regarded as the primary source of inebriety.[790] By the last two decades of the century, however, opium, morphine, cocaine and other drugs attained a new place of prominence among specialists.[791] While temperance organizations targeted alcohol, succeeding in imposing controls and blue laws in various counties and states, other drugs were left behind. But the professional call to ban drugs was soon heard loud and clear.

Many experts in the 19th century subscribed to the idea that race was a vital factor for addiction to develop. For example, opium, when smoked by Chinese, was more hazardous than morphine, consumed by white women. After all, white women outnumbered male habitués in the United States,[792] and they could not have been immoral.[793]

In 1915, Williams, a professor of medicine claimed that American Jews were all but immune to the effects of alcohol, and were 80 times less likely to develop a drinking disease than an American, and 300 times less likely to develop a disease than a European. Thus he concluded: Jews

---

Medizin 63 (1906), 786-803, reproduced and translated in Terry and Pellens, *The Opium Problem*, 186-192.

788 Stewart Paton, *Psychiatry: A Text-book for Students and Physicians* (Philadelphia, 1905), quoted in Terry and Pellens, *The Opium Problem*, 185.

789 Edward H. Williams, *Alcohol, Hygiene and Legislation* (New York, 1915), 10-13.

790 The first article to mention opium as an inebriant was published under the auspices of the *American Association for the Cure of Inebriates* in 1874, but the matter became more seriously developed in the decades to come. See Hickman, *The Secret Leprosy of Modern Days*, 47-49.

791 Arnold Jaffe, *Addiction Reform in the Progressive Age: Scientific and Social Responses to Drug Dependence in the United States, 1870-1930* (New York: Arno Press, 1981 [1976]), 41.

792 Earle, "The Opium Habit," 442-446; Kane, *Drugs that Enslave*, 24-26.

793 Not all experts agreed. J. B. Mattison asserted that opium smoking, though a vice, probably caused less severe cases of addiction than morphine. See J. B. Mattison, "A Case of Opium-Smoking," *Philadelphia Medical Times* 16:6 (1885), 197-199.

acquired immunity, whereas other races did not. According to Williams, race could also provide selective immunity to the same essential substance. For example, Peruvians were immune to cocaine addiction when chewing the coca leaves, but were susceptible to the disease if given the alkaloid cocaine.[794]

Moral degeneration and neurasthenia resonated with the understanding of addiction, as it had with alcoholism. In 1881, Harry Hubbell Kane, one of the leading experts on drug addiction in New York, opened his book *Drugs that Enslave* with: "A higher degree of civilization, bringing with it increased mental development among all classes, increased cares, duties and shocks, seems to have caused the habitual use of narcotics, once a comparatively rare vice among Christian nations, to have become alarmingly common." So alarming was the degeneration that "nine-tenths of us neither eat, sleep, exercise, bathe, or procreate in the proper way. It is all hurry and turmoil; little rest and much care."[795]

Kane, like others who followed him, discounted the hereditary nature of addiction. Following Eduard Levinstein's thesis,[796] Kane asserted that the morphine disease was not hereditary. Instead, physicians were responsible for spreading the disease, as they were ignorant of the vice, and gave habitués syringes to inject drugs in their absence.[797]

Thomas Crothers demonstrated in a talk held in Philadelphia in February 1892 that children born to morphine addicts were either unwittingly addicted to the drug, or succumbed to addiction at a later point in their lives. Their condition was not necessarily caused by heredity, but rather a 'neurotic diathesis,' or a propensity that had no biological cause.[798]

In October, Dr. T. J. Happel of Trenton, Tennessee claimed that alcoholism often replaced morphinism in children of addicts; thus, the children of alcoholics often developed a morphine addiction, or vice versa. Children born addicted to whiskey or opium had to be weaned carefully, not reducing the dosage too rapidly. Treatment aside, he finally concluded, "It

---

794 Williams, *Alcohol, Hygiene and Legislation*, 10-13.

795 Kane, *Drugs that Enslave*, 17.

796 Eduard Levinstein, *Die Morphiumsucht: Eine Monographie nach eigenen Beobachtungen* (Berlin, 1877).

797 Kane, *Drugs that Enslave*, 18-26.

798 Thomas D. Crothers, "Some New Studies of the Opium Disease," *The Journal of the American Medical Association* 18:8 (1892), 277-233.

is still an undecided question in my own mind, however, whether, considering the good of the child alone, it were not better to allow it to die."[799] The idea of ending life not worth living took root early among American physicians, not just their German counterparts.

The speed of drug withdrawal remained the major point of contention between German and American physicians. Whereas Levinstein believed in the immediate withdrawal of morphine, allowing the addict to suffer the sickness, known as 'cold turkey,' without alleviating the symptoms,[800] Kane believed that a gradual withdrawal was in order, finding alleviations in baths, and substitutions to the drug if possible.[801] Passing judgment on Levinstein's treatment, he wrote: "however well this plan may answer for the Germans and Chinese, it certainly is a dangerous and barbarous practice when applied to American and English people."[802]

Were Americans softer than Germans? Perhaps; but, unlike their German counterparts, American addicts went into sanatoria to be healed, paying out of their own pockets, and retaining the right to go in and out of treatment at will. Who, after all, would pay to suffer in a hospital? The American physical constitution, therefore, was weak because of the American pocket. In contrast, Levinstein's patients had usually forgone their right to leave the sanatorium until deemed fit, and were usually insured after Bismarck's health insurance reform in 1883, allowing their doctor to afford a harsher treatment.

Alcoholism and drug addiction were understood to be similar in physical terms, but not all doctors agreed that the two diseases shared a common moral strain. Kane, for example, wrote in 1882:

> Between opium-smoking and chronic alcoholism there can be no comparison. The latter is by far the greater evil, both as regards its effects on the individual and on the community. The opium-smoker does not break furniture, beat his wife, kill his fellow-men, reel through the streets disgracing himself or friends, or wind up a long debouch comatose in the gutter. He is not unfitted

---

799 T. J. Happel, "Morphinism in its Relations to the Sexual Functions and Appetite, and its Effect on the Offspring of the users of the Drug," *The Medical and Surgical Reporter* 67 (1892), 406-407.

800 Levinstein, *Die Morphiumsucht.*

801 Kane, *Drugs that Enslave*, 130-148.

802 Ibid., 129. See also J. B. Mattison, *The Treatment of Opium Addiction* (New York, 1885), 4.

for work to the same extent that an inebriate is. True organic lesions rarely follow.[803]

The moral depravity of the drunkard was far worse than drugs. Kane concluded: "As compared with other ways of using the drug habitually, there is no question in my mind but that in smoking (1) it takes longer to form a real habit, (2) it works less physical and mental injury when once formed, and (3) it is much easier to cure."[804]

In 1885, Jansen Mattison pushed the disease concept of addiction even further, claiming that doctors should refer to an opium addiction, rather than to the opium habit. A habit implied that the user controlled his behavior, but addiction made it clear that the patient consumed drugs uncontrollably. Heavily influenced by German doctors, Mattison adopted German nomenclature of dubbing addicts according to their drug, thus a morphine user was denoted a morphinist, and a cocaine user a cocainist. Addiction was a form of functional neurosis, which had very little to do with vice; the drug attacked the nervous system, causing the disease.[805]

Theories upon theories piled up as physicians struggled to define and treat addiction. George E. Pettey, a member of the *American Medical Society for the Study of Alcohol and Other Narcotics*, claimed in 1913 that addiction was nothing more than a form of toxemia of intestinal origin, basing his findings on clinical observation. He wished to correct his fellow physicians by insisting on a distinction between morphinism and morphinomania, which they, in their ignorance, used interchangeably.

According to Pettey, morphinism was caused by a prolonged use of opiates by a person of any type or character. It neither caused nor was the cause of a mental disease, and certainly did not attack the nerves directly. It presented no less than 75 percent of addiction cases in America. Morphinomania, on the other hand, was enmeshed with a mental disease, which existed either before or during addiction. The patient, therefore, should not bear any moral responsibility for his condition.[806]

---

803 Kane, *Opium-smoking in American and China*, 74-75.

804 Ibid., 80.

805 Mattison, *The Treatment of Opium Addiction*, 1-3; idem, *The Mattison Method in Morphinism: A Modern and Humane Treatment of the Morphin Disease* (New York, 1902), 7-40.

806 George E. Pettey, *The Narcotic Drug Diseases and Allies Ailments: Pathology, Pathogenesis, and Treatment* (Philadelphia, 1913), 4-10; an earlier explanation of

Pettey conceded that moral cowardice, self-centered life, softness and overindulgence by parents were but a few other reasons for addiction. After all, an individual with a strong character should be able to stand against the pain that would otherwise be treated with morphine.[807] Here, too, a moral condemnation of the patient was handed, even though Pettey professed to absolve his patients from the sin of addiction. As if he were a Prussian, Pettey claimed that patients should bear the pain, unless they were mortally wounded or suffered from inoperable cancer.

Unsurprisingly, Pettey's treatment was less merciful than most of his American counterparts. Since opiates poisoned the cells, the goal of any treatment of addiction was to clean the cells from the toxin; consequently, he adopted the 'cold turkey' treatment. Strychnine was to be used, when necessary, to revive the body after it was depleted by the drugs, and in some cases the limited administration of scopolamine could ease the subject's withdrawal symptoms when necessary.[808]

Ernest S. Bishop (1876-1927), one of Pettey's followers, wrote in 1920 that anyone, of any color or social class, could potentially become an addict, if enough of the drug entered his system. Therefore, every physician who administered opiates should be warned against the dangers of addiction. When taken internally, opiates caused intoxication, a process termed autointoxication. Similar to the opinions of the German psychiatrist Eugen Bleuler, Bishop believed that the reason why the human organism could tolerate larger doses of opiates was a result of an antitoxin produced by the body to deal with the poisoning.[809]

Men of medicine, who wished to reform the drug laws and treatment of addicts, espoused Bishop's theory. It was even popularized to the public, assuring citizens that a cure to the opium disease was at hand, if only the budget would be given to municipal boards of health.[810] Yet, neither Pettey nor Bishop could establish their theory in the laboratory, basing

---

toxemia could be find in Charles W. Carter, "What is the Morphine Disease?" *Journal of Inebriety* 30 (1908), 28-33, reproduced in Musto, ed. *Drugs in America*, 239-244.

807 Pettey, *The Narcotic Drug Diseases and Allies Ailments*, 17-22.

808 Ibid., 11, 51-57; Morgan, *Drugs in America*, 84-85.

809 Ernest S. Bishop, *The Narcotic Drug Problem* (New York, 1981 [1920]). See also Eugen Bleuler, *Lehrbuch der Psychiatrie* (Berlin, 1916), 208.

810 See William C. Hassler (Health Officer for the City and County of San Francisco), "'The Hop-Heads' a Great Truth from the 'Dope' World," in Williams, *Hop-Heads*, 119-129.

their research on clinical observations and logic. They insisted on the non-psychological factors of addiction.[811]

Addiction as a form of autointoxication did not hold water, and was proven wrong in a series of experiments conducted in the fall of 1919, and published soon after and in 1924. No anti-toxins were found in the bodies of addicts. This revelation, considered as a disproval of the physical theory for addiction, paved the way to other theories on addiction.[812]

After studying case files of addicts, Lawrence Kolb (1881-1972), a U.S. Public Health Service psychiatrist, concluded in 1925 that addicts could be divided into five personality types: accidental addicts, individuals with a psychopathic-diathesis or predisposition, psychoneurotics, psychopathic personalities who suffered from no psychoses, and addicts with inebriate personalities, or people who were drunk before becoming addicted. Since physicians were more careful in prescribing drugs, the number of accidental addicts was on the decline.

Psychopaths and neurotics were the addicts who potentially were the most problematic. Neurotics used drugs to relieve symptoms of other mental problems, and psychopaths' behavior bordered on antisocial in an attempt to feel more important than others. Individuals who suffered from a psychopathic predisposition, however, were somewhat different from other psychopaths in the sense that they believed their drug use would help them cope with their lives.[813]

Most drug addicts sought the pleasure in drugs. In fact, one of the driving forces of the psychopathic addict was to relive the first experience of pleasure under the influence of drugs. When drugs were first used, the pleasure attained was greater than normal, but as the individual became addicted, the pleasure threshold declined and addicts were forced to use drugs to attain a sense of normalcy.

Euphoria was the problem. Normal people, who received narcotics, were not as susceptible to the euphoric effects of drugs, whilst the

---

811 Jaffe, *Addiction Reform in the Progressive Age*, 42-43.
812 Musto, *American Disease*, 82-83, 335-337n. 40; Acker, *Creating the American Junkie*, 34-42, 46.
813 Lawrence Kolb, "Types and Characteristics of Drug Addicts," *Mental Hygiene* 9:2 (1925), 300-313. See also, Lawrence Kolb and William F. Ossenfort, "The Treatment of Addicts at the Lexington Hospital," *Southern Medical Journal* 31 (1938), 914-920; Lawrence Kolb, "The Narcotic Addict: His Treatment," *Federal Probation* 111:3 (1939) at NARA Acc #170-73-1 box 42.

psychopaths sought it out.[814] Though Kolb himself favored medical treatment for addicts rather than incarceration,[815] policemen and politicians had no patience for the fine points of a psychiatrist, thinking that there was no real difference between a psychopath and a sociopath, and that both deserved to rot in jail.[816]

Kolb's theory, however, was not only adopted and misconstrued by agents of law enforcement, but was also accepted by many physicians. It was, however, a honey trap. Kolb absolved physicians of their past behavior, as it finally cleansed physicians' culpability for addicting their patients.[817] But in return doctors lost control over most of them.

In the late 1930s, sociologists, such as Bingham Dai and his fellow graduate student Alfred Lindesmith (1905-1991), dissented; stressing that social class, anxieties and other causes for addiction should be explored.[818] Lindesmith in particular questioned Kolb's theory that certain personality types were susceptible to addiction. Instead, he argued that addiction caused addicts' manipulative behavior, since they learned that their painful withdrawal symptoms could be alleviated with a single dose of the drug. As a result, they were compelled to addiction to avoid agony.[819]

Fearing that Lindesmith's theory would lead to legal leniency and perhaps compassion to the addict, the Federal Bureau of Narcotics often

---

814 Lawrence Kolb, "Pleasure and Deterioration from Narcotic Addiction," *Mental Hygiene* 9:4 (1925), 699-724; Musto, *The American Disease*, 84.

815 Nancy D. Campbell, *Discovering Addiction: the Science and Politics of Substance Abuse Research* (Ann Arbor: University of Michigan Press, 2007), 16-17; Acker, *Creating the American Junkie*, 50.

816 Sarah W. Tracy and Caroline Jean Acker, "Psychoactive Drugs—An American Way of Life" in *Altering American Consciousness: The History of Alcohol and Drug Use in the United States, 1800-2000*, ed. Sarah W. Tracy and Caroline Jean Acker (Amherst: University of Massachusetts Press, 2004), 16-17.

817 Acker, *Creating the American Junkie*, 141-154, 213; Hickman, "The Double Meaning of Addiction," 190-191.

818 Bingham Dai, *Opium Addiction in Chicago* (Montclair NJ: Patterson Smith, 1970 [1937]).

819 Alfred R. Lindesmith, *Addiction and Opiates* (Chicago: Aldine Publishing Company, 1968 [1947]); Tracy and Acker, "Psychoactive Drugs – An American Way of Life," 16-17.

harassed him as early as 1939. The bureau remained firm in the stance that the only proven treatment of addicts was incarceration.[820]

In the United States addiction was defined in 1929 as: "that condition of mind or body induced by drugging which requires a continuation of that drug and without which a serious physical or mental derangement result." Another definition from 1937 claimed that addiction "embraces three intimately related but distinct phenomena; namely, tolerance, habituation and dependence. These phenomena which make up the psycho-somatic complex known as addiction are intricately interwoven and interdependent."[821] A different definition, devised in 1935 claimed that "Addiction is a state of bondage to a masterful drug, usually but not always of the narcotic class, and is manifested by craving, tolerance, intense discomfort of a specialized character on withdrawal of the drug, and tendency to relapse. Its origin lies in a defect of the personality which may be of varied kind but is most commonly of the nature of an inability to stand up to reality."[822]

In a series of studies conducted at the narcotic wards of the Philadelphia General Hospital in 1930, several observations on the addict were made, creating the following profile: The average addict was a man, aged 24, of a poor background, usually involved in criminal activities. He might honestly want a cure for his addiction; but once the effect of the drug had subsided, he became untrustworthy and would use any means possible to get a hold of the drug. "He is disgusted with his slavery to drugs; he desires temporary refuge from the police, or for financial reasons he wishes to reduce the amount of his daily dosage or obtain free maintenance for a time." Addicts "will agree to any sort of experimentation as long as it promises their immediate or early acceptance for treatment. This

---

820 John F. Galliher, David Keys and Michael Elsner, "Lindesmith v. Anslinger: An Early Government Victory in the Failed War on Drugs," *Journal of Criminal Law & Criminology* 88:2 (1998), 661-682.

821 A. L. Tatum, M. H. Seevers and K. H. Collins, "Morphine Addiction and its Physiological Interpretation based on Experimental Evidence," *Journal of Pharmacology and Experimental* Therapeutics 36 (1929), 447, quoted in Nathan B. Eddy, *The National Research Council Involvement in the Opiate Problem, 1928-1971* (Washington DC: National Academy of Science, 1973), 1-2.

822 C. K. Himmelsbach & L. F. Small, "Clinical Studies of Drug Addiction" *Public Health Report*, (1937) suppl. 125; E. W. Adams, "What is Addiction?" *British Journal of Inebriety* 31 (1935), 1.

apparent desire on their part to cooperate must not be taken seriously, as we will point out later."[823]

The drug addict, usually a criminal, was deemed untrustworthy, only confirming what journalists and the public had been saying for years: "a dope user is invariably the biggest liar on earth."[824] No compliance should be expected, since addiction prevented the addict from curing himself. In fact, the procurement of more drugs turned into the primary purpose of an addict's existence. Once the addict secures his supply, he "becomes amenable. His behavior is excellent, and he desires to cooperate in any experiment which does not interfere with his daily dosage. This cooperative attitude on the part of the addict is real and sincere but lasts only as long as the effects of the drug persist, usually a matter of hours. When the effects of the drug pass off, all the sagacity and ingenuity on his part are brought into play as only those who have been associated with this type of person can appreciate." Consequently, "the addict cannot be trusted, for he will probably try smuggling drugs into the ward in any way or means possible. Contacts from the outside world may try to smuggle drugs into the ward, as in the example of one case of a letter addressed to the addict and "have been written on a paper previously saturated with the drug, dried, ironed, and then inscribed with a harmless message."[825]

In the 1930s, general practitioners and surgeons hardly received any education about addiction during their studies.[826] The little a general practitioner or a surgeon would know about addiction came from the textbooks of the time. Two major categories of the disease appeared in them, intoxication and chronic addiction. Intoxication often occurred among the chronic addicts, and those who received opiates for medicinal purposes. Opiates such as heroin, morphine and dilaudid were the most common addictive substances in America, all malefic to the user's personality:

---

823 Arthur B. Light and Edward G. Torrance, "The Conduct of the Addict in Relation to Investigative Study" in Arthur B. Light and Edward G. Torrance (eds.), *Opium Addiction* (Chicago, 1930), 7-12.

824 Williams, *Hop-Heads*, 80.

825 Light and Torrance, "The Conduct of the Addict in Relation to Investigative Study," 7-20.

826 Conversation with Dr. Carlisle B. Hughes, who attained his medical degree in surgery at Richmond College in 1938, which took place two weeks before his death in Autumn, 2008.

The opium habit has many features in common with chronic alcoholism. There is also a certain amount of interrelation between addiction to these two substances. Opium has been used extensively in the Orient for centuries, and there is suggestive evidence that its chronic use in small amounts for smoking has no detectable deleterious effect on personality. The use of opium and its derivatives in the western hemisphere, however, represents not only a significant medical, but also a serious sociological problem.[827]

Chronic addiction was not only a disease, but was also a pernicious social phenomenon; thus, it had an etiology, but one which depended on the character of the addict:

Opium and its derivatives are usually taken in order to assure euphoria, or for the purpose of abolishing or escaping unpleasant reality. The more powerful the analgesic and euphoric effect, the more apt a drug is to cause addiction. In an appreciable percentage of cases the subject has taken the drug first for therapeutic purposes, on the prescription of a physician or through the use of 'patent medicines.' In another group, however, the initial motive has been a desire for euphoria. Closely allied to the latter factor are the personality and the occupation of the addict. Certain unstable and psychoneurotic individuals come to contact with these drugs either through their friends or though their occupation (physicians and nurses), and subsequently acquire the habit. Many drug addicts are persons of superior intelligence who acquired the habit during adolescence before character had become stabilized. Drug addiction is primarily a social and neuropsychiatric problem.[828]

Medical students learned that the etiology of cocaine was similar to the opium habit. It could originate from a contact with a habitué or from nasal sprays given by physicians. However, unlike morphine, criminals used cocaine to boost their courage.[829]

Physicians were taught in the late 1930s that "relapse is particularly apt to develop among psychopathic patients, for reasons which are often identical with the original cause of addiction. The inebriate impulse, memory associations and nervous or physical defects in coping with daily activities are the usual cause of relapse."[830] Not only were addiction and

---

827 Soma Weiss, "Definition of Acute and Chronic Opium Intoxications," in *A Textbook of Medicine by American Authors*, ed. Russel L. Cecil and Foster Kennedy, 3rd edition, (Philadelphia, 1938), 566-571.

828 Ibid.

829 Soma Weiss, "Cocaine Intoxication," in *A Textbook of Medicine by American Authors*, ed. Russel L. Cecil and Foster Kennedy, 3rd edition, (Philadelphia, 1938), 564.

830 Soma Weiss, "Definition of Acute and Chronic Opium Intoxications."

psychopathy linked to one another, but addicts developed antisocial behavior:

> Addicts tend to become egocentric and selfish, and grow increasingly careless about their bodily habits. Often they are intensely unhappy and have a strong sense of inferiority. They are apt to resent the stigma placed on them by society. The deterioration of personality and character is further intensified by the fact that addicts are in constant conflict with the social order and usually are forced to keep in contact with the underworld. In order to secure drugs they have to lie, cheat and often commit misdemeanor and crime. In spite of these changes in character, addicts retain a full insight to their difficulties. Some of the changes in character cannot be attributed to morphine. Addicts whose initial constitutions were normal and who are able to acquire the drug regularly show a lesser degree of deterioration.[831]

Similar to morphine, cocaine addiction led to a deterioration of the personality. Addicts became careless and irresponsible – in other words, antisocial.

Although cocaine, unlike morphine, had no withdrawal symptoms, cocaine addicts were willing to do anything to procure the drug. "The tendency to relapse is great. This is due primarily to personality defects. Many of the addicts are inferior personalities who cannot resist the craving for renewal of their past experience with the drug."[832]

Medical texts remained dispassionate with little moral condemnation of the addict, only hinting at the antisocial nature of addiction; yet, the definition could hardly be called scientific, since cause and effect were confused. Psychopaths who took drugs would turn into addicts, but an addict was a psychopath by definition. This tautology should not come as a surprise in light of the evolution of addiction in America. From the work of Alonzo Calkins in the mid 19th century to Thomas Crothers at the turn of the century, the same paradox existed: were drugs responsible for addiction, or were weak personalities more susceptible to addiction? This question was not solved conclusively, and so medical students in 1938 were taught that both caused addiction. Lawrence Kolb's answer that addicts were psychopaths almost solved the question, but it also spelled out the physicians' loss of control over the patient in favor of the prison guard and the policeman.

---

831 Ibid.
832 Weiss, "Cocaine Intoxication," 565-566.

10. Age of Prohibition

In the early days of the republic, alcohol featured prominently in everyday society. Men and women, laymen and men of the cloth, businessmen and laborers, all drank, either in public or in private. Contemporary voices cried out against the United States becoming a republic of drunkards. The people had a taste for spirits, ciders and other beverages with high alcohol content, drinking comparatively little beer or wine.

The rate of alcohol consumption in America peaked in 1830, at nearly 15 liters of pure alcohol per capita, a level that has not been repeated since. America's consumption, based on such numbers, exceeded that of England and France, but was lower than that of Sweden.[833]

For much of the late 18th century and early 19th century, distilled spirits were perceived to be both nutritious and healthy. The belief was not entirely without reason, if one considers the hygienic conditions of that era. The water supply in most cities was hopelessly polluted, and nutrient-rich milk, to begin with only sporadically available, had only a short shelf life before becoming a potentially dangerous source of disease. The most available form of milk available to the public was the brownish swill milk, whose taste was not palatable to most. In contrast, Alcohol was considered a cure for centuries. In addition, Americans subsisted on a generally salty and oily diet, which heavy spirits helped to digest.[834] In a country where alcohol was already widely popular, the belief in its healthy properties only helped to increase its appeal.[835]

Economic considerations, specifically production and distribution, also help explain the popularity of distilled spirits over other alcoholic beverages. Beer and wine, which are made out of, respectively, fermented grains and fruits, spoiled quickly. The grains and fruit out of which alcohol was made spoiled even faster. But by converting them into

---

833 W. J. Rorabaugh, *The Alcoholic Republic: An American Tradition* (Oxford: Oxford University Press, 1979), 6-11.

834 James A. Morone, *Hellfire Nation: The Politics of Sin in American History* (New Haven: Yale University Press, 2003), 283-284. Rorabaugh, *The Alcoholic Republic*, 95-98, 117.

835 Ibid., 25.

alcohol, distillers were able to preserve indefinitely unpreserved produce. Brandy, rum and whiskey kept well over time; in fact, their quality improved, making these spirits easier to transport. Thus, as one historian deftly put it, "distilling rendered perishable crops imperishable."[836]

Prior to the American Revolution, the only beverages served at the dinner tables of the rich and mighty were alcoholic. It was only after the war that water began to be offered to guests as well. Talk of temperance and abstention from spirits, though not yet from wine or other fermented alcohol, was first heard in earnest in the late 18th century.

In 1814 Lyman Beecher (1775-1863), a famous orator and Presbyterian minister, spoke out against what he saw as the two great dangers to American society, slavery and drunkenness. He declared that total abstention, not mere temperance, was required for salvation. His sermons on the drink and society's other ills were reprinted across the country, and found receptive audiences for the duration of the 19th century.[837] That is not to say, of course, that drinking was not deemed immoral before Beecher's time. More than once, alcohol appeared as a convenient pariah in blue laws enforcing religious standards. In fact, in 1789, the first order of the day in the newly established House of Representatives was, after solving matters of procedure, the question of taxing alcohol. Revenues from the sale of alcohol were expected to pay for the deficit incurred during the Revolutionary War, as well as to serve as a moral chastiser to the people.[838]

Scientific claims that alcohol was indeed harmful were widely repeated, to the point of masking moral prejudice against alcohol in medicinal language, even though many physicians often prescribed spirits against all manner of diseases. Benjamin Rush (1746-1813), a signer of the Declaration of Independence and the first surgeon general of the Continental Army, was particularly concerned with the fact that ardent spirits, as

---

836 David T. Courtwright, *Forces of Habit: Drugs and the Making of the Modern World* (Cambridge MA: Harvard University Press, 2001), 12-13.

837 Lyman Beecher, "Six Sermons on the Nature, Occasions, signs, Evils and Remedy of Intemperance, (1828 [1814?])" reproduced in David F. Musto (ed.), *Drugs in America: A Documentary History* (New York: New York University Press, 2002), 44-86.

838 *Annals of Congress-House of Representatives*, first Congress, first session, (8 April 1789), 106-108.

opposed to beer, wine or opium, kept the drunkard from meeting his moral obligations, such as paying his debts.[839]

This morality-influenced attitude toward medicine was for the most part accepted in America well into the 20th century. This was especially the case when the unmet moral obligations of a drunkard hampered the financial order of society. Indeed, it is a likely explanation for why the American Medical Association deemed inebriety a moral disease in 1876.[840]

Contemporary industrialists listened to science, in the hopes of maximizing profits. Although in retrospect, it ought to have been viewed as bad for business. Controlling alcohol implied a loss of revenue from the trade of a product that at the time enjoyed tremendous popularity. In addition, restricted access to alcohol could incite agitation among laborers, who had grown accustomed to seeking strength from the drink or drowning their sorrows in it. Yet the entrepreneurs, industrialists and merchants of the day did not, as might have been expected, wield their tremendous influence on legislators to keep their alcoholic wares free from state control. One reason may be found in a view of workers as old as the country itself. Since the dawn of the Republic, wealthy American farmers and industrialists viewed their laborers as a commodity that should be harnessed, as well as protected from their inherent chaotic tendencies. Inebriation was viewed as a threat that could lead to a loss in production and other negative economic consequences. The fear of losing money helped tilt America's upper class toward imposing controlling measures on alcohol.

The first manifestation of the upper crust's suddenly acquired class-consciousness was the formation of the American Temperance Society in 1826. The society was the first organization to seek total abstention, and not just regulation, among workers. It was not coincidence that during this time it was discovered that the productivity of dry workers was higher than that of wet ones.[841]

---

839 Benjamin Rush, *An Inquiry into the Effects of the Spirituous Liquors upon the Human Body, and their Influence upon the Happiness of Society* (Edinburgh, 1791), 5-7; idem, *Essays, Literary, Moral & Philosophical* (Philadelphia, 1798 [1796]), 258.

840 Sarah H. Tracy, *Alcoholism in America from Reconstruction to Prohibition* (Baltimore: Johns Hopkins University Press, 2005), 26.

841 John J. Rumbarger, *Profits, Power, and Prohibition: Alcohol Reform and the Industrializing of America, 1800-1930* (Albany: State University of New York Press, 1989), 3-20.

Churches were urged to mobilize against the use of ardent spirits. Their efforts, however, met with only limited success, not least because wine was required for the eucharist. Reformers, many of whom were preachers, recognized that their self-serving goals would not be popular among workers. They anticipated that churches would be reluctant to risk alienating their flocks. They therefore concluded that for the temperance movement to gain support, it had to draw its moral appeal from "an agency not associated with the churches."[842] And so, in 1833, the American Temperance Society convened its members and took upon itself to be that agency, christening it the United States Temperance Union. "The traffic in ardent spirit as a drink, and the use of it as such, are morally wrong, and ought to be abandoned through the world," the newly formed union declared.[843] In 1836, it was renamed the American Temperance Union, and its members gathered at a convention in upstate New York to advocate for teetotalism.

During the mid-19th century, other temperance societies appeared like mushrooms after rain, some with a religious bent, others secular. To be sure, there were plenty of potential souls to save. The lower classes drank. And the new immigrants, especially the Irish during the great famine and the Germans, drank even more heavily.[844]

The immigrants and the poor wished to continue drinking, and the middle and upper classes were equally determined, each for their own reasons, to force the lower orders to conform to a new ethic. The industrialists, with the exception of the brewers and distillers, were interested in preventing the loss of revenue they perceived to be caused by alcohol. And wealthy temperance conservatives, after prohibitionists failed to form a coherent political party in the 1890s, began to prod middle-class prohibitionists toward alcohol control, appealing to their morality-driven concerns.[845]

The old aristocracy, industrialists, landowners and Nativists, such as the secretive Know-Nothings advocated temperance, with the latter also

---

842 Ibid., 14. In other words, the society was not a branch of the certain church, but was supposedly neutral. It was, however, co-founded by Lyman Beecher, himself a minister in the Presbyterian Church.
843 Ibid., 16.
844 John C. Burnham, *Bad Habits: Drinking, Smoking, Taking Drugs, Gambling, Sexual Misbehavior, and Swearing in American History* (New York: New York University Press, 1993), 54, 59-60; Alfred Heggen, *Alkohol und Bürgerliche Gesellschaft im 19. Jahrhundert* (Berlin: Colloquium Verlag, 1988), 88-89.
845 Rumbarger, *Profits, Power, and Prohibition*, 89.

opposing slavery, which was often equated with drunkenness.[846] Temperance itself was not an American invention, but the New World proved to be an excellent breeding ground for new ideas to control alcohol. The Washingtonians, founded in 1840, was a society of reformed drunkards who preached against alcohol. They appealed to the hearts of their listeners, with spectacles of mass meetings, marches and lectures filled with descriptions of the vice.[847] They talked about how drunkards progressed "from the first glass to the grave."[848] They held confessions, replete with accounts of repentance to scare off potential drinkers.

Ever so slowly, the campaign against the drink shifted from temperance to prohibition, and from ethics to law. Whereas in the beginning the American Temperance Union and the Washingtonians appealed to the morality of men, the Friends of Prohibition, as they became to be known, sought to stamp out drinking by law.

Not yet strong enough or inclined to tackle prohibition on the national level, temperance societies targeted cities and states. In 1851, Maine was the first state to enact a statewide dry law. It would be only the first of many laws to follow in the ensuing decades, as the tide of prohibition ebbed and flowed across the country, culminating in the 18th Amendment.[849] "Wet vs. Dry" politics played out in state after state, resulting in laws, and law breaking, wherever strict regulations on alcohol were imposed.

Probably the best known of the temperance societies was the Woman's Christian Temperance Union, or WCTU. It was founded in 1873 to persuade men to stop drinking, and became a national organization the following year. It also promoted women's rights, as well as advocated for laws against prostitution, for the protection of labor, and for world peace.

The tactics used by the union were non-violent, and were aimed at appealing to men's consciences. As the guardians of the home and family, these women argued, they ought to receive the wages earned by men, rather than the saloon and the drink. The WCTU leveraged the power of

---

846 John Kobler, *Ardent Spirits: The Rise and Fall of Prohibition* (New York: Putnam, 1973), 83, 88. Morone, *The Hellfire Nation*, 189-200, 286.

847 Andrew Sinclair, *Prohibition: The Era of Excess* (Boston: Little, Brown, 1962), 57-58.

848 John W. Crowley, ed. *Drunkard's Progress: Narratives of Addiction, Despair, and Recovery* (Baltimore: Johns Hopkins University Press, 1999), 1-19.

849 Kobler, *Ardent Spirits*, 76-91.

the family, much as London women had done more than a century before, when they petitioned against coffee in 1764, complaining that it caused men's seed to be as dry as the desert.[850] Women would go to saloons, stay outside, kneel, sing and pray for the souls inside. Embarrassment led many saloonkeepers to close their businesses. As the WCTU grew, its target changed from the individual saloonkeeper to the entire industry.[851]

Not all Christian denominations, however, espoused prohibition. The Catholic Church, advocating temperance, avoided calling for total abstinence. Relying on the many instances in the Old and New Testaments of wine drinking, the Church insisted that a devout Catholic could choose to drink or not at his or her discretion, as long as drinking was temperate. Catholics insisted that the freedom to drink should be upheld at all costs, lest prohibition turn into tyranny, and rejected the idea that the abolition of slavery could be equated with prohibition of alcohol. Instead of prohibition on either the national or local level, the Church advocated a licensing system. The Catholic Church insisted its proposal was not the "legalizing of evil," as many prohibitionists claimed, but rather the regulation of a trade that would otherwise invite illegal traffic and its associated problems.[852]

The few industrialists and landowners who did support the Wet cause were producers of alcohol. Americans drank like fish, and saloons, bars and restaurants all served alcohol. Indeed, it could be argued that alcohol was woven into the very history of the Republic. During the American Revolution, the saloon was known to be a place of freedom where anti-monarchist sentiments ran high.[853] Public meetings were often held in the saloon or the bar. In one early 19th century frontier town in Illinois, for

---

850 Wolfgang Schivelbusch, *Tastes of Paradise: A Social History of Spices, Stimulants, and Intoxicants* (New York: Vintage Books, 1993), 37.

851 Richard F. Hamm, *Shaping the 18th Amendment: Temperance Reform, Legal Culture, and the Polity, 1880 -1920* (Chapel Hill: University of North Carolina Press, 1995), 24-25.

852 See, for example, J. A. Homan, *Prohibition-The Enemy of Temperance: An Exposition of the Liquor Problem in the Light of Scripture, Physiology, Legislation and Political Economy. Defending the Strictly Moderate Drinker and Advocating the License System as a Restrictive Measure* (Cincinnati, 1910).

853 Rorabaugh, *The Alcoholic Republic*, 34-35. For a short list of taverns where revolutionary activity took place, see Eric Burns, *Spirits of America: A Social History of Alcohol* (Philadelphia: Temple University Press, 2004), 7-8.

example, the saloon was the only chamber large enough to hold important court cases.[854]

Money was to be made from alcohol, and money translated into power. And when the Industrial Revolution reached the distillery, the production of alcohol was concentrated into the hands of a relatively small number of industrialists, translating into even more money and power for the lucky few. In 1825 there were no less than 1,129 small distilleries licensed in New York; by 1860, just 77 dominated the market.[855]

And the market was unquestionably booming. In 1896, approximately 58 million bushels of corn were devoted to the production of alcohol. In addition, 11.27 percent of the rye and 40.44 percent of barley consumed in the United States went to the drink. The distilleries produced more than $250 million worth of alcohol, with nearly $1 billion invested in the liquor traffic; and perhaps most importantly, at least to a broad swathe of Americans, the industry provided employment to some 364,000 people, not including farmers and transportation agents.[856]

The economic power derived from the production of alcohol strengthened the political position of industrialists, but to what degree is rather difficult to ascertain.[857] What is certain, however, is that American distillers could only envy the political influence their German colleagues held. American distillers had a lobby, but so did the prohibitionists, whose lobby was more effective and more energetic.[858]

In the long run, alcohol industrialists in America slowly but surely lost the not inconsequential amount of power they had acquired. Saloon owners and alcohol distillers found themselves in an increasingly untenable position as more states and counties enacted blue laws and prohibitions in the late 19th century and early 20th century. With the passage of the 18th Amendment, the weakening of the industrialists' might was undeniable. Indeed, it was not the alcohol industrialists who drove the repeal of

---

854 Lawrence M. Friedman, *A History of American Law* (New York: Simon and Schuster, 1985), 162-163.

855 Burnham, *Bad Habits*, 53.

856 Committee of Fifty, *The Liquor Problem: A Summary of Investigations, 1893-1903* (New York, 1970 [1905]), 104-106, 127-128.

857 Burnham claimed that industrialized had, indeed, strengthened the industry, see *Bad Habits*, 53-56.

858 David E. Kyvig, *Repealing National Prohibition* (Chicago: University of Chicago Press, 1979), 5-19.

Prohibition. By the time the 21st Amendment was passed in 1933, the industry was, for all sense and purposes, politically broken.

American alcohol manufacturers only owned their distilleries, and had to buy the grain to produce alcohol. When World War I broke out and the need arose to conserve grain for bread, the American producer of alcohol – as well as the consumer – came under fire for collaborating with the Kaiser, who aimed to deplete America of its grain storages.[859] When America entered the war in 1917, it came to share what British Prime Minister Lloyd George (1863-1945) later called the "three great enemies, Germany, Austria and Drink, and... the greatest of these enemies was Drink."[860]

The alcohol industrialists were on the wrong side of an era noted for widespread reforms aimed at improving public welfare. During this progressive period, varied campaigns were launched against business monopolies, child labor, poverty and slum housing, among other causes. Progressive politicians advocated for minimum wages, public education and transportation, food standards, and honest elections. They did not shy away from limiting personal liberties, however, when it went toward the common good, such as advocating for the prohibition of alcohol and drugs, the imposition of immigration quotas and limitations, or a ban on prostitution, obscene literature and gambling.

A prime example of Progressive thought is embodied in the five-volume report published in 1905 by the Committee of the Fifty for the Investigation of the Liquor Problem. It was a privately financed research group that was commissioned 12 years earlier, and which provided one of the most detailed accounts of the drinking problem in America. The report, not incidentally, elucidated the opinions of wealthy industrialists who sought state control of alcohol.[861]

The Committee was composed of four subcommittees, and counted among its members physicians, lawyers, academics and industrialists. Its professed mission was to seek a rational solution to American workers' drinking problem.[862] Steeped in Progressive ideals, the committee's report

---

859   Charles Merz, *The Dry Decade* (Seattle, 1969 [1930]), 27.
860   Quoted in Ernest Hurst Cherrington, *America and the World Liquor Problem* (Westerville, OH., 1922), 30-31.
861   Harry G. Levine, "The Committee of Fifty and the Origins of Alcohol Control" in *the Journal of Drug Issues* 13 (1983), 95-116.
862   Committee of Fifty, *The Liquor Problem*, 3-11.

urged moderation, rather than prohibition, and steered away from the moral condemnations issued by America's temperance societies.

Drunkards and drinking presented a danger to both society and the individual alike, the committee warned, as continuous drinking caused cirrhosis of the liver and other diseases, including inherited or acquired inebriety and chronic alcoholism.[863] And intemperance was largely responsible for poverty and crime, two social ailments that had to be reckoned with in a functioning social welfare system.

The subcommittee on economics examined race's influence on the drinking disease, concluding that Russians were least susceptible to crime caused by alcohol, while "a Negro under the influence of liquor is much more apt to commit some impulsive crime than a white man. He is, however, less apt to become permanently a slave of the habit and thus to sink into pauperism."[864] More worrisome still was the deteriorating financial situation of women, who were more susceptible to pauperism caused by drunkenness because alcohol rendered their husbands and fathers unable to hold jobs and support their families.[865]

In a prescient warning, the Committee argued that total prohibition would lead to corruption and disregard for the law.[866] Prohibition was possible only in communities that were in favor of it, noting how some counties in Maine and Iowa – two states that adopted prohibition in the 19th century – were in open rebellion against the law.

In 1897, more than 20 years before Prohibition, the legislation subcommittee issued a warning that came to pass in the bootlegging 1920s:

> The liquor traffic, being very profitable, has been able, when attacked by prohibitory legislation, to pay fines, bribes, hush-money, and assessments for political purposes to large amounts. This money has tended to corrupt the

---

863 Ibid., 24-25; W. O. Atwater, John S. Billings, H. Bowditch, R. H. Chittenden, and W. H. Welch (Sub-Committee of the Committee of Fifty to Investigate the Liquor Problem), *Physiological Aspects of the Liquor Problem*, vol. 2 (Boston, 1903), 365-372.

864 Committee of Fifty, *The Liquor Problem*, 108-125.

865 John Koren (an investigation made for the Committee of Fifty under the direction of Henry W. Farnam), *Economic Aspects of the Liquor Problem* (Boston, 1899), 23-24, 43, 46, 104-105.

866 Levine, "The Committee of Fifty and the Origins of Alcohol Control," 95-116.

lower courts, the police administration, political organizations, and even the electorate itself.[867]

The Committee's warning, however, fell mostly on deaf ears, and its conclusions for control were espoused; morality won the day first locally, and later nationally.

At the turn of the century, local control, and not national prohibition, was believed to be the solution for the drinking problem. Municipal governments were perceived as being more attuned to local needs, and in the eyes of temperance industrialists, perhaps easier to manipulate. Efforts to curb drinking locally were directed via the National Municipal League. One early success was found in Minneapolis in 1884, when the powers of the mayor were enhanced at the expense of the city council with the purpose of controlling alcohol. Calls were made for the Minnesotan example to be emulated elsewhere, but municipal alcohol reform was soon abandoned, as the problem appeared far greater than the municipalities' ability to develop a solution. The industrialists who had thrown their weight behind municipal reform shifted their support to nationwide efforts.[868]

The Committee of Fifty identified the key to dissuading potential drinkers in education, namely teaching children and adults that alcohol was both dangerous and a waste.[869] Education alone, however, was deemed to be insufficient. The rowdy saloons of the 19th century were where the leisure time of the working class was shaped, and as such were the focus of the interest of the wealthy. Afraid of social chaos and the possibility of socialist agitation springing from the saloons, the committee sought to impose controls over them as well. They did not, however, attempt to ban them outright or at any cost, recognizing that the saloon was important to the lives of many laborers.[870]

---

867 Frederic H. Wines and John Koren (an investigation made under the direction of Charles W. Eliot, Seth Low and James C. Carter sub-committee of the committee of fifty to investigate the liquor problem), *The Liquor Problem in Its Legislative Aspects*, (Boston, 1897), 4-6.

868 Rumbarger, *Profits, Power, and Prohibition*, 109-122.

869 Committee of Fifty, *The Liquor Problem*, 35-42.

870 Raymond Calkins (an investigation made for the Committee of Fifty under the direction of Francis G. Peabody, Elgin R. L. Gould and William M. Sloane), *Substitutes for the Saloon* (Boston, 1901), 1-24.

That is not to say that the committee's recommendations were without teeth. Restrictions on drinking were to be imposed, starting with barring alcohol from being served to minors, the intoxicated or the habitually drunk. Saloons, the committee concluded, should be closed on Sundays and other holidays and should not serve as a place of entertainment, be it for music, billiards, cards or dice tables. No theaters or concert halls were to be allowed to operate in saloons, or in a place where alcohol was served. The windows of saloons should not be obstructed, allowing a clear view from the street. Limits were to be put on the number of hours when liquor could be sold, and the number of female bartenders was to be restricted.

Notably, the committee urged that such restrictions only be enacted in communities that were ready to accept them. Control measures in a Wet community would only result in complete disregard for the law. In such locales, the committee argued, it was better for the state to run the bars, rather than leave such a sensitive location in private hands.[871]

During the 19th century the penal codes of most states steadily grew, with crimes pertaining to public morality among the most prominent additions. Gambling, pimping, prostitution and public indecency all became illegal. Bans on specific aspects of the sale and consumption of alcohol went on the books as well. In 1881 Indiana made it a crime to sell liquor on Sundays. By 1887, Iowa, Kansas, Maine, New Hampshire, Rhode Island and Vermont had all passed liquor control laws making them dry states at least on paper, since they were unable to to control the interstate alcohol trade without federal intervention.[872]

The South was particularly temperate, arguably in an attempt to reclaim the moral high ground after the Civil War. As one historian would later put it, "If the North had abolished chattel slavery in the South, the South would retaliate by abolishing rum slavery in the North."[873] Soon after the fall of the Confederacy, the temperance movement succeeded in putting its stamp on politics. Fearing that the Prohibition Party would divide the Democratic Party in 1869, Southern Democrats diverged from their Northern counterparts and supported Prohibition, which was espoused by many Progressive Republicans in the North.

---

871 Committee of Fifty, *The Liquor Problem*, 62-63, 71, 125-127.
872 Friedman, *A History of American Law*, 583, 586.
873 Sinclair, *Prohibition*, 49.

The Prohibition Party, which sprang from smaller state parties into national politics, never succeeded in achieving its goal, but did manage to create an alcohol-centered split within both of the major parties. It drew in Wet Democrats in Northern cities and Dry Democrats in the rural South, as well as Republicans in the Northeast and Midwest.[874]

With proponents of prohibition on the rise, it is perhaps no wonder that soft drinks were introduced in the South as a replacement for hard liquor. Tellingly, the recipe for Coca-Cola was invented in 1886, the same year that Atlanta went dry. At the time, the fact that it was the cocaine in soft drinks that was replacing alcohol troubled few.[875]

Other national organizations calling for prohibition soon arose. The Intercollegiate Prohibition Association, established in 1901, quickly became the largest in the United States. It advocated national prohibition, and sponsored all manner of publications against the drink, often adopting Progressive rhetoric devoid of moral condemnation of drinking but nonetheless promoting prohibition in the name of the greater good, as in the words of Harry S. Warner, the secretary of the Association:

> It is their effects upon the community as a whole, upon the health, happiness and morality of large masses of people, and upon the permanency of the nation, that condemn the drink habit and traffic. It is not so much that harm comes to the individual user, as that others must bear so large a burden of undeserved consequences, that calls for action on the part of organized society.
>
> It may not be inherently wrong to drink a glass of liquor or to manufacture in response to a pre-existing call for intoxicants, for occasional use. But the consequences of the drink habit and the saloon, the impossibility of preserving such moderation that no evil will result, and the active creation of a new demand, produce a deep-seated wrong that strikes at the foundation of community and nation life.
>
> It is an absurdity and a contradiction of the purposes of government that an institution which is a danger to public welfare should receive the sanction of law – the only method by which the whole of society speaks authorita- tively.[876]

---

874 Ibid., 50, 66, 100-103; Hamm, *Shaping the 18th Amendment*, 23-24.
875 Joseph F. Spillane, *Cocaine: From Medical Marvel to Modern Menace in the United States, 1884-1920* (Baltimore: Johns Hopkins University Press, 2000), 75-79.
876 Harry S. Warner, *Social Welfare and the Liquor Problems: Studies in the Sources of the Problem and How They Relate to its Solution* (Chicago, 1916 [1908]), 275.

Various states tried to enact their own prohibitions and restrictions on alcohol, but the results were often divisive. South Carolina attempted to monopolize the sale of alcohol in 1892, but the endeavor proved rocky. Prohibitionists were displeased because dry counties could host state dispensaries. Wets were unhappy, because county and municipal taxes on liquor stores were imposed on alcohol. Moreover, governmental dispensers depended on sales, which only strengthened the interest of the state in alcohol sales, and as a result attracted the ire of prohibitionists.[877]

To make matters worse, South Carolina was unable to stop the importation of alcohol from other states and to prevent private dealers from selling alcohol on the black market. Furthermore, the fate of the temperance law itself was uncertain as the state Supreme Court threatened to declare the law unconstitutional. Attempts to modify the law in 1893 and 1894 led to riots, and even the threat of civil war, with state constables armed with rifles employing force to enforce the law. The law, meanwhile, made its way through various state and federal courts, eventually reaching the United States Supreme Court.[878]

From Ohio came the Anti-Saloon League, which began as a state society in 1893 but within two years had expanded into a national movement. Unlike the Woman's Christian Temperance Union, the Prohibition Party and other predecessor organizations, the Anti-Saloon League focused its efforts on passage of federal legislation against alcohol, concentrating its effort in lobbying. It steered clear of partisan politics, sticking to its sole issue, in what was effectively the birth of modern lobbying practices.

At the time, Prohibitionists viewed the federal government with suspicion. Federal taxes were imposed on the liquor industry, but the government refused to divulge information regarding distilleries, in an effort to protect its source of revenue from states with dry laws. The Drys argued that the taxation of alcohol amounted to the government's tacit complicity with immoral drinking. One of the Anti-Saloon League's first successes was a push towards Federal tax laws reforms with the 16th amendment in 1913, which led to weaning the Federal government off the liquor tax.[879]

Flush with momentum, the league went on to steer passage of the 18th Amendment to the Constitution, passing the necessary legislation through

---

877 Committee of Fifty, *The Liquor Problem*, 71-72.
878 Wines and Koren, *The Liquor Problem in Its Legislative Aspects*, 147-162.
879 Hamm, *Shaping the 18th Amendment*, 101-107, 184, 190-191.

Congress despite a presidential veto. The United States formally became a Dry country in 1920. To judge by contemporary reports, the ban on alcohol had more than a few supporters, among them many doctors.

The year after Prohibition became the law of the land, Dry politicians turned to regulation of dispensing alcohol to medical patients. In November 1921, the Willis-Campbell Act was passed; limiting the amount of alcohol doctors could prescribe to their patients. Some physicians lamented the legislation, but the majority of the medical community appeared willing to accept the will of the people. In a poll conducted by the American Medical Association in 1921, 60 percent of the 30,000 physicians surveyed were in favor of Prohibition and limiting the prescription of alcohol.[880]

Prohibition also found supporters among the many Americans who believed the ban on alcohol would promote economic improvement. A telling example appeared in a 1922 article in *The New York Times*, with the owner of a beauty parlor explaining:

> It is very easy to trace the growth of the beauty parlor business to prohibition. When men drank, they were not so critical. Their wives and sweethearts looked attractive to them without the assistance of beauty parlors. Now, however, men remain clear-eyed all evening and notice wrinkles, pallor, straight hair and unsparkling eyes. As a result, the women are clocking to beauty parlors and we have to turn many away every day.[881]

Who could argue with that logic? Prohibition would rid society of its drunkards and be good for business, and to boot would make America's women more beautifully kept. Within a decade, however, the onset of the Great Depression would put to rest any remaining hopes that the ban on alcohol was good for business.

A major pitfall of Prohibition was the belief that as an engine for economic growth, it would effectively pay for itself. Congress, it was believed during passage of the 18th Amendment, would not be required to appropriate large sums of money to enforce the ban. Over the course of the 1920s, as the price of enforcing Prohibition steadily increased, the Wets used the burden on the public purse as a weapon against the Drys.[882]

---

880 Kyvig, *Repealing National Prohibition*, 33-34; David F. Musto, *The American Disease* (Oxford: Oxford University Press, 1999), 213.
881 *New York Times*, (13 April 1922), quoted in Merz, *The Dry Decade*, 180.
882 Merz, *The Dry Decade*, 179, 185-207.

With the stock market crash of 1929, an economically broken America took an even harsher view of Prohibition's costs.

Proponents of Prohibition also promised, in addition to economic growth, lower crime rates. The government's own figures, however, dispelled any such notions. According to the federal Census Bureau, in 1910, 32.3 persons in 100,000 were imprisoned in state or federal institutions. By 1923, three years into Prohibition, the rate had increased to 34.6. By 1926, the rate had risen to 41.8 persons in 100,000. In addition, rumrunners, bootleggers, moonshiners, smugglers, and organized crime all flourished in the wake of the 18th amendment.

Debate raged throughout the decade over whether the substantial increase in the prisoner population was due to Prohibition. The Wets regarded the increase as proof that the Volstead Act promoted crime; the Drys denied any connection between imprisonment rates and Prohibition.[883] The truth probably lay somewhere in between, but on either side of the ideological divide, few still believed in the promise of a crime-free, dry America.

By the beginning of the 1930s, efforts began to mount into a campaign to repeal Prohibition. As they had earlier in the Dry campaign against alcohol, women were at the front of the campaign to repeal Prohibition. The Women's Organization for National Prohibition Reform was formed in an effort to save the youth from being incarcerated for what was perceived to be an ineffective law. For their part, industrialists such as Pierre du Pont were worried that the complete disregard for the law promoted other criminal activity and disillusionment from the state as a whole – the same concerns raised by the Committee of Fifty 30 years earlier.

Public sentiment quickly turned against the ban. In late 1931, The New York Times reported that "prohibition is criticized as scientifically, morally and economically unsound," going on to note that "prohibition in the United States has led to a tremendous increase in the use of narcotics and other excitants."[884] The Wets formed their own lobby, which exerted substantial pressure on Congress while the Dry lobby mostly rested on its laurels. So confident were the Drys that Senator Morris Sheppard of Texas (1875-1941), the leading Prohibitionist in Congress, felt no compunction

---

883 Ibid., 176-177.
884 *New York Times*, 23 December 1931. Reproduced in:http://users.lycaeum.org/~sp utnik/Ludlow/NYT/122331.html

in claiming in March 1931: "There is as much chance of repealing the Eighteenth Amendment as there is for a hummingbird to fly to the planet Mars with the Washington Monument tied to its tail."[885]

Just two years later, Prohibition was repealed with passage of the 21st amendment. It took only eight months to usher the legislation through Congress, the fastest passage of an amendment to the Constitution in American history. As would be expected from a government bureaucracy that wished to preserve its resources and influence, the Prohibition Bureau fought alcohol to the bitter end, at least rhetorically. As late as February 1933, the chief of the bureau, Amos W. W. Woodcock (1883-1964), claimed that his men would uphold the law,[886] even though by then it was quite clear that the 18th amendment would be repealed.

The 18th and 21st amendments were unquestionably watershed moments in the development of American society, the former signifying the beginning of Prohibition and the latter its end. Their constitutional importance, however, might lead to the faulty conclusion that a political and cultural rift existed between the Dry America of Prohibition and the Wet America that preceded and followed it, as if American society dramatically changed between 1920 and 1933.[887]

This simplified dichotomy of Wet versus Dry might result in a myopic view of a wide palate of shades of gray that was peculiar to the temperance and prohibition movements in America. The public discourse on the negative moral aspects of alcohol was prevalent in American history long before Congress passed the 18th amendment, dating as far back as Anthony Benezet's moral tirades against the drink in the early 18th century or Benjamin Rush's warning against the immorality of drunkards in the early 19th century.

Furthermore, the prohibitionist discourse hardly went silent with the repeal of Prohibition in 1933. Indeed, the Woman's Christian Temperance Union and eight other prohibitionist and temperance organizations are still active today. For example, Mothers Against Drug Driving, or MADD, is a non-profit organization founded in 1980 that employs a powerful lobby in Washington to keep alcohol control in the political limelight. Other organizations exist as mere shadows of past glories, such as the Prohibition

---

885 Merz, *The Dry Decade*, ix.
886 "Federal Dry Tasks Big Pending Repeal," *New York Times*, (23 February 1933), 4.
887 For such a claim, see Burnham, *Bad Habits*, 269.

Party, which managed to draw only 643 votes in the 2008 presidential election.

Prohibition existed in many states long before the Volstead Act in 1919, and its vestiges still exist today in many dry counties across the country. At the municipal, county and state levels, various restrictions on alcohol are still imposed, including bans on underage drinking and drinking in public, the licensing of the sale of alcohol, and a long list of other laws, rules and ordinances pertaining to liquor. The United States was not a country where alcohol was freely available prior to Prohibition, and it is not one today.

The 18th amendment certainly signified a change in American society, but it was neither dramatic nor revolutionary. Instead, it was the result of various political forces successfully banding together to temporarily impose their will on the public on the national level. Whether Americans gained or lost their sense of respectability after World War I, as more than a few historians have debated, had little to do with the ban on alcohol and drinking. Nor, for that matter, did the repeal of Prohibition signify America's sudden change from respectable society to counterculture.

Convenient as the narrative might be, the United States was not more or less Puritan before or after Prohibition. Even after repeal Wets and Drys continued to struggle against each other, both peppering their arguments with hypocritical fervor, trying to harness science and medical knowledge to suit their goals. It is perhaps fitting that their efforts were often marked by agenda-driven hypocrisy. After all, the Founding Fathers, who expressed serious concern about the intemperate drinking of the masses, themselves drank alcohol and even financially benefited from the liquor trade.

11. Fighting the Drug Trade

Prohibition divided America, with Wets and Drys struggling mightily against each other in the courts and in Congress. Little public outcry, however, greeted the government's introduction, during the very same era, of a far more enduring form of prohibition – what is today, a century later, known as the war on drugs.

The first anti-drug law passed by the federal government was the Smoking Opium Seclusion Act in 1909, followed five years later by the Harrison Act. The legal crackdown on drugs shared several important features with the national prohibition on alcohol passed later that decade. To begin with, many Americans morally condemned both alcohol and drugs. In both cases, the government's efforts to enact prohibition were driven at least in part by an interest in controlling public behavior. And, more importantly, given public sentiments at the time, most doctors backed a ban on both alcohol and drugs.

The anti-drug laws, and more broadly America's national drug policy, were inextricably intertwined with the country's foreign policy in the late 19th century and early 20th century. As a rising world power, America was eager to flex its muscles abroad, and a crusade against the twin scourges of drugs and alcohol provided a welcome opportunity.

In early 1901, the Senate adopted a resolution submitted by Henry Cabot Lodge (1850-1824), the esteemed senator from Massachusetts, calling for a ban on selling alcohol to uncivilized races, as non-whites were described at the time:

> That in the opinion of this body the time has come when the principle, twice affirmed in international treaties for Central Africa, that native races should be protected against the destructive traffic in intoxicants should be extended to all uncivilized peoples by the enactment of such laws and the making of such treaties as will effectively prohibit the sale by the signatory powers to aboriginal tribes and uncivilized races of opium and intoxicating beverages.[888]

---

888 "Resolution, Adopted by the Senate January 4, 1901, Relative to the Protection of Uncivilized Peoples Against the Destructive Traffic in Intoxicants," *56th Congress, 2nd Session* (1901), *Senate Document 159*, quoted in Arnold H. Taylor, *American Diplomacy and the Narcotic Traffic, 1900-1939: A Study in Interna-*

It was the duty of the United States – indeed, the white man's burden – to keep the natives away from alcohol and opium. Ironically, Lodge's own family profited from the 19th century opium trade in China like so many other Brahmin families. Be that as it may, America's benevolent calls for keeping Africa intoxicant free were, for all sense and purposes, new only in their geography. The American colonists of the 17th century and 18th century, realizing that the natives in the New World were unaccustomed to ardent spirits, had prohibited the sale of alcoholic beverages to them.[889] At the turn of the century, the domestic policy of protecting America's natives was adopted to include natives abroad as a foreign policy priority.

The United States, perhaps in an attempt to assert itself with the traditional powers, followed the European example set in the Brussels General Act of 1889, according to which the European powers limited the sale of alcohol to Africa and aimed at restricting slavery on that continent.[890] Morality-driven considerations were never far off from policymaking. Religious lobbies, such as the Woman's Christian Temperance Union and the General Convention of Baptists of North America, pressured the government to intervene in favor of prohibition in Africa. In perhaps the most glaring example, a German company was dissuaded from building a distillery in Liberia in 1913 by Secretary of State William Jennings Bryan (1860-1925), whose wife happened to be a member of the temperance union and who had given the lobby access to her husband.[891]

The changing balance of power from Europe to North America also opened doors in Washington for anti-drug campaigners. In 1898, the United States declared war against Spain. In a few swift military maneuvers lasting less than five months, America acquired its first real colonies, gaining control over Guam, the Philippines and Puerto Rico, as well as installing a friendly government in Cuba in 1902. The Philippines was of

---

tional Humanitarian Reform (Durham: Duke University Press, 1969), 27. (Also known as: Resolution on protection of uncivilized races of Africa against liquor traffic and opium.).

889 Rorabaugh, *The Alcoholic Republic*, 155.

890 Robin Room, "Addiction Concepts and International Control," *The Social History of Alcohol and Drugs* 20:1 (2006), 279-280. For a contemporary account of the treaty, see Franz von Liszt, *Das Völkerrecht systematisch dargestellt* (Berlin, 1902), 262-263.

891 Ian Tyrrell, *Woman's World, Woman's Empire: The Woman's Christian Temperance Union in International Perspective, 1880-1930* (Chapel Hill: University of North Carolina Press, 1991), 160.

particular economic and strategic importance to Washington as it brought the United States closer to China. But, the control of the colony came with control of its lucrative opium monopoly.

Like many other colonial powers in East Asia, the Spanish government managed a system through which Chinese people native to the Philippines could only buy opium from colonial wholesalers. The policy enriched the colony's coffers, while delivering a regular supply of opium to addicts.[892] To certain segments of American society, assuming control of the Philippines presented an opportunity for a rising Washington to enact a new policy in East Asia. Foremost among them were American missionaries, who had been urging the government to take a stance against opium for much of the 19th century. The political weight of these missionaries should not be underestimated. They were among the first to urge President William McKinley (1843-1901) to annex the Philippines, arguing that the United States had a responsibility to educate the natives, uplift them and instill Christianity in them.[893] Banning the opium trade abroad also fit well with the idealistic notions of the Progressive movement and temperance advocates. If drugs were gone, the reasoning went, drug addiction as a disease would disappear as well.[894]

And perhaps most importantly, at least in the eyes of America's foreign policy leaders, the opium problem in the Philippines was deeply linked with China. Addressing the opium monopoly allowed the United States to meddle in Chinese affairs in the guise of a benign, humanitarian-oriented open-door policy.[895]

Despite the overwhelming interest back home in cracking down on the opium trade, during the first two years America controlled the Philippines, little was done to the opium monopoly. For the most part, the American administration gave the matter scant thought, debating only the rate at

---

892 Anne L. Foster, "Models for Governing: Opium and Colonial Policies in Southeast Asia, 1898-1910," in *The American Colonial State in the Philippines: Global Perspectives*, Julian Go and Anne L. Foster (Durham: Duke University Press, 2003), 92-117; idem, "Prohibition as Superiority: Policing opium in South-East Asia, 1898-1925," *International History Review* 22:2 (2000), 255.

893 McKinley's words are quoted in J. W. Wheeler-Bennett, "Thirty Years of American-Filipino Relations, 1899-1929," *Journal of the Royal Institute of International Affairs* 8:5 (1929), 503-521.

894 Arnold H. Taylor, "American Confrontation with Opium Traffic in the Philippines," *Pacific Historical Review* 36:3 (1967), 309.

895 Ibid., 309.

which opium ought to be taxed. The Chinese residents of the Philippines were considered by the Americans to be expert smugglers as well as prodigious opium smokers, and therefore attempts to impose high tariffs were expected to cause an illicit trade that would be difficult to control. Consequently, Washington opted for what appeared as a pragmatic policy of treating opium as just another commodity.[896]

American missionaries were appalled, decrying the country's involvement in what they lambasted as an immoral practice. America's federal tax on alcohol was a sign of complicity in the alcohol trade, they argued, and a tax on opium was no different, particularly given that several states had already imposed restrictions on opium. Nevertheless, contrary to the wishes of the then-civilian governor of the Philippines and future president of the United States, William Howard Taft (1857-1930), prohibitive taxes were imposed on opium in the early days of occupation. He wished to keep the functioning Spanish monopoly, but to no avail. Once more, morality won the day.

As Taft and others warned, the tax policy proved ineffective. The total amount of opium entering the Philippines through both legal and illegal channels tripled between 1899 and 1903.[897] In 1903, the opium policy in the Philippines was summarily sent back to the drawing board. Various proposals were raised in Washington, including the reestablishment of the opium monopoly, the establishment of "opium farms" in the Philippines, and restricting the sale of the drug to full-blooded Chinese over 21 years of age. None of the proposals, however, fit with the enlightened colonial rule that Americans expected from their government.[898]

"I feel very sure that [a licensing system] would do good, and it would bring us a good revenue," Taft wrote to then-secretary of war Elihu Root (1845-1937), "but it is difficult to reconcile the religious people of the United States to any system which in the slightest degree recognizes the fact that opium is smoked in spite of whatever prohibition is sought to be imposed."[899] In the end, President Theodore Roosevelt ordered a halt to all plans regarding the reinstatement of the opium monopoly in the Philip-

---

896 Foster, "Models for Governing," 95-96.
897 Taylor, "American Confrontation with Opium Traffic in the Philippines," 311.
898 Foster, "Models for Governing," 97-98.
899 Quoted in Joseph Michael Gabriel, "Gods and Monsters: Drugs, Addiction, and the Origins of Narcotic Control in the Nineteenth-Century Urban North" (Ph.D. Dissertation, Rutgers University, 2006), 507-508.

pines.[900] The colonial government remonstrated, but to no avail. Washington had decided.

Shortly before resigning as civilian governor, Taft commissioned an investigation on opium in Asia that would inform a better, more moral policy in the Philippines. He appointed the Episcopal bishop of the Philippines, Charles Henry Brent (1862-1929), to head the commission, thereby signaling his own evolving view on the opium monopoly, of which Brent had often spoken of as a vice.[901]

After surveying the region from Japan to Java, the commissioner recommended in 1905 the establishment of a time-limited government monopoly over supplying opium to registered drug users, to be replaced no later than March 1908 by outright prohibition. As The New York Times reported at the time:

> The commission recommends an exclusive monoply [sic], the right of importation and sale being limited to the Government. It says the exercise of this Governmental function should be intrusted [sic] to upright, intelligent, honorable, and well-recommended persons, following the practice observed in Java, with the object of eliminating from such a responsible trust all personal and commercial interests which would tend to extend the sale of the drug. The recommendation is also made that the monopoly be replaced as soon as practicable by absolute prohibition. [In three years time.] A system of registration and licensing for all chronic smokers is urged, limiting the right to procure opium in definite quantities to them. As a corrective and educative measure all Filipino opium habitués are to be deprived of the right of franchise, and to be ineligible for any public office, municipal, provincial, and insular. Gratuitous treatment of all habitués wishing to free themselves from the opium vice is to be provided in the hospitals at Government expense.[902]

The prohibition of opium in the Philippines indeed became the law of the land in 1908. From the day it went into effect until the end of American colonial rule in 1946, opium prohibition proved to be woefully ineffective.

---

900 Taylor, "American Confrontation with Opium Traffic in the Philippines," 313-315.

901 Ibid., 106-107; Taylor, "American Confrontation with Opium Traffic in the Philippines," 316. See also Christopher Allen Morrison, "A World of Empires: United States Rule in the Philippines, 1898-1913," (Ph.D. dissertation, Georgetown University, 2009), 115-154.

902 "Our Government may Sell Opium to Filipinos," *New York Times* (22 September 1904), 9. For the full report, see "Use of Opium and Traffic Therein, Message from the President of the United States," Senate Doc. 265, 59th Congress, 1st Session, (Washington D.C., 1906).

Occasionally the ineptitude bordered on the comical. In 1913 the Philippines welcomed a new governor general, Francis Burton Harrison (1872-1957). Upon his arrival in Manila, two trunks full of opium were discovered in his baggage, planted there by audacious smugglers. It was the same Harrison who lent his name to the American drug law of 1914.[903]

Two decades after Harrison's embarrassment, smuggling continued unabated. In a report submitted to the League of Nations in 1933 by the United States, it was disclosed that Chinese ports, particularly Amoy (Xiamen), Shanghai and Hong Kong, supplied the Philippines with opium and other prepared drugs. Seizures of opium, morphine and cocaine in the Philippines had reached nearly four tons, or roughly 3,600 kilograms, in a country with a population of less than 16 million.[904] By comparison, 213 kilograms of raw opium were seized in Germany in 1933, in a country with 65 million people.[905]

Charles Brent, the influential Episcopal missionary bishop of the Philippines, realized early on that an opium prohibition could not be enforced by American colonial rule alone. In July 1906, he urged President Theodore Roosevelt to persuade the European powers to limit the opium trade in their own backyard.[906]

By the next year, Roosevelt began laying the groundwork for a global anti-opium conference. It came to be known as the International Opium Commission, and was convened in Shanghai in February 1909. The goal of the opium commission, according to the American State Department, was to investigate how governments could cooperate in limiting the use of and traffic in opium. The key to success, according to Secretary of State Elihu Root, was to persuade the colonial powers to assist China's efforts to eradicate the evil from its empire.[907]

---

903 Foster, "Prohibition as Superiority," 253-254.
904 League of Nations-OAC, "Reports from Governments on the Illicit Traffic in 1933," (7 November 1934), NARA RG 170, Acc# 170-174-0005, box 116, file 1230-1. The population of the Philippines reached 16 million in 1939, according to the census conducted on 1 January 1939: http://www.census.gov.ph/census200 0/index_history.html (Last access: 23.1.2016).
905 Ibid.
906 Foster, "Models for Governing," 110.
907 E. W. Thwing, "The Opium Question" (February, 1909), 11-12 at the Library of Cogress, CLC RM. 41, *Drugs*; Hamilton Wright, "The International Opium Commission," *The American Journal of International Law* 3:3 (1909), 648-673.

No important agreements were reached in Shanghai, but the conference was hardly a failure for Washington. First, it was made clear to the world that the United States strongly desired an international drug treaty. Second, the members of the Shanghai commission were confronted, in stark terms, with the dangers of morphine, heroin and cocaine.[908] And two years later, after on-again, off-again deliberations, the *Convention Internationale de l'Opium* was signed in The Hague, codifying many of the findings of the International Opium Commission.

Washington's strong support for the Shanghai commission was driven by multiple motives. To begin with, the United States saw an opportunity to demonstrate moral superiority over the wicked European powers who continued to poison the Chinese with opium. Washington also saw an opportunity to curry favor with the Chinese as part of America's open-door policy with China.[909] At the time, anti-Chinese sentiments were running high in America, and a crusade against the opium trade seemed like a cheap way to gain appreciation in East Asia.

Furthermore, few Americans dealt in opium. The great American opium houses of the 19th century, such as Russell & Co. and Augustine Heard & Co., folded in the 1870s and 1880s.[910] In a sense, the United States was implementing the same policy it had enacted with Japan half a century earlier, forgoing opium in the hope of gaining greater economic access to the country's market.[911]

Yet, arguably the motive that most drove the United States to push for the Shanghai commission was the belief that America's drug problem was foreign in nature. If the opium trade were to be halted, so went the

---

908 William B. McAllister, *Drug Diplomacy in the 20th Century* (London: Routledge, 2000), 28-33.

909 Taylor, "American Confrontation with Opium Traffic in the Philippines," 323-324. David Musto, *The American Disease*, 3-4.

910 Mira Wilkins, "The Impacts of American Multinational Enterprise on American-Chinese Economic Relations, 1786-1949" in *America's China Trade in Historical Perspective: The Chinese and American Performance*, ed. Ernst R. May and John K. Fairbank (Cambridge MA: Harvard University Press, 1986), 261-262.

911 Bob Tadashi Wakabayashi, "Opium, Expulsion, Sovereignty. China's Lessons for Bakumatsu Japan" *Monumenta Nipponica* 47:1 (1992), 18-19. See also: "Treaty with the Empire of Japan, 29 July 1858" in *Public Acts of the Thirty Sixth Congress of the United States*, 1st session, 1055, at memory.loc.gov/cgi-bin/ampage?collId=llsl&fileName=012/ llsl012.db&recNum=1108. The treaty was ratified on 22 May 1860. (Last access: 23.1.2026).

thinking, a ban in the Philippines would work. If the vile narcotic traders stopped carrying their wares with impunity, the United States would not have so many problems with drug smuggling. If opium production were limited to medicinal purposes, addiction would be eradicated.

On February 9, 1909, days before the International Opium Commission opened in Shanghai, the US Congress passed America's first federal law against drugs, the Smoking Opium Exclusion Act. The law was unnecessary, since the Pure Foods and Drugs Act passed by Congress in 1906 already allowed the government to ban the importation of any drug deemed harmful to public health.

For the State Department, however, the Smoking Opium Exclusion Act was important, as the legislation offered a face-saving demonstration of America's commitment to curbing the opium trade.[912] In the words of Hamilton Wright (1867-1917), a member of the American delegation to Shanghai, the law "was an urgent and necessary act if the American Government was to appear in the International Opium Commission at Shanghai with fairly clean hands."[913]

A year after the Shanghai conference, Taft, by now the President of the United States, called on Congress to enact additional laws against opium. Among other requests, the president asked for $25,000 to be appropriated for international conferences, as well as for an expansion of Washington, D.C.'s 1906 anti-narcotic laws to other consular districts abroad, especially China, where Americans enjoyed ex-territorial status. To accommodate the agreements reached in Shanghai in 1909, Taft recommended that Congress regulate medicinal opium in the United States with "acts… to govern interstate traffic in habit-forming drugs, and an internal revenue law taxing out of existence manufacturers of opium products for other than medicinal use."[914]

Congress, for its part, had already devoted some floor time to the issue of opium. In 1909, Wright approached Representative James R. Mann of Illinois (1856-1922), chairman of the House Committee on Interstate and Foreign Commerce, with a proposal for a tax act that would curb interstate

---

912 Musto, *The American Disease*, 34-35.
913 Hamilton Wright, "Report on the International Opium Commission and on the Opium Problem as seen within the United States and its Possessions" in *Opium Problem: Message from the President of the United States*, U.S. Senate Doc. 377, 61st Congress, 2nd session, (21 February 1910), 54.
914 Ibid.

traffic, limit drug dealers to a select few who would pay a small tax, and force vendors to record all drug transactions. Mann, who had failed to pass an anti-narcotic bill in May 1908, declined to support the legislation, forcing Wright to look elsewhere in the House of Representatives. He found a more receptive ear in Representative David Foster of Vermont (1857-1912), chairman of the Committee on Foreign Affairs, and the bill was introduced in April 1910.[915]

As a domestic tax bill written by a diplomat specializing in tropical diseases and introduced into the House's committee on foreign affairs, the Foster Bill could strike some as a rather incongruous piece of legislation. But if one considers the international implications of the drug trade, as seen at the time from the State Department, the anti-opium bill was nothing more than a manifestation of Washington's determination to stamp out the drug scourge.

The Foster Bill, however, ran up against significant resistance from drug-industry lobbyists, who declared its burden on business to be too onerous. The National Wholesale Druggist Association argued that forcing vendors to keep records of every transaction involving opiates, cocaine, chloral hydrates and cannabis, regardless of quantity, would be prohibitively expensive. The legislation did earn the support of the American Pharmaceutical Association, which sought to protect pharmacists from quacks and their patent medicines, but ultimately the bill failed to pass.[916]

Denied legislation by Congress, Wright turned to the court of public opinion, embarking on a campaign to rouse public anger against drugs. He declared that it was the money-driven drug industry, with annual profits exceeding $100 million, that had dissuaded Congress from enacting the law.[917] He also took full advantage of the press. "Uncle Sam is the Worst Drug Fiend in the World," screamed the headline of a 1911 New York Times article featuring Wright as the primary source.

Among other claims reported in the article, the United States, with a population of 90 million, imported 300,000 pounds of opium. The European empires of Austria-Hungary, Italy, Germany, Russia and the Nether-

---

915 Musto, *The American Disease*, 41-44.
916 Ibid., 44-48.
917 Edward Marshall, "Uncle Sam is the Worst Drug Fiend in the World," *New York Times* (12 March 1911), SM12.

lands, meanwhile, with a combined total population of 155 million, imported barely one-tenth of what America brought in.

Wright was scathing in his attacks, sparing no one. Doctors prescribed drugs liberally, the drug industry sold nostrums containing opiates, and pharmacists convinced their customers to buy narcotics. "Our prisons and our hospitals are full of victims of [opium]," he said, "it has robbed ten thousand business men of moral sense and made them beasts who prey upon their fellows, unidentified it has become one of the most fertile causes of unhappiness and sin in the United States, if not that cause which can be charged with more of both than any other."[918]

After making his case to the American public, Wright embarked for The Hague for the third annual meeting of the International Opium Commission, to which he served as America's representative. Taft, meanwhile, turned his attention to Congress, prodding senators and representatives to seize the historic moment:

> Since the passage of the opium-exclusion act, more than twenty States have been animated to modify their pharmacy laws and bring them in accord with the spirit of that act, thus stamping out, to a measure, the intrastate traffic in opium and other habit-forming drugs. But, although I have urged on the Congress the passage of certain measures for Federal control of the interstate and foreign traffic in these drugs, no action has yet been taken. In view of the fact that there is now sitting at The Hague so important a conference, which has under review the municipal laws of the different nations for the mitigation of their opium and other allied evils, a conference which will certainly deal with the international aspects of these evils, it seems to me most essential that the Congress should take immediate action on the anti-narcotic legislation to which I have already called attention by a special message.[919]

Try as they might, however, Taft and Wright could not convince Congress. America had missed an opportunity to set an example to the other world powers.

The Hague conference resulted in the International Opium Convention, which upon signing in January 1912 became the first international drug treaty. All signatory countries were to enact laws controlling raw opium cultivation and trade. Signatories were also to impose trade controls on prepared opium, with the eventual goal of complete prohibition. Other substances addressed by the treaty included manufactured drugs, such as medicinal opium, morphine, heroin and cocaine.

---

918 Ibid.
919 Ibid.

As expected, Germany strongly objected to curtailing the production of and trade in manufactured drugs. German pharmaceutical companies dominated the drug manufacturing industry at the time, and Berlin simply refused to give up the international market as well as one of the most important medicines known to man. During negotiations in The Hague, Germany managed to exclude from the list of controlled substances lucrative drugs such as codeine, a popular opiate still in use today. It also succeeded in taking some teeth out of the enforcement of the treaty, softening the language to a tame demand that governments make "their best efforts" to enact the relevant measures regulating the manufacture of drugs.[920] Essentially, this was the adoption of the German practical foreign policy towards the international drug control: each country to itself.[921]

Yet, in spite of the German moderate position, article 20 of the treaty became the first international measure to explicitly call for a ban on drugs: "The contracting Powers shall examine the possibility of enacting laws or regulations making it a penal offence to be in illegal possessions of raw opium, prepared opium, morphine, cocaine, and their respective salts, unless laws or regulations on the subject are already in existence."[922]

The International Opium Convention was unquestionably a historic treaty, but it would be nearly another decade before the agreement had any practical effect. During the final stages of negotiations in The Hague, Germany, supported by France, frustrated the vitality of the treaty by insisting that even minor producing countries would need to ratify it before entering into force.[923] After objecting, modifying and castrating any operative measures in the treaty, Germany never willingly ratified it. As a result, the treaty did not enter into force as scheduled. Three conventions were called to mend the situation, but all failed. Then World War I broke out, and negotiations were halted.

It would only be after Germany's defeat in 1918, and the inclusion in the Treaty of Versailles of Article 295, which required accession to the

---

920 McAllister, *Drug Diplomacy in the Twentieth Century*, 34

921 Germany did not wish to appear as a naysayer to drug control, and so tried to play the national interests of other countries against each other, hoping that the conference would end with no result. See Annika Hoffmann, *Drogenkonsum und –kontrolle: Zur Etablierung eines sozialen Problems im ersten Drittel des 20. Jahrhunderts* (Wiesbaden: VS Verlag, 2012), 38-54.

922 *International Opium Convention*, 23 January 1912 at http://www.vilp.de/Enpdf/e 175.pdf. (Last access: 23.1.2016).

923 McAllister, *Drug Diplomacy in the Twentieth Century*, 34-35.

Hague Treaty, that the United States and Britain were able to force Germany into compliance.[924] Once ratified, the treaty became hailed as a stunning international success. By the 1930s, its effects were widespread. The Dutch East Indies opium trade to China was more than halved, from 35 million Guilders in 1914 to 17 million in 1932. Indian trade to China suffered even more, dropping from 7.5 million pounds in 1914 to 2.5 million in 1932.[925]

The success of the international control regime, however, was hardly a given when the International Opium Convention was signed back in 1912. Indeed, when Wright returned home that January, the United States did not yet have a national law controlling drugs, and would remain without one for another two years.

In 1914, Congress passed the Harrison Act sponsored by the then representative Francis Burton Harrison before he left to Manila with a trunk full of opium. It was a piece of tax legislation that effectively banned drug use. The act set three legal requirements for producers and distributors of opiates and cocaine: Registration with the federal government, record-keeping of all sales and transactions, and paying a purchase tax. Unregistered persons could purchase drugs only with a prescription from a physician who prescribed it in good faith and in the pursuit of his professional practice. A fine of $2,000, or five years imprisonment, or both, awaited any person who broke the law.

The Harrison Act was designed to restrict trade between states and to limit drugs to professional use. Drug use itself was not defined as a federal offense, but rather the drug trade. Drug prohibitionists were therefore left to rely on individual states to enact their own anti-narcotic laws.

Notably, the Harrison Act barely expressed concern for the health of patients, other than the vague statement that drugs could be dispensed only for "acceptable medicinal purposes." And who was to define these accept-

---

924 *Der Vertrag von Versailles: Der Friedensvertrag zwischen Deutschland und den Alliierten und Assoziierten Mächten nebst dem Schlussprotokoll und der Vereinbarung betr. die militaerische Besetzung der Rheinlande*, (Berlin, 1924), 292-294. The United States expressed its desire to force Germany to ratify the treaty, whereas Britain suggested adding the ratification requirement to the peace treaty. See Home Office, *International Opium Convention, 1912: Statement of Action taken by the British Government* (London, 1922), 5-6 at Library of Congress, CLC RM 41 *Drugs*.

925 Petrus C. van Duyne and Michael Levi, *Drugs and Money: Managing the Drug Trade and Crime-Money in Europe* (London, 2005), 24.

able medicinal purposes? Not physicians, but the Treasury Department and the courts.[926]

According to an internal government memorandum from 1914, the government's primary goal was "to safeguard public health and morality by restricting the distribution of these drugs to legitimate channels of trade."[927] Little thought was given to the fact that the laws themselves did not mention health. They were actually tax laws, according to guidelines laid out by Taft in 1910.

The lack of concern for the public's health, in fact, was one of the chief criticisms leveled against the law. "There is no doubt that Congress has no power to legislate directly for the purpose of safeguarding the health and morals of the public, nevertheless, the Harrison Law, as I understand, had primarily in view those very same principles besides the question of a revenue measure," a leading psychiatrist wrote several years after its enactment. "As to the latter, the law had to be drawn as a revenue measure in order that it might be constitutional and enforceable by the courts. But so far, has it accomplished its primary purpose? Has it actually placed in the power of the country a prophylactic measure to prevent moral and intellectual degeneration which, indeed, should be its chief aim?"[928] The answer to the rhetorical question, of course, was no.

Shortly after passage of the Harrison Act, a series of cases regarding doctors and the terms of the national prohibition on drugs made their way through the courts. The deliberations eventually reached the Supreme Court. The first such case before the highest bench, *United States v. Jin Fuey Moy* in 1916, pertained to the case of a doctor who prescribed

---

926 For a partial reproduction of the Harrison Act, see Musto, ed. *Drugs in America*, 253-255.; Jim Baumohl, "Maintaining Orthodoxy: The Depression-Era Struggle over Morphine Maintenance in California," in *Altering American Consciousness: The History of Alcohol and Drug Use in the United States, 1800-2000*, ed. Sarah W. Tracy and Caroline Jean Acker (Amherst: University of Massachusetts Press, 2004), 225-266; Musto, *The American Disease*. See below regarding the case of *Webb et al. v. United States* and the court's decision on acceptable medicinal uses of drugs.

927 "Memorandum of Drs. Wilbert and Motter (Hygienic Laboratory) forwarded to the Chief Division of Customs by the Surgeon General (27 April 1914)," NARA (DC) RG 36 Customs Case Files 1909-1938, box 960, file 101688.

928 Alfred Gordon, "The Relation of Legislative Acts to the Problem of Drug Addiction," *Journal of the American Institute of Criminal Law and Criminology* 8:2 (1917), 212.

morphine to an addicted patient. In a lower court, the government claimed that the doctor, Jin Fuey Moy, conspired with his patient to procure drugs, thus breaking the terms of the law that enabled physicians to prescribe drugs only "in good faith."

A district judge immediately dismissed the charges brought against the patient, claiming that he had not tried to "import, produce, manufacture, deal in, dispense, sell or distribute" morphine, but rather was only interested in consuming it.[929] The Supreme Court found in favor of the doctor in a 7-2 ruling, arguing that the Harrison Act was not clear on whether the requirement to prescribe drugs in good faith was indeed grounds for prohibition. So long as a physician paid the appropriate taxes, prescribing drugs, even to an addict, was not illegal.[930]

The Supreme Court decision threatened to undercut the federal ban on drugs, prompting Treasury officials to quickly ask Congress to amend the law. A new legal tool was found: Since the Harrison Act required a tax stamp on drugs; the lack of a stamp could be used as evidence of illegal possession. This measure allowed federal prosecutors to indict patients, but the question of what was to be done with physicians remained unanswered.

In 1919 the government appealed once more to the Supreme Court to reverse a drug-related ruling by a lower court. The defendant in the case was a physician practicing in San Antonio, Charles T. Doremus – a known "dope doctor" – who dispensed large amounts of drugs to addicts. The Supreme Court, in a 5-4 decision, agreed with the government, effectively reversing the ruling it had made in 1916.[931]

On the same day the Supreme Court settled the Doremus case, it turned to address the practice of the medical profession regarding drugs in *Web et al. v. United States*. The plaintiffs in the case believed it was beneficial to wean addicts slowly, or not at all, providing them with a sufficient amount of drugs to lead a normal life. A doctor and a pharmacist from Memphis, Tennessee, prescribed and filled morphine prescriptions to addicts as part of a drug maintenance program. In yet another 5-4 decision, the court concluded: "Prescribing drugs so that an addict could be 'comfortable'

---

929 Musto, *The American Disease*, 128-130.
930 Morgan, *Drugs in America*, 110; Hickman, *The Secret Leprosy of Modern Days*, 129.
931 Musto, *The American Disease*, 130-131. For a substantial excerpt of the case, see Musto, ed. *Drugs in America*, 256-260.

and maintain 'his customary use' was a 'perversion' of the law, said the court."[932]

In the wake of the Supreme Court cases of 1919, maintenance clinics closed one after another, most notably in New York City; Jacksonville, Florida; and Shreveport, Louisiana. Although a dwindling number of physicians, scrupulous in their beliefs, still believed that drug maintenance should be a legitimate practice, by 1923 the threat of federal prosecution led to a nationwide end to the practice.[933]

Just nine years after passage of the Harrison Act, a federal ban on drugs had been imposed across the United States, with only the slight hiccough of the Supreme Court's 1916 ruling slowing its adoption.

With the ban came increased power and money to enforce it. In 1920, Congress established a Narcotics Division within the Bureau of Prohibition, headed by a retired army colonel and pharmacist, Levi G. Nutt (1866–1938). The new federal officers wasted little time in putting Americans behind bars for narcotics violations. By 1925, they had made no less than 10,297 arrests, or roughly 5.5 arrests per day since the creation of the Division.[934]

The tenacity of the narcotic agents earned them a rather dubious reputation. A telling example is a 1930 letter sent from the secretary of the Colorado Pharmaceutical Association, Charles Clayton, to that state's two senators in Washington. There is a regional narcotic agent named Bradshaw, Clayton complained, who "seems to be out to make a record for himself with respect to the amount of penalties collected through 'offers in compromise,' for he has reported violations in many instances, which were merely technical and of trivial and inconsequential character [...]. He has carried these practices so far that we cannot avoid the feeling that they have come to a stage bordering on blackmail."

Clayton also suggested that the Colorado narcotics agent was acting on orders from above. He noted that rumors were circulating that the Collector of Internal Revenue in Denver had assigned a quarterly quota of $35,000 that agents had to collect from companies.[935] The Colorado sena-

---

932 Lawrence M. Friedman, *American Law in the 20th Century* (New Haven: Yale University Press, 2002), 106. See also Musto, ed. *Drugs in America*, 260-261.

933 Ibid., 140-141, 151-182.

934 Friedman, *American Law in the 20th Century*, 107.

935 Charles J. Clayton (Secretary of the Colorado Pharmacal Association) to Lawrence C. Phipps (United States Senator), 20 March 1930; Charles J. Clayton

tors dutifully forwarded the letters to Nutt, but by the time the matter was dealt with, Nutt himself had effectively been replaced and the future of the Narcotics Division itself was uncertain.[936]

Charges of corruption dogged the Narcotics Division from the beginning. The final blow came in November 1928, when an unknown assailant murdered Arnold Rothstein, a Jewish crime boss in New York City with interests in gambling, liquor and drug smuggling. Among his papers was evidence that none other than Levi G. Nutt's son and son-in-law had represented Rothstein before the tax authorities. A subsequent investigation found no criminal violations, but caused a public uproar that forced Nutt out of office.

Congress came to the realization that maintaining the Narcotics Division within the legal framework of Prohibition was unsustainable, and that it had to do something to restore both public and international confidence in its ability to enforce the country's drug laws. Representative Stephen G. Porter (1869-1930), just before his death in office in 1930, pushed for the separation of the Narcotic Division from the Bureau of Prohibition, leading to the creation of the Federal Bureau of Narcotics. The Bureau of Prohibition was transferred to the Department of Justice, while the Bureau of Narcotics remained under the umbrella of the Treasury.[937]

To fend off all allegations of corruption, an outsider was chosen as the head of the newly established Federal Bureau of Narcotics. Harry J. Anslinger was a professional diplomat who served first in the Netherlands and later in the Bahamas. While in the Caribbean he managed to convince Britain to sign a treaty curtailing rum-running operations. Anslinger was subsequently sent to negotiate similar treaties with Canada, Cuba and France.

In 1928 Anslinger was loaned for a month by the State Department to the Treasury, but his new superiors were so impressed with his organiza-

---

(Secretary of the Colorado Pharmacal Association) to Charles W. Waterman (United States Senator), 21 March 1930, NARA RG 170, Acc# 170-73-1 box 44 file 0145 folder Assoc.

936 H. J. Anslinger (Assistant Commissioner of Narcotics) to Charled W. Waterman (United States Senator), 27 March 1930, NARA RG 170, Acc# 170-73-1 box 44 file 0145 folder Assoc.

937 Musto, *The American Disease*, 206-208; John C. McWilliams, *The Protectors: Harry J. Anslinger and the Federal Bureau of Narcotics, 1930-1962* (Newark: University of Delaware Press, 1990), 37-42.

tional skills that he was kept on staff. He was assigned to head the Bureau of Prohibition's foreign control division, where his hawkish opinions became more pronounced.[938] When it became clear that Nutt would be forced to resign, the secretary of the Treasury chose Anslinger – who happened to have been married to his niece – to be the interim commissioner of the Narcotics Division. From there, the path was paved for him to become the head of the new Bureau of Narcotics in 1930.[939]

The Federal Bureau of Narcotics quickly and aggressively expanded. Within a year of its establishment, the bureau could boast 426 office employees and 271 field agents, to go along with an annual budget of $1.7 million. It covered the breadth and depth of the United States, from Alaska in the north to Texas and the Panama Canal Zone in the south, from Puerto Rico in the east to Hawaii in the west. It divided the country into 15 districts, along the same lines drawn for federal appeals courts.[940]

The Bureau of Narcotics was smaller than J. Edgar Hoover's United States Bureau of Investigation, but not by much. The agency that would later become the FBI had less than 500 special agents, with only 30 field offices for the entire country.[941] Thus, in essence, Hoover's police force was about twice the size of Anslinger's, but was responsible for enforcing all manners of crimes, from liquor violations, white slavery and murders to petty theft against federal property.

The Bureau of Narcotics, by contrast, was dedicated to enforcing one crime and one crime only. And while in Washington it may have been overshadowed by Hoover's burgeoning bureaucracy, in the eyes of officials at drug-enforcement agencies elsewhere in the world, the Federal Bureau of Narcotics was very large indeed.

Aside from its task as a law enforcement agency, the Narcotics Bureau lobbied Congress, pursued a foreign policy independently of the State Department, and maintained contact with various organizations and associations whose agenda was to eradicate the drug threat within the United States. The bureau also kept a close eye on associations that advocated for

---

938 Ibid., 31-33.
939 Ibid., 42-45.
940 Ibid., 46-47. See also *Minutes of the Nineteenth Session of the Opium Advisory Committee* (15-28 November 1934), NARA RG 170, Acc# 170-74-0005, box 116, file 1230-1.
941 Shahid M. Shahidullah, *Crime Policy in America: Laws, Institutions, and Programs* (Lanham: University Press of America, 2008), 68.

the legalization of drugs, or which pursued a more liberal approach to drug enforcement.

Perhaps the most peculiar practice of narcotics agents at the time was the recording of "confessions" from addicts. Bureau agents regarded the confessions as a key tool for keeping tabs of those on the streets. Although proclaimed to be personal statements, the confessions followed a template that made them almost indistinguishable from one another, save for the name of the addict.

The confessions of two addicts from Clarksburg, West Virginia, Roxie Deem and Charles Vannort, offer a telling example. Deem and Vannort both confessed to a narcotics agent named F. Elmer Niebuhr on the same day. Both wrote their letter in exactly the same format, using the same words to describe who they were, how they got addicted, how long they had been addicted, and when they got caught. Both explained that they had gone through several cures in hospitals, but the only effective treatment they had undergone was that provided by Dr. A. J. Kemper in the Harrison County Jail.

According to the confessions, the addicts had not relapsed because of the high price of drugs and because the physicians in Clarksburg had refused to prescribe narcotics unless extreme conditions warranted the treatment. Vannort added in his letter that he was afraid of surveillance by the law enforcement agencies, which he said kept a close eye on him.[942] Considering that some sentences were repeated word for word in both letters, one cannot avoid the impression that Niebuhr, the narcotics agent, was in fact the one behind the letters, perhaps in an effort to impress his superiors. Or, perhaps, impress Congress of the bureau's effectiveness, stressing the fact that incarceration is the only trusted cure for addiction.

The Federal Bureau of Narcotics kept a meticulous archive of drug offenders. The index of names was kept in albums, each numbering at least 360 pages and measuring roughly 30 centimeters in width and 20 centimeters in length. Each drug offender received his own page, with a short biography, a photograph and a fingerprint, as well as an FBI serial number when available. Smaller binders featuring key information and pictures were also available for field agents.

---

942 Roxie Deem to F. E. Niebuhr (Narcotic Agent), 24 May 1940, and Charles Vannort to F. E. Niebuhr (Narcotic Agent), 24 May 1940, NARA RG 170, Acc# 170-73-1 box 42 file 0120-28 folder Daily Dosage of Addicts.

The district office in New York went even further, supplying its agents with a binder on more than 200 drug offenders known to live in the district. The binder was divided into several categories, among them "suspected Mafia members believed to be engaged in the narcotic traffic," "suspected 'Chinese' narcotic traffickers," "national list of persons known to be or suspected of being engaged in the illicit traffic in narcotics drugs," "fugitives" and "international list."[943]

The Federal Bureau of Narcotics also kept track of former addicts after their release from treatment. A substantial number of hospitals and institutions collaborated with the bureau, providing the authorities with patients' personal information. Others, however, were less cooperative. The United States Public Health Service, for one, refused to share the medical profiles of its patients, though it on occasion divulged names.

The bureau was tenacious in its mission, and by the end of the 1930s it was claiming success in the crackdown on drugs. Examples surfaced across the country. The chief narcotics official for Ohio and Michigan, Ralph Oyler, declared that illegal drugs were scarce in his district. Oyler noted the poor quality of heroin seized from drug smugglers in his district, such as in the arrest of Chas Jaffe and Harry Greeson in 1940, which was taken as evidence that the drug supply had been sharply curtailed. Addicts were reportedly claiming that street heroin had become useless, and were turning to barbiturates, paregoric and medicinal-grade drugs.[944]

That same year, Oyler received a report from one of his field agents, George O. Wilson, spelling out just how tight the faucet had been closed:

> Since the last two years there has been no morphine to amount to anything, the last I saw were large 'cubes' which had turned dark. Heroin has been cut to 2% and they are asking $50 apiece for it. I doubt whether there is any heroin except in Chicago or New York, with the exception possibly of the West Coast, and I don't know anything about that. I have not been in Detroit or Toledo in seventeen years, except on one occasion, to change trains. The stuff I had came out of Chicago, to tell you who it was would do no good as he has nothing now; I was to pay $50 an ounce for it; You can go to bed as far as this racket is concerned unless something comes in from Japan. The last

---

943   NARA RG 170, Acc# 170-74-4, box 175, file 0250.

944   "Memorandum, Scarcity file from District 8 (Ohio and Michigan)," (April 1940), NARA RG 170, Acc# 170-73-1 box 42 file 0120-28 folder Daily dosage of addicts.

loophole was Brussels and now the Germans have that; as far as opium is concerned a toy is about $25, if you can get it.[945]

The drug supply in Tennessee and Kentucky had similarly gone dry. The district supervisor there warned that illegal drug "dealers were besieging country physicians for morphine and are supplementing what supply can be obtained in that manner with paregoric purchased at drug stores. Several cases were reported involving such violations on the part of the registered dealers."[946]

To the Federal Bureau of Narcotics, such reports were hard evidence that the federal ban on drugs was working, and well. And arguably it did, at least in some respects. This was certainly the case when world trade practically stopped during the World War. However, at least some of the credit goes not to the Bureau of Narcotics, but to another branch of the Treasury Department: the United States Customs Service. The Customs Service, which employed agents at various ports of entry into the United States, played an often overlooked role in the fight against drugs. This lapse is significant due to the long-held belief in the American government that the drug problem was foreign in nature.

Although opium tariffs had been adopted as early as 1842, and a ban on the importation of opium had been in place since 1909, customs agents required time to adapt to the Harrison Act of 1914. The first recorded case of a successful seizure took place in Blaine, Washington on October 30, 1915. Thirty-seven ounces of morphine and 50 ounces of cocaine were seized from a Canadian automobile trying to cross the border from Vancouver, British Columbia. Since the cocaine container bore the label of Mallinckrodt Chemical Works of St. Louis and New York, the lead customs agent in Seattle suspected a smuggling ring, suggesting that they exported drugs to Canada and smuggled them back into the United States in order to circumvent the Harrison Act.[947] The press ran stories on how

---

945 G. O. Wilson (Narcotic Agent) to R. H. Oyler (District Supervisor), May 25, 1940, NARA RG 170, Acc# 170-73-1 box 42 file 0120-28 folder Daily Dosage of Addicts.

946 Excerpt from the Progress Report for the month of June, 1940, District No. 7, (undated), NARA RG 170, Acc# 170-73-1 box 42 file 0120-28 folder Daily Dosage of Addicts.

947 "G. E. Hamming (Special Agent in Charge) to the Secretary of the Treasury, 5 November 1915" and "A. B. Hamer (Special Inspector) to the Secretary of the Treasury, 5 November 1915" in NARA (DC) RG 36, Customs Case Files 1909-1938, box 447, file 90956.

companies such as Powers-Weightman-Rosengarten of Philadelphia, The New York Quinine and Chemical Co. of New York City, and the English firm Burroughs and Welcome manufactured cocaine legitimately in the United States for shipment to Mexico or Canada, yet the cocaine somehow found its way back to America. Dope rings, particularly strong in Canada, bought cocaine and smuggled it back across the border "wrapped tightly about the bodies of men and women and even children."

By then Canada had already gotten a name as the source of illegal liquor in the United States. It soon became associated with illicit cocaine as well. The cost of manufacturing cocaine, according to one journalist, was $2 to $3 an ounce. In Canada, the smuggling rings bought the drug for $80 to $90 an ounce wholesale, and retailed it back in the United States for $200 to $300 an ounce. By the time the drug reached the street, it was worth $480 to $500 an ounce.

As the drug made its way through the supply chain, it was adulterated to maximize profits. In the South, Mexican rings dealt with lower grades of opiates. Low-grade opium from Mexico wholesaled for $90 a tin containing less than half a pound of the drug. High-grade opium wholesaled for $147 to $200 for half a pound, and retailed for $350. Since one required more opium to attain the same high than with morphine or heroin, opium was far more expensive. Thus, the ashes of the smoked opium, or yen shee, were sold to poorer smokers.[948]

The vibrant drug trade became a thorn in Washington's side. The United States aspired to be the world leader in the fight against drugs, yet drugs manufactured by American companies were finding their way into the illicit world market. Testimony given to the Senate Committee on Finance in December 1920 made clear the extent of the problem. Chinese authorities, according to the testimony, had singled out three American companies as being the primary producers of morphine smuggled into China, usually via Japan: Powers-Weightman-Rosengarten Co., New York Quinine and Chemical Co., and Merk & Co.[949]

Porous borders and incessant smuggling forced Congress to pass the Narcotics Drugs Import and Export Act in 1922. Also known as the Jones-Miller Act, the legislation, which made it more difficult to export cocaine

---

948 Fred V. Williams, *The Hop-Heads: Personal Experiences Among the Users of 'Dope' in the San Francisco Underworld* (San Francisco, 1920), 104-112.

949 "Exportation of Opium," *Hearings before the Committee on Finance of the United States Senate*, 66th Congress, 3rd Session, (11 December 1920), 4-5.

and morphine to Canada and other countries with the intent of importing the drugs back into the United States. The act also created the Federal Narcotics Control Board. Although three Cabinet members sat on the board, it was an infective body that delegated all decisions to the Treasury Department's Narcotic Division.[950] The Jones-Miller Act was credited, along with the Supreme Court's 1919 decision prohibiting narcotic prescriptions to addicts, with causing a hike in the price of morphine and subsequent switch by many addicts to heroin.[951]

History has shown time and again that wherever and whenever tariffs are imposed on legal trade, smugglers will try to make a profit on the black market. The demand for drugs in the United States during the 1920s was no exception. As the government cracked down, first on opium and later on morphine, cocaine and eventually heroin, the price of drugs skyrocketed, and availability caught up with customer's desires. Smugglers developed their wares to meet the demands of the market. At first they sought out smaller and more potent drugs to offer to their addicted clientele. With time, they also learned to dilute the drugs in order to maximize profit.[952]

The rising price of drugs and their declining potency could arguably serve as concrete evidence of the government's success in its crackdown. The opposite argument, however, could just as easily be made – namely, that demand caused both the quality and price of drugs to shoot up. Since no irrefutable data is available regarding the number of users at the time, or the true size of the drug market, both arguments remain plausible, with sufficient evidence available to back up both assertions. What is certain is that Americans clearly had an enduring appetite for drugs, and even if the government wielded an iron fist at home, the financial incentives to meet that demand from abroad were too great for smugglers to ignore.

As early as 1916, United States Customs Service officials in El Paso, Texas expressed concern about increasing attempts to smuggle Chinese smoking opium into the United States via Mexico. Torn by war and general political discord, Mexico, despite efforts by the Carranza govern-

---

950 Musto, *The American Disease*, 197.
951 Courtwright, *Dark Paradise*, 242 n.131.
952 Addicts, who were interviewed in the early 1980s, recalled the tricks dealers did in order to cut the drugs. See David Courtwright, Herman Joseph, and Don Des Jarlais, *Addicts Who Survived: An Oral History of Narcotic Use in America, 1923-1965* (Knoxville: University of Tennessee Press, 1989).

ment, had little ability to enforce a durable cross-border crackdown on the drug trade. As one Texas customs agent put it in a 1917 report on a smuggling ring of Germans operating on the Mexican border: "I do not see how anything can be accomplished through bringing this situation to the attention of the Mexican government. Unless [there] is a law recently enacted, I know of no federal law in Mexico prohibiting the dealing in opium. Several of the states in Mexico have such laws but under existing conditions they are not being enforced."[953]

The smuggling of drugs and alcohol from Mexico was based in the states of Baja California, Sonora and Chihuahua, with the border cities of Tijuana, Mexicali and Ciudad Juárez serving as regional hubs. As the drugs went north, American dollars flowed south, supporting the war-stricken provinces of Mexico. With corruption rampant, the money also padded the bank accounts of governors and other officials.

American temperance lobby groups tried to convince the Mexican government to enact dry laws, but to little avail. After the passage of the Harrison Act, the State Department pressured Mexico to impose stricter drug laws and conform to the international treaties it had signed, but again little success was found.[954] Smuggling continued unabated, eventually expanding into production as well.

With Mexico unwilling or unable to enforce a stricter drug policy, border states in America took matters into their own hands. Their efforts had perhaps their greatest impact when it came to marijuana. By the 1920s, most had laws on the books against the drug. The most important border state, California, outlawed marijuana – the drug associated with Mexicans – in 1913, as part of a broader drug control law.[955]

The federal government, however, did not match efforts at the state level. Contrary to common perception, the United States was a relative latecomer to marijuana prohibition. Marijuana was not included in the

---

953 "J. Brighton (Special Agent in Charge) to the Secretary of the Treasury," (24 March 1917), NARA (DC) RG 36 (customs case files), 1909-1938, box 447, file 90956.

954 Gabriela Recio, "Drugs and Alcohol: US Prohibition and the Origins of the Drug Trade in Mexico, 1910-1930," *Journal of Latin American Studies* 34:1 (2002), 21-42.

955 Dale H. Gieringer, "The Forgotten Origins of Cannabis Prohibition in California," *Contemporary Drug Problems* 26:2 (1999), 237-288. The first state to enact an anti-marijuana law was actually Massachusetts in 1912, but other states from the Northeast followed suit only in the 1920s and 30s.

Harrison Act of 1914, although several drafts of the bill listed marijuana as a narcotic. Hashish and marijuana, in fact, remained legal until 1937.

The first push for a ban on the drug came far from America's shores. In 1911, South Africa passed laws against marijuana. That same year Italy acquired Libya as a colony, and at the 1912 Hague conference it proposed banning cannabis, to little success. More than a decade later, South Africa again took the lead in calling for a ban. In 1923 it appealed to the League of Nations in Geneva to add cannabis to the list of controlled substances, a call echoed a year later by Turkey and, importantly, Egypt.

The Egyptian representative to Geneva adamantly insisted that no less than a third of mental cases in Egypt were the result of hashish. He based his claim on a 1903 report by John Warnock, at the time the medical director of the Egyptian hospital for the insane, stating that 27 percent of his patients were hashish smokers. The figure was subsequently inflated to as high as 60 percent. More reliable statistics recorded between 1909 and 1913 by the Egyptian government put the percentage of hashish smokers among mental hospital inmates at 11 percent to 15 percent, with the figure even lower in official reports published after 1920.[956]

The Egyptian representative at first had the support of Britain, which was eager to show both concern for and authority over the international drug trade. The Americans, by contrast, displayed complete indifference in Geneva toward cannabis, even questioning whether the drug should be discussed at all. But as deliberations dragged on through 1924 and into 1925, London and Washington found their roles reversing. Britain lost its enthusiasm for banning marijuana because of its profitable hemp policy in colonial India, while the United States turned on the drug in the pursuit of more stringent controls on the international drug trade.[957]

On February 19, 1925, the League of Nations voted to include marijuana and hashish on the list of controlled substances. During the negotiations, nine states voted in favor, seven against. Britain and the Netherlands abstained. Germany voted in favor of the ban only after securing a deal with Egypt for the sale of manufactured drugs. The United States, though

---

956 Liat Kozma, "Egyptian Cannabis Prohibition 1880-1939: From Local Ban to the League of Nations," *Middle Eastern Studies* 41:3 (2011), 443-460.

957 James Mills, *Cannabis Britannica: Empire, Trade, and Prohibition 1800-1928* (Oxford: Oxford University Press, 2003), 165.

not a member of the league, was also invited to vote, which it did in favor of the Egyptian proposal.[958]

Its vote, however, was only symbolic. The American representative to the talks, Pennsylvania congressman Stephen G. Porter, walked out of the talks when the terms of the international mechanism for controlling the drug trade were deemed to be unacceptable to Washington. The United States was left outside the purview of the treaty, and therefore had no international obligation to enact a national ban on cannabis when the International Opium Convention was signed and ratified by other powers in 1925.[959]

America had too much invested in the fight against drugs to remain silent on the international stage, and eventually two forums for letting America's voice be heard were created within the League of Nations, even though it was never a member of the organization. The Opium Advisory Committee and the Permanent Central Opium Board were established in 1920 and 1925 respectively with a mandate to direct the international effort to curb drug trafficking. Washington was invited to send representatives to the Permanent Central Opium Board, and often sent independent representatives to the Opium Advisory Committee.

Back home, marijuana was not yet seen as a threatening drug menace. The soft gloves with which America handled marijuana is, at first glance, somewhat perplexing. A country that harshly condemned drugs and made control of the drug trade a key foreign policy priority took its time when it came to banning marijuana. One explanation may be that relatively few Americans used the drug in the 1920s. Another explanation may have been the concern, as elucidated by Harry Anslinger, about banning a crop that was native to the United States.[960]

Whatever the reason for its initial recalcitrance, by the 1930s the United States had unquestionably turned against cannabis. The press was rife with stories of marijuana-induced crimes and other sordid societal ills caused by the "killer weed." Marijuana, which already had a bad name among

---

958 Westel W. Willoughby, *Opium as an International Problem: The Geneva Conferences* (Baltimore, 1925), 374-384; Sebastian Scheerer, "North American Bias and Non-American Roots of Cannabis Prohibition," at http://www.bisdro.uni-bremen.de/boellinger/cannabis/04-schee.pdf. (Last access: 23.1.2016).
959 McAllister, *Drug Diplomacy in the Twentieth Century*, 69-78.
960 "Roosevelt asks Narcotic War Aid," *New York Times*, (22 March 1935).

Americans for its association with Mexicans, sparked yet another drug panic in the United States.

Anslinger, attuned to the mood on the street as well as in Washington, changed his tune and came out strongly for a ban on marijuana. In March 1937, several months before Congress passed America's first federal law against cannabis, the Bureau of Narcotics chief warned of a rising tide of marijuana-driven crime. "Despite the fact that medical men and scientists have disagreed upon the properties of marihuana, and some are inclined to minimize the harmfulness of this drug, the records offer ample evidence that it has a disastrous effect upon many if its users," Anslinger said in a speech. "Recently we received many reports showing crimes of violence committed by persons while under the influence of marihuana.... The deleterious, even vicious, qualities of the drug render it highly dangerous to the mind and body upon which it operates to destroy the will, cause one to lose the power of connected thought, producing imaginary delectable situations and gradually weakening the physical power. Its use frequently leads to insanity."[961]

Others in government took a more moderate approach, including Surgeon General Thomas Parran Jr. (1892-1968), who argued in a report in June of that year to the League of Nations that marijuana was not addictive like opium, but rather habit-forming like alcohol, sugar and coffee.[962] But Anslinger's argument, based in part on the data collected in Egypt three decades earlier, won the day.

On August 2, 1937, Congress passed the Marihuana Tax Act.[963] The mechanics of the anti-cannabis legislation were nearly identical to those of the Harrison Act of 1914, with one notable exception. It was understood that the government would not issue tax stamps that would allow physicians to prescribe cannabis to their patients, thereby circumventing the legitimate medical use tenet of the Harrison Act. The drug would be illegal for all. After passage of the Marihuana Tax Act, Dr. R. P. Walton and other physicians urged the federal government to refrain from restricting research on cannabis and its potential medical uses, arguing that

---

961 "Marihuana, speech by commissioner H. J. Anslinger," NARA RG 170, Acc# 170-73-1, Box 44, file 0145 gen., folder #1.

962 Bonnie and Whitebread, *The Marijuana Conviction*, 152.

963 Ibid., 164-174. Please note the contemporary spelling of the drug using an 'h' instead of a 'j'.

there was no evidence whatsoever that medicinal use of cannabis caused addiction.[964] Their calls, however, fell on deaf ears.

Medical research on cannabis in the United States came to a halt, and remained so for years to come. The workings of the drug were so shrouded in mystery that it was not until the 1960s that the alkaloid of the drug was isolated – notably, not in the United States, but in the tiny country of Israel. As research into the drug went down, arrests for dealing it went up, eventually becoming the dominant cause for federal drug-related arrests. In 1938, the year after passage of the Marijuana Tax Act, less than one-quarter of those arrested on federal drug charges were booked for marijuana. By 1950, marijuana crimes accounted for no less than 73 percent of federal drug prosecutions.[965]

---

964 R. Walton, *Marijuana: America's New Drug Problem* (Philadelphia, 1938), 151-157.

965 Kenneth J. Meier, *The Politics of Sin: Drugs, Alcohol, and Public Policy* (New York: M. E. Sharpe, 1994), 38.

12. Treatment vs. Incarceration

During the first two decades of the 20th century, debate grew in Washington over whether incarceration or treatment offered a better chance of curing the drug ills plaguing American society. The heavy hand of the law would prevail, proving too entrenched to be reformed by calls for more medically-based approaches. But for a brief number of years in the 1930s, prison was not the predetermined fate of those caught with illicit drugs. Though hardly available to all, medical treatment was offered to few drug addicts, with the full backing of the federal government, as an alternative to incarceration.

The change in policy had its roots during the mid-1920s, when James V. Bennet (1894-1978), at the time working for the Bureau of Efficiency, conducted an investigative tour of America's federal prisons. Bennet, who would go on to direct the Bureau of Prisons from 1937 to 1969, reported that no less than 2,000 of the prisoners he came across were drug addicts. He warned that they lacked medical attention in custody, and recommended that two institutions be established where addicts could be treated away from the general prison population.[966]

In 1928, Representative Stephen G. Porter took up Bennet's recommendation, introducing a bill in the House calling for the establishment of two "Narcotic Farms." Porter claimed that the Narcotic Farms would help alleviate the overcrowding of federal penitentiaries that had occurred since the enactment of the Harrison Act and other federal criminal laws. Since 1915, he noted, the prison population of federal penitentiaries had increased fourfold, with more and more addicts being sent to jail. The congressman's concern was hardly only with the intolerable conditions in prisons. Just as strong was the fear that addicts would infect other prisoners with their disease – namely, drug use.[967] Porter, one of the more experienced members of Congress on drug policy, wrote in a letter to the

---

966 J. V. Bennett, *I Chose Prison* (New York: Knopf, 1970), 84, 94; Nathan B. Eddy, *The National Research Council Involvement in the Opiate Problem, 1928-1971* (Washington DC: The National Academy of Science, 1973), 25.

967 "Statement of Representative Stephen G. Porter, [undated, probably 1928]," NARA RG 170, Acc# 170-73-1, box 40, file 120-5, folder #3.

secretary of the Treasury that in all his years on the Hill he had never seen such strong approval for a bill.[968]

Porter stressed that addiction was not only a vice, but also a disease. And if cured of their disease, drug addicts would stay away from a life of crime, because they would have no addiction to finance. He proposed creating "farms" where the addicts could be placed for an extended stay, away from other prisoners who might be susceptible to drugs. The legislation was intended to serve as a model for individual states to imitate.[969]

Porter's bill had the backing of the Prohibition Bureau's Narcotic Division. The head of the Narcotic Division, Levi G. Nutt, commended the legislation, in particular for allowing known criminals to enter the farms for treatment.[970] Yet Nutt was clear that many drug addicts deserved to be punished by the full extent of the law. "Many of these addicts have been and continued to be guilty of selling narcotic drugs unlawfully," Nutt warned, "and it is assumed it will be agreed that this class must be required to suffer the punishment imposed upon them for their crimes, with the understanding, of course, that they will incidentally be offered proper medical treatment in the penal institution to which they are sentenced, whether such institution be a penitentiary or a special place of imprisonment designed for the purpose."[971]

His endorsement of such special places of imprisonment, however, came with an unequivocal qualification:

> So far as the bill will operate to separate narcotic drug addicts from other prisoners, and to give them necessary care and attention, it recommends itself to favorable consideration. However, this office does not wish to be understood as admitting that a permanent cure may be expected in the case of this type of drug addict, since it is estimated that 95% of narcotic drug addicts sent to the penitentiaries are or will be recidivists, having psychopathic complications that preclude any hope of permanent cure.[972]

---

968 Humphrey Porter (Congressman) [sic] to Andrew Mellon (Secretary of the Treasury), 27 February 1928, NARA RG 170, Acc# 170-73-1 box 40 file 120-5 unmarked folder.

969 Ibid.

970 "Statement made by Col. Nutt before Judiciary Committee, 26 April 1928," NARA RG 170, Acc# 170-73-1, box 40, file 120-5, folder #3.

971 "L. G. Nutt (Deputy Commissioner) to Charles R. Davis (U.S. District Judge, Eastern District of Missouri), 10 March 1928," NARA RG 170 Acc# 170-73-1, box 40, file 120-5, folder #3.

On January 29, 1929, Congress approved the establishment of two institutions for treating addicts. The description of them in Washington as "Narcotic Farms" quickly drew public ridicule, and in short order the two institutions became known as the more generic "United States Health Service Hospitals." They were designed to house drug addicts found guilty by federal courts for "offenses against the United States," in the words of the then-assistant commissioner of narcotics, Will S. Wood.[973] The purpose of the farms was to rehabilitate addicts, restoring their health and training them to be self-supporting and self-reliant.[974]

Due to lack of zeal it took another five years before ground was broken on the first federal farm. Construction finally began in mid 1934 in Lexington, Kentucky, and a year later the hospital opened its doors, with capacity for 1,000 patients.[975] The farm began operating under the directorship of leading psychiatrist Lawrence Kolb.[976]

The second federal farm was built in the vicinity of Fort Worth, Texas. Originally the Lexington farm had been intended for men and the Fort Worth farm for women, but both came to be used for men. Lexington served addicts from the eastern part of the country, while Fort Worth treated those from the western half.

It would take until 1939 for a women's ward to be established in Lexington.[977] Until then, women were sent to the Federal Industrial Institution for Women in Alderson, West Virginia, or to other private institution such as the Women's Prison Association of New York and the Isaac T. Hopper Home. Women addicts were not perceived to pose as great a threat

---

972 "L. G. Nutt (Deputy Commissioner) to S. Lowman (Assistant Secretary of the Treasury), 2 March 1928," NARA RG 170 Acc# 170-73-1, box 40, file 120-5, folder #3.

973 "Will S. Wood to Dr. M. K. Cole (January 2, 1935)," NARA RG 170, Acc# 170-31-1 box 40 file 0120-5 Gen. The term was used also in the "Regulations Governing the Admission of Persons to a United States Narcotic Farm (April 1, 1935)," NARA RG 170, Acc# 170-31-1 box 40 0120-5 Gen.

974 *New York Journal* (October 11, 1934), clipping found in NARA RG 170, Acc# 170-31-1 box 40 0120-5 Gen.

975 "Assistant Surgeon General, Division of Mental Hygiene to Miss Isabelle S. Fosler (June 4, 1934)," NARA RG 170, Acc# 170-31-1 box 40 0120-5 Gen.

976 "Invitation for the Dedication of the Narcotic Farm in Lexington (May 20, 1935)," NARA RG 170, Acc# 170-31-1 box 40 0120-5 Gen.

977 "Medical Officer in Charge of the U.S. Public Service Hospital, Fort Worth, Texas to District Supervisor Joseph Bell (November 4, 1938)," NARA RG 170, Acc# 170-73-1 Box 42 file 0120-21 Gen. Circ. #3.

to society as men. In the words of the prison association's director, Rachael Hopper Powell, most offenses committed by women were "social" rather than "criminal" in nature.[978]

Addicts convicted by a federal court were eligible for treatment in Lexington or Fort Worth for the duration of their confinement. Inmates who wished to extend treatment beyond their term of incarceration could petition the surgeon general for approval. Addicts who had been sentenced to probation by any federal court were likewise eligible for treatment, until they had been determined to be cured by the surgeon general. Voluntary patients were also admitted to the farm if there was space, so long as they paid $1 a day for treatment and had secured approval from the surgeon general. Drug addicts sent to Lexington on probation were usually pronounced cured after nine months, while patients who entered the hospital of their own volition were encouraged to stay for at least six months.[979]

The regulations governing admittance to the narcotic farms departed in some notable instances from the laws on the books at the time. An addict was defined as any "person who habitually uses a habit-forming narcotic drug so as to endanger the public morals, health, safety, or welfare, or who is or has been so far addicted to the use of habit-forming narcotic drugs as to have lost the power of self control with reference to his addiction." The regulations not only defined opium, cocaine and their alkaloids, derivatives, salts and preparations as narcotic drugs, but also Indian hemp (cannabis sativa) and peyote,[980] which were not listed in the Harrison Act and were not proscribed in the United States at the time.

The Lexington facility looked, at least upon arrival, much like a prison, down to the gates, fences and locks. The effect was intentional. The large Art Deco building was grand in scale, with tall brick pillars and a large courtyard that was designed to instill fear in newcomers. The towering

---

978 *Ninety-Fourth Annual Report of the Women's Prison Association of New York and the Isaac T. Hooper Home* (October 1, 1937-September 30, 1938) NARA RG 170, Acc# 170-31-1 box 42 file 0120-23 Female addiction.

979 Michael J. Pescor, "A Statistical Analysis of the Clinical Records of Hospitalized Drug Addicts," *Public Health Reports* (Washington, 1938), supplement no. 143, 1.

980 "Regulations Governing the Admission of Persons to a United States Narcotic Farm (April 1, 1935)," NARA RG 170, Acc# 170-31-1 box 40 0120-5 Gen.

administrative building reminded one contemporary observer of a "temple of rehabilitation."[981]

Upon arrival, patients were repeatedly required to reconstruct their drug history. As noted by then-assistant surgeon general Michael J. Pescor (1904-?), there was a singular purpose to demanding addicts recount their experience with addiction first to an admitting officer, and subsequently to a ward physician and a psychiatrist, as well as to a chief supervising guardian and a social service representative: "Thus the patients [had] ample opportunity to contradict themselves if they [were] not careful."[982]

Lawrence Kolb, who in addition to directing the Lexington farm also served as its chief medical officer, put a primacy on rehabilitating the personality traits that caused addiction. To that end, he deemed labor in shops or out in the fields as suitable endeavors for the inmates. Addicts in Lexington were sent to milk cows, build chairs and even work as servants in the homes of the medical staff – conditions that inmates in regular prisons could only dream of. The narcotic farm, despite being run by physicians and more humane treatment, was not a holiday resort. Barred windows, menacing appearance, discipline, experiments and searches were the order of the day.

In the Lexington farm – or Narco, as it was sometimes called, for "Narcotic Colony" – district supervisors in the Federal Bureau of Narcotics sensed an opportunity to send their addicts to faraway Kentucky. Occasionally their efforts to clean up their districts overstepped jurisdictional boundaries, leading to public infighting between bureau headquarters in Washington and its field offices.

In July 1935, the district supervisor for New England, William E. Clark, informed the press that his office was accepting applications from addicts interested in being treated at the narcotic farm. Articles subsequently appeared in Boston's main newspapers reporting that the Lexington institution had 100 empty beds for voluntary patients, and that Clark himself was selecting candidates for admission.

---

981 Nancy D. Campbell, J. Olsen and Luke Walden, *The Narcotic Farm: The Rise and Fall of America's First Prison of Drug Addicts* (New York: Abrams, 2008), 14.

982 Michael J. Pescor, "A Statistical Analysis of the Clinical Records of Hospitalized Drug Addicts" *Public Health Reports* (Washington D.C., 1938), supplement no. 143, 2.

Upon hearing the news, Federal Bureau of Narcotics head Harry J. Anslinger dispatched an angry letter to his New England district supervisor, forbidding him from contacting the press without explicit approval from headquarters. The bureau chief argued that Clark's misstep attracted undue media, and furthermore gave the mistaken impression that addiction was a disease with a cure, rather than a crime.[983] But what caused Anslinger perhaps the greatest concern was that the Federal Bureau of Narcotics simply lacked the authority to accept candidates for drug rehabilitation at the narcotic farm in Kentucky.

That authority, as Anslinger well knew, belonged to the Public Health Service. Moreover, under the conditions laid down by Congress in 1929, when the narcotic farms were legislated into existence, federal prisoners were explicitly given precedence over voluntary patients, a mandate that was clearly challenged by Clark's call for addicts to voluntary submit their candidacies for Lexington.

New England was hardly the only jurisdiction where Federal Bureau of Narcotics agents employed suspect methods in attempting to place drug addicts in the narcotic farms. The Maryland district office cultivated informants among drug addicts by promising to secure them a bed in Lexington, free of charge. A 1935 report submitted to District Supervisor Boyd M. Martin by a field agent offers a telling example. An informant named Alonzo Roscoe Meyers was told that if he provided to the bureau the names of four drug suppliers, he would be found a place at the narcotic farm and have his $1-per-day fee covered. A contract was even signed with the local district attorney.[984]

Upon hearing of Meyers' contract, however, the surgeon general informed Anslinger that such a practice was illegal. A patient had to be voluntarily admitted to the narcotic farm, and an informant who had been pressured by the bureau hardly met the definition of voluntary. Anslinger promptly ordered that all field agents cease submitting applications on behalf of their informants, instructing instead that the informants were to contact the surgeon general directly.[985] This bureaucratic process,

---

983 "H. J. Anslinger to William E. Clark (August 1, 1935)," NARA RG 170, Acc# 170-31-1 box 40 file 0120-5 Gen.

984 "Robert E. Meeds to District Supervisor B. M. Martin (December 14, 1935)," NARA RG 170, Acc# 170-31-1 box 40 file 0120-5 Gen.

985 "H. J. Anslinger to B. M. Martin (December 24, 1935)," NARA RG 170, Acc# 170-31-1 box 40 file 0120-5 Gen.

however, led many addicts to lose interest in voluntary treatment at the narcotic farms.

While the debate over the legality and efficacy of drug rehabilitation unfolded during the early decades of the 20th century, the number of drug addicts being sent to jail continued to rise; and, with the rise in imprisoned addicts came, not surprisingly, a major influx of drugs into America's prisons. According to L. L. Stanley, the resident physician at San Quentin prison near San Francisco, half of the inmates used drugs from 1915 to 1928, with the figure above 60 percent in 1915 and again from 1924 to 1926.[986] All manner of methods were used to smuggle drugs inside prison walls. Foodstuffs were often used to transport the contraband. Lawyers took advantage of their clients' right to legal consultation to slip them the goods. Drugs were found saturated into the paper of letters sent to prison, and in the mouths, anuses and vaginas of prisoners' spouses visiting their loved ones in jail.[987]

Prison officials on the far side of the country were telling similar stories. Amos Osborne, the chief physician of Sing Sing prison in New York, was outspoken in warning about the rise of drug addicts in jail. At Sing Sing, the percentage of new inmates who were drug addicts jumped from 0.4 percent in 1917 to 9.1 percent in 1922, more than a 20-fold increase in just five years.[988]

Whether in prison or in institutional treatment, there was widespread acceptance among politicians, law enforcement officials and physicians – who otherwise rarely agreed on much when it came to controlling drug addiction – that drug users needed to be isolated from the general population, lest they infect others with their disease. It was hoped that over time, addicts would die off in isolation from respectable society, freeing America once and for all from the drug scourge. Such hopes, however, were hardly grounded in firm evidence. Indeed, the narcotic farms were arguably the government's sole reliable source of information on the nature of addiction, and the evidence gleaned from Lexington and Fort

---

986 Chart prepared by L. L. Stanley in "Harry V. Williamson (Narcotic Agent in Charge) to L. G. Nutt (9 February 1929)," NARA RG 170, Acc# 170-31-1 box 40, file 0120-5, folder #3.

987 "L. G. Nutt (Deputy Commissioner) to HR John J. Cochran, 23 April 1928," NARA RG 170, Acc# 170-73-1, box 40, file 120-5, folder #3.

988 Amos Osborne, "The Influence of Narcotic Drugs on Crime" (1924) *Drugs Pamphlets*, Library of Congress, CLC RM 41, No. 33.

Worth gave the lie to the belief that isolating addicts would rid the country of the drug menace.[989]

In 1938, Pescor, the assistant surgeon general, published a report on the nature of addiction. According to the study, 80 percent of the patients at the three-year-old narcotic farm in Lexington had become addicted to drugs after the passage of the Harrison Act. Drug users, in short, were getting younger, with an average age lower than that found in 1925 research by Lawrence Kolb. Pescor concluded that drug addiction had clearly not been isolated from general society, but was at a loss to pinpoint a specific cause:

> Propaganda about the evils of drug addiction not only spreads a knowledge of its existence, but may backfire, arousing curiosity in place of dread. Better organization of drug dealers with more efficient methods of procuring new habitués may be another factor. Economic unrest and lack of occupational opportunity with its attendant discouragement, is still another possibility. Or it may be simply another manifestation of the increasing sophistication of the younger generation.[990]

It was clear that federal legislation attempts to curb drug addiction had failed. Drug addicts were not isolated, drugs were available, and addicts were getting acquainted with drugs at a younger age. The most common reason addicts gave for getting involved with drugs, according to Pescor, was curiosity and the urge to associate with "undesirable companions." What caused that curiosity and urge was left unanswered. Pescor appeared inclined to accept Kolb's belief that addicts were psychopaths in nature, but was dismissive of Kolb's claims during the late 1920s that medical addicts used drugs for their analgesic effect.[991] Seeking out drugs to relieve pain, Pescor argued, was hardly a satisfactory explanation for addiction:

> On the face of it [pain relief] is more substantial excuse than mere curiosity. Nevertheless, there are very few individuals who have an incurable, painful disease necessitating the continuous administration of narcotic drugs. The majority of therapeutically addicted individuals find that the drug supplies something that has been missing in their lives, so that even when the original

---

989 Campbell, *Discovering Addiction*, 1-11.
990 Pescor, "A Statistical Analysis of the Clinical Records of Hospitalized Drug Addicts," 2-3.
991 Lawrence Kolb, "Drug Addiction: A Study of Some Medical Cases" *Archives of Neurology and Psychiatry* 20:1 (1928), 171-183; idem, "Types and Characteristics of Drug Addicts," 300-313.

physical cause for addiction has been removed and the patients withdrawn from drugs, they relapse in order to 'feel normal.'[992]

Pescor was equally dismissive of another reason commonly given for drug use, to relieve alcohol-induced hangovers. "Ostensibly alcoholism is the cause of drug addiction in these instances, but what precipitated the alcoholism?" he questioned. He also cited relief from fatigue and environmental stress, as well as performance enhancement, as causes of addiction.[993]

Pescor's report was replete with facts and figures. The average period of addiction was 12.5 years, with the majority ranging from five to ten years. The shortest case lasted one year, and five had been addicted for 40 years or more. One patient had been addicted for 59 years without undergoing a rehabilitation program so much as once; he had a steady income, which allowed him to pay for his habit without resorting to criminal activity.[994]

Morphine was the drug of choice, according to Pescor's report, followed by opium smoking and heroin. Only a small percentage of addicts began their drug habit with cocaine:

> Several patients started with marihuana, one with hashish (genuine Indian hemp), two with pantopon, one with codeine, and one with dilaudid. The majority of the patients used more than one narcotic drug. However, one-fourth of the patients used morphine exclusively, 7.4 per cent heroin exclusively, 2.7 per cent opium exclusively; one patient used pantopon only, one dilaudid only, and one confined himself to marihuana. Two individuals boasted they had used or tried every form of narcotic drug…. Morphine is… most likely to be the first drug used, the drug of choice, and the last drug used. Heroin is used chiefly when morphine is unavailable or when it sells cheaper than morphine.[995]

Pescor found the ratio of morphine addicts to heroin addicts to be nearly equal, a fundamental shift from Kolb's finding a decade earlier that addicts were six times more likely to use morphine than heroin.[996] In raising a red flag about the spread of heroin use, Pescor found himself aligned with the head of the Federal Bureau of Narcotics.

---

992 Pescor, "A Statistical Analysis of the Clinical Records of Hospitalized Drug Addicts," 3-4.
993 Ibid., 3-4.
994 Ibid., 5.
995 Ibid., 4.
996 Ibid.

In a 1938 memorandum to the assistant secretary of the Treasury, Anslinger stated that the bureau seized five times more heroin than morphine, discounting foreign seizures. The figures led Anslinger to conclude that the illicit use of heroin had become greater than morphine. He declared that for each morphine addict there were five heroin addicts, and that because morphine was difficult to obtain, heroin use had spread from its New York City roots across the country.[997]

Pescor and Anslinger, however, were hardly on the same page, as became clear that November after Anslinger requested comment on Pescor's study from A. L. Tennyson, the Federal Bureau of Narcotics' chief counsel.[998] "I note a significant statement 'two-thirds of the voluntary patients failed to stay the required length of time for an optimal cure,'" Tennyson reported back to Anslinger. "I have long had the impression – of course as a layman – that the government could not look for much lasting benefit to the voluntary patient, for this very reason. The last paragraph of the study immediately preceding the 'Acknowledgment' is pessimistic but very frank. It seems to emphasize the need for social service work with the cured addict, after his release from the institution, but this perhaps should be a function of the authorities of the state where the addict is to reside."[999]

Tennyson was generally approving of the report, in particular what he saw as its justification for stricter laws and enforcement and the placing of responsibility for rehabilitation on individual states. To Anslinger, however, the study was dangerously misguided. Two assertions in particular troubled the bureau chief. The first was Pescor's claim that "most of the alcoholics are better off on drugs than they were on alcohol."[1000] The second was the claim that addicts were not, in fact, anti-social, a conclusion based on the finding that three-fourths of the patients at Lexington

---

997 H. J. Anslinger (Commissioner of Narcotics) to Gibbons (Assistant Secretary of the Treasury), 21 November 1938, NARA RG 170, Acc# 170-73-1 box 40 file 0120-5 Lex. folder "Pescor, Michael J., M.D."

998 H. J. Anslinger (Commissioner of Narcotics) to A. L. Tennyson (Chief Counsel), 4 November 1938, NARA RG 170, Acc# 170-73-1 box 40 file 0120-5 Lex. folder "Pescor, Michael J., M.D."

999 A. L. Tennyson (Chief Counsel) to H. J. Anslinger (Commissioner of Narcotics) 12 November 1938, NARA RG 170, Acc# 170-73-1 box 40 file 0120-5 Lex. folder "Pescor, Michael J., M.D."

1000 Pescor, "A Statistical Analysis of the Clinical Records of Hospitalized Drug Addicts," 8.

had no history of delinquency or anti-social behavior prior to addiction.[1001] The Federal Bureau of Narcotics moved quickly to discredit Pescor's findings. "This theory is not supported by authorities known to the Bureau," Anslinger derided Pescor's suggestion that alcoholics would be better off on drugs, perhaps reflecting a fear that addiction would be taken less seriously. "I do not know the basis for the conclusion."[1002]

To counter Pescor's claim that the vast majority of addicted inmates had no history of delinquency prior to addiction, Anslinger dispatched a memorandum to the assistant secretary of the Treasury detailing the bureau's analysis of 500 "run of the mill" cases in the Northeast. More than 78 percent were first arrested for violations of non-narcotic offenses, the bureau chief stated, presenting the Treasury official with a breakdown of cases by state and, in New York, by region:

First Criminal Offenses of Narcotic Law Violators

State	Number of Addicted Defendants	Nature of First Offense	
		Narcotic Laws	Other Laws
Maine	18	5	13
Massachusetts	162	33	129
Rhode Island	7	0	7
New Hampshire	1	1	0
Connecticut	37	7	30
Eastern New York	44	10	34
Northern New York	28	4	24
Southern New York	176	40	136
Western New York	27	7	20
Total	500	107	393
Cases in which first offense was under Narcotic Laws 21.4 percent.			
Cases in which first offense was under Other Laws 78.6 percent.			

1001 Pescor, "A Statistical Analysis of the Clinical Records of Hospitalized Drug Addicts," 8.

1002 H. J. Anslinger (Commissioner of Narcotics) to Gibbons (Assistant Secretary of the Treasury), 21 November 1938, NARA RG 170, Acc# 170-73-1 box 40 file 0120-5 Lex. folder "Pescor, Michael J., M.D."

Nor did the Federal Bureau of Narcotics stop there. Two days after the publication of Pescor's report, the bureau publicly declared that the addiction rate in the United States was just two per 10,000 people, down five-fold from 14 years earlier.[1003] Contrary to Pescor's claims, Anslinger declared, the federal system for incarcerating drug felons was working; whether that was indeed the case remains open to debate.

At a minimum, there is reason for doubt, to judge by information gleaned from the narcotic farms' female equivalent in Alderson, West Virginia. According to a report on the status of female inmates discharged from the Federal Industrial Institution, of the 547 discharged women who had served time for narcotics-related crimes, just 89 remained cured, a success rate of less than one in six.[1004]

The writing, however, was on the wall. By the end of the decade, the heavy hand of the law had won the drug addiction debate. Law enforcement officials and doctors alike had come to the conclusion that the type of treatment found in Alderson, Lexington and Fort Worth was an ineffectual remedy for the drug ills that plagued American society.[1005]

1003 *Los Angeles Times* 13 November 1938.
1004 "Present Status of Females Reported Discharged from the Federal Industrial Institution for Women at Alderson, West Virginia, after having served Sentences for Violation of the Narcotic Laws," (4 January 1939), NARA RG 170, Acc# 170-73-1 Box 42 file 0120-21 folder Gen. Circ. #3.
1005 Baumohl, "Maintaining Orthodoxy: The Depression-Era Struggle over Morphine Maintenance in California," 255.

Conclusions

Why were the Nazis so convinced, that addiction was not a racial pollutant, and why were Americans so eager to maltreat their own addicts? The answers to both questions lie in the respective role of physicians and medicine in each country in the 19ᵗʰ century.

The birth of addiction in the early 19ᵗʰ century revealed two different national approaches to medicine. In Germany, C. von Brühl-Cramer's drinking disease left the treatment of drunkenness firmly in the hands of physicians as the habit turned from a vice to a disease. Germans, who were less inclined to chastise drunkards than Americans, rarely turned to religion or moral figures to treat this hidden disease.

All attempts to rouse the German public against drinking utterly failed. Although the temperance movements received the blessing of the Kaiser, the public and the Reichstag refused to ban alcohol. Laws controlling drinking in Germany were few and far between and never reached the same intensity as Prohibition in the United States or the measures taken in Sweden or even Britain. Pubs and restaurants kept on serving alcohol, and Germans continued to drink to their hearts' content. The only dents in the rising drinking rates in Germany were caused by periodical economic crises, rather than intervention by the state. The United States, by contrast, was wary of alcohol. From the early days of the Republic, Americans both consumed and feared alcohol, as excessive drinking was deemed a moral vice plaguing a defective individual. Even when American physicians sought to imitate their German counterparts by insisting that alcoholism was a disease like any other, they could not shake off the notion that it was also a sign of moral failing, thus producing the medical hybrid of a "moral disease." Prohibition was the culmination of a moral panic rather than a medical idea. As a matter of practicality, American doctors allied themselves with the temperance movement to achieve a common goal: a reduction or cessation of alcohol consumption in the United States. But in the process, their voice of reason and science was dimmed by the preaching of moralists.

Alcoholism was only the first hidden disease to be indentified by physicians. By the end of the 19ᵗʰ century, opium, morphine and cocaine were included to the list of agents that caused similar diseases. German doctors, for their part, managed to retain their monopoly over treatment, to the point of convincing the courts that the disease could excuse criminal activity. In a sense, the more drugged or drunk a person was, the less likely he was to bear criminal liability in Germany.

The same could not be said about the United States. Drunkenness or drug use only aggravated the punishment a criminal could expect from the court. American physicians had no inclination to plead in favor of drug users before judges, as they, too, were influenced by racial and moral biases against users. In fact, many physicians simply refused to treat addicts, leaving policemen and jailors to arrest them.

Drug addiction in Germany, first identified with opium and soon recognized with morphine and cocaine, shared a similar evolution to the drinking disease and alcoholism. Both were seen as specific diseases. Both were considered chronic, with very little chances of a cure. However, they also differed. Drug addiction did not cause crime and was not hereditary. As Eduard Levinstein concluded, anyone who took drugs would eventually develop the disease. Drugs, in a sense, served the same role as bacteria. Just like a germ would cause tuberculosis, drugs caused addiction. No matter who was exposed to the drug, an addiction could develop over time.

Unlike in Britain, France and the United States, there was no German public panic regarding drugs. The German public did not fear that foreigners would try to seduce Germans to smoke, inject or sniff drugs. Germany enjoyed the protection of being a latecomer in attaining colonial possessions, and consequently avoided the immigration of Indians, Chinese and Mexicans and their foreign habits. Hamburg, probably the only German city with a significant Asian population, experienced brief spells with such fears, but nothing that lasted long or that swept the entire country into a panic.

Physicians, not troubled by a panicking public, could concentrate on drugs and the disease they caused without being influenced by hysteria, applying what they deemed cold and objective judgment. They concentrated on the source of the disease, rather than the patient's moral failings. As such, the German drug laws reflected the medical understanding of addiction well into the Third Reich and after.

Alcoholism and drug addiction were necessary medical concepts for the implementation of substance prohibition in the 20th century. In the new age of reason, hard scientific facts had to be the basis of policy, at least in theory if not in practice. If physicians did not regard drugs as unhealthy and addictive, no politician or policeman would have been able to pass the necessary legislation to ban drugs. Whereas the word "health" might be missing from the Harrison Act of 1914, the ideal behind it was to protect society from a menace that was ostensibly medical in nature. Thus, physicians' discourse was essential to the drug panic that seized America. Yet, if one scratches the surface of the American medical discourse, one discovers that all manner of biases led to the condemnation of alcoholism and drug addiction.

The Golem of drug control took on a life of its own, and once Americans understood the dangers of the drug, physicians were no longer needed or even heeded in the quest to quash the problem. In some instances, physicians could only blame themselves for their inability to influence the drug policies. Some refused to treat addicted patients, since the quintessential picture of an addict was that of a poor, dirty criminal who lacked willpower to quit. Addicts tended to relapse and disregard medical advice, a fact that angered many physicians. Lack of unity weakened the stance of physicians over policy even further. The inability to identify and isolate addiction as a physical disease as well as the inability to provide an effective remedy or cure rendered doctors impotent. Doctors were vague, and theories on addiction replaced one another rapidly.

American morality prompted Prohibition and the understanding that alcoholism and drug addiction were moral diseases, but it had also saved alcoholics from a grim fate. German physicians believed that addiction and alcoholism were physical in nature, or mental diseases with a strong physical component. These beliefs regarding drug addiction and alcoholism survived the Kaiser, the two presidents of the Weimar Republic and even the Führer. By the end of the 19th and beginning of the 20th centuries, most German doctors sought the cure for the drinking disease in heredity. Since alcohol was believed to mutate an individual's germ plasm, alcoholism presented a threat to society as a whole, potentially infecting healthy offspring. With the National Socialist rise in 1933, physicians were finally given the power to implement their theories.

Nazi ideology was based on racial and biological models of reality. Society and culture were not the keys to understanding reality or politics. In their stead, race and biology held the kernel of truth. Severe alcoholism as defined by law was perceived as a biological deficiency, and the National Socialist sentence was forced sterilization. Since German physicians never considered drug addiction as a hereditary disease, but only a physical disease, drug addicts were safe from Nazi persecutions. While the eugenic theories and beliefs in the United States, England, Scandinavia and other countries led to a similar outcome, the sheer number of victims in a short period of time was unique to the Nazi regime. Alcoholism was condemned in the United States and in Germany, but American physicians never received free reign to dispose of alcoholics as they saw fit, as was the case in the Third Reich, and so alcoholics might have suffered humiliation and other difficulties, but they rarely underwent physical harm.

Drug addiction was never a criminal offense in Germany, nor was drug use. In the Third Reich, drug addiction and severe alcoholism were not seen as equal threats to the racial purity of Germany. The political police expressed an interest in alcoholism, but mostly ignored drug addiction. The criminal police spared only eleven police officers to coordinate the enforcement of the drug laws nationwide. In comparison to the American Federal Bureau of Narcotics, the German drug unit was miniscule, with less than 5 percent of the manpower of the American bureau. The number of German policemen corresponded to the number of addicts thought to be in each country, with about 5,000 addicts in Germany and anywhere between 100,000 to 1 million in the United States.

Lawrence Kolb defined most addicts as psychopaths in 1925. This was crucial for the seclusion of addicts from society in the United States. Undoubtedly psychopaths were a menace to society, and they themselves were at fault. Addiction was a mental condition, not a physical one. Therefore, there was something wrong with the addict himself rather than with the drug, or manner of consumption. Furthermore, morality played a role in the condemnation of the addict, as well as the accusation that addicts lost their liberty to a substance.

As American physicians refused to treat or plea on the behalf of addicts, lawmen filled the void with zeal. Some, such as Harry Anslinger and the Federal Bureau of Narcotics, saw the drug peril a bureaucratic bonanza to increase their power. The panic caused by physicians and racial stereotypes only strengthened the earnestness of the government to stop the menace at all costs. The menace had to be stopped, and the full brunt of the law was required.

What was true with drugs was also true with alcohol. Americans drank much, and drank hard. Physicians distrusted their alcoholic patients who did not comply with medical reason to stop drinking. They agreed that temperance, if not total abstention, was necessary for a sound mind and body. The majority of physicians, as well as a large segment of the American public, supported Prohibition. The ban on alcohol promised so much, from better breeding to a better economy, but with the economic crash of 1929 and the continual disregard of the law by Wets, proved that Prohibition could not answer the country's woes. All this was simply absent from the discourse in Germany.

In conjunction with the medical fears that addiction would spread in society like a disease, drugs and drug use were seen through racist lenses in America: Chinese smoked opium, Mexicans smoked marijuana, and blacks snorted cocaine. These racial stereotypes certainly affected physicians when they started condemning drug use, but also affected the general public, which was now afraid of violent black cocaine fiends or seductive Chinese opium dens that would rob a white man of his free will.

Once more, lawmen rather than physicians were required to keep the disease from spreading. While physicians had no cure, lawmen were able to stop the immigration into America and put in jail those who threatened the citizens. In Germany, even during the Third Reich, drugs were rarely associated with race, or even social outsiders. The regime did not view drug use or addiction as anti-social behavior, but rather as a disease in need of treatment in hospitals. In the United States, when the government decided to treat addicts, it had sent them to either prisons, or prison-hospitals.

Racial fears went well with the authorities' maxim that the drug problem in America was foreign in nature. Foreigners brought drugs to America, and they also smuggled drugs into the country. This was also true with American possessions overseas; thus, the problem in the Philippines was not the addicted population that was supported by the Spanish monopoly until 1898, but the fact that other countries, in particular the other European colonial powers, allowed the drug trade to flourish, thus encouraging smuggling.

Drug use was immoral, and it was as if the addicts of the Philippines wanted to adhere to the new American law and stop drugs deep in their souls, but the international market and incessant smuggling prevented the addicts from ridding themselves of this colonial yoke. This belief led the United States to turn to international politics, and devise an international control regime over drugs. After all, the United States thought it knew how to implement and enforce laws, even if they were prohibitory, even if the consumers still craved their drugs, even if these laws were not always popular. American policymakers could not admit that the failures of these policies were due to a false understanding of the drug problem, or to assigning the wrong people to stamp out the menace, as in the decision to hand authority for treating addiction to policemen instead of physicians. Instead, foreigners, smugglers, and seducers were all blamed.

Science and technology marked German drug policy, whereas a moralistic attitude prevailed in the United States. Together with the advancement in drug production, German physicians enjoyed tremendous prestige among their peers and were considered leaders in an art that turned into science. German doctors developed a certain understanding of what addiction was, one that influenced their American counterparts, and yet remained distinct. Furthermore, as the prestige of doctors climbed in Germany, doctors were privileged as politicians and judges sought their advice as professionals. It was believed that an informed opinion, unbiased and non-political, was the manner in which policy had to be developed.

In the United States, the role of the physician in policymaking was hardly clear, resulting in a struggle between lawmen and doctors over what was to be done with drug addicts. Xenophobia, coupled with international obligations, only complicated policy. Whereas policymakers paid lip service to science, their actions and policy only sometimes reflected up-to-date medical research, and seemed to echo moral convictions regarding crime, individual social obligations and notions of free will.

What was the difference between drugs and alcohol? To ban alcohol, the Constitution had to be amended. Drugs required no such thing. To ban alcohol, it was necessary to claim that drunkenness resulted in an economic loss to society. Alcoholics and drunkards clogged the almshouses and hospitals of America, and the ban on alcohol promised to solve a moral and an economic problem. Prohibition was repealed to a large extent because many Americans did not adhere to the new law, but also because the punitive venture of banning alcohol proved to be economically untenable. The Dries promised America that Prohibition would bring a dawn of a new age of prosperity, and no crime. Then, the Great Depression came, resulting in increase of crime and poverty.

The ban on drugs never promised a better America. It was a convergence of three forces that led to drug prohibition. The first was the internal pressure to keep foreigners at bay. The second was the attempt to stop the addiction disease from spreading. The notion that drug addiction was a disease, and drugs themselves were the agents that caused the disease came from the realm of medicine. However, it was taken out of the hands of doctors and adapted into a punitive system in which addicts were treated as criminals, rather than sick people. The third was to satisfy

America's international obligations. A federal ban on drugs was enacted as a direct result from the opium problem the United States inherited from Spain after acquiring the Philippines.

The fear of drugs coming from abroad proved as a catalyst to a wider phenomenon. The United States, in a sense, attributed its drug problem onto others. American authorities and doctors blamed foreigners for polluting the people with the foreign practice of smoking opium or cannabis. After the laws against importing drugs were enacted in 1909, and drug use was controlled in 1914, the United States turned its attention to stop the international trade in drugs, which was responsible for drug smuggling into the country. The logic behind this policy was clear. America could handle its own internal problems, but it could not trust other countries, not even the Western powers such as the corrupt British Empire that still made money off the opium in India or Germany, which continued to sell its manufactured drugs abroad with no regulations. The demand at home was mostly ignored as the only viable method to treat addicts was incarceration. The two federal hospitals that were reserved for treatment and research had too few beds to provide an answer. The American policy was essentially blaming others for its problem.

Prohibiting drugs proved easier than prohibiting alcohol. The former was consumed by those considered racially inferior, such as blacks, Chinese and Mexicans. Many Americans, some natives and other European immigrants, consumed the latter. Numbers as well as racial biases might explain why it was easier to ban drugs. Even if one assumes that there were one million drug users in America during the early years of the 20th century, the number of drinkers and drunkards eclipsed anything of that sort, even during Prohibition. Many physicians refused to treat addicts, and law enforcers picked up the slack. Addicts and drug felons had to be segregated from the streets, or else they would spread their disease among the general population. The few physicians who were willing to treat addicts, encountered difficulties from state and federal authorities, who were now armed with a Supreme Court decision that forbade maintenance. Although physicians helped to shape the understanding of what was addiction, in the final analysis they failed in treating the disease.

Germany, unlike the United States, was never a maritime power, militarily or commercially. German merchants rarely visited China in the 19th century and if they took part in the opium trade their contribution could not have been great, try as they might.[1006] Chinese, Indians or Malays, in turn, rarely came to Germany and so the practice of opium smoking was almost unheard of in Imperial Germany. Experience with opium and cocaine was either reported by travelers, the most famous of which were Alexander von Humboldt, Ernst von Bibra, and Ferdinand von Richthofen, or seen among foreigners who came to Germany. For example, in 1884, Hsiü-Chin-Cheng, the Minister to Germany opened the Chinese legation in Berlin. He hired for his daughter a private German tutor. The two were never left alone; instead the Minister stayed in the room, sitting with his legs under him like a Turk, and smoked his opium pipe during the lesson.[1007] The father's interest in his daughter's education was as foreign to the tutor as the opium he had smoked. Yet, opium smoking was not necessarily portrayed as a vice in the 19th century, but as a habit that all Chinese partook, similar to the queue they wore and their women's small feet.[1008]

Other German observers wagged their fingers at the British traders, who were poisoning the Chinese nation with opium.[1009] The drug was regarded as a poison, first and foremost, not as a vice. Mild moral condemnation, however, did not escape some of the German travelers. For example, Richthofen commented on the population of Liaotung peninsula in his travel log written at the turn of the 19th century: "The population … has no needs except for opium and gambling. These two vices, which are very common here, seem to be the main reason why a constant form of prosperity prevails in Liaotung, but not opulence."[1010] If opium caused constant prosperity, instead of opulence, it could not have been that bad of a vice. In some twisted way, it could have even suited the Protestant ideal of financial moderation.

1006   To date, no one has researched the German opium trade in China, if it had existed at all. Perhaps German merchants took part in the trade, or invested in it. See Bernd Eberstein, *Hamburg-China Geschichte einer Partnerschaft* (Hamburg: Christians, 1988), 190.

1007   Erich Gütinger, *Die Geschichte der Chinesen in Deutschland: ein Überblick über die ersten 100 Jahre ab 1822* (Münster: Waxmann, 2004), 137.

1008   Liu Jing, "Wahrnehmung des Fremden: China in deutschen und Deutschland in chinesischen Reiseberichten vom Opiumkrieg bis zum Ersten Weltkrieg," (Ph.D. dissertation, Albert-Ludwigs-Universität zu Freiburg, 2001), 2.

1009   Ibid., 119-121.

1010   Ferdinand von Richthofen, *Ferdinand von Richthofen's Tagebücher aus China*, Vol. 1, edited by Ernst Tiessen (Berlin, 1907), 219.

Opium was far and away from the German empire, consumed somewhere in mysterious and obscure lands such as China or Malaya. The vice of smoking the drug was unknown at home, and the public trusted the physicians who prescribed opium or its derivatives as medicine. German physicians enjoyed a degree of prestige unknown in America. The state entrusted them with securing the health of the people, and the health insurance scheme introduced by Bismarck only strengthened the position of physicians, who turned into the ultimate arbiters of all things medical. Professional doctors and psychiatrists enjoyed an esteem that allowed them to poach in fields previously reserved to lawyers and policemen. Drug dispensing and medical techniques remained in the realm of doctors and no one seriously considered the possibility of tampering with their authority.

Modern warfare changed the experience of war from exhilaration to trauma. Soldiers, who looked for honor in the battlefields, now sank into depression or sobering self-revelations.[1011] Physicians claimed that soldiers were introduced to morphine in field hospitals and continued their habits after their discharge. If they were not wounded in battle, veterans sought out drugs to alleviate their mental stress. As one war followed the other, new waves of addicts appeared. Drug specialists could blame the American Civil War as a catalyst for the drug epidemic in the United States, which turned into a firm belief that wars spread drugs and caused addiction.[1012] Since then, nearly every European or American war brought with it a fear from addiction, whether real or imagined. The German victories in the wars of unification in 1864 – 1871 brought with them the widespread use of morphine in field medicine. And so the morphine disease suddenly appeared and troubled physicians, who were quick to blame themselves for causing it; but without a panic, or public fervor. Policy makers were not required to address the issue. Instead, addiction was deemed a medical problem.

Industrialized drugs, such as chloral hydrates, cocaine, morphine and heroin, were mass-produced in Germany by the growing drugs and dye industry that dotted the Rhine and its tributaries. After the wars of unification, the attempts of the Imperial Health Office to regulate medicine and

---

1011 Yuval. N. Harari, *The Ultimate Experience: Battlefield Revelations and the Making of Modern War Culture, 1450-2000* (Basingstoke: Palgrave, 2008).

1012 David T. Courtwright, *Forces of Habit: Drugs and the Making of the Modern World* (Cambridge MA: Harvard University Press, 2002), 15-17, 26, 33.

drug manufacturing were met with resistance, which led to limited state intervention in the manufacture and sale of drugs. As long as high quality standards were kept, the authorities rarely interfered. The Health Office, however, was not a rubber stamp, and represented the interests of the government and the people to keep the companies in line, and produce the best possible products.[1013]

German authorities dealt with a phenomenon that was less pressing than in the United States. The number of addicts in Germany was significantly lower than was the case across the Atlantic. Extrapolating from the number of addicts, one can also conclude that drug use in Germany was not as common, especially without medical supervision. While talk about marijuana as the "Assassin of Youth" was common in the United States,[1014] cannabis was virtually unknown in Germany. Morphine, cocaine and heroin use in Germany was low by all counts. Officials declared that Germany had no drug problem, even though they were only concerned with what would happen after the end of World War II. Even in the gay years of Weimar, when the country was awash in decadent parties and supposedly widespread cocaine use, German consumption was never close to the consumption levels in the United States.

Medicine and medical theory dictated German policy. With the rise of National Socialism, physicians were given the opportunity to realize a medical utopia, selecting those who were worthy of living, and those were to be sterilized or exterminated. The laws governing the undesirables were designed by doctors, and, for the most part, implemented by them. Yet, none of the German drug laws adopted the racial or hygienic rhetoric. Not even the penal code reform, which enabled the commitment of habitual criminals to concentration camps, was used against addicts. Save for a few confirmed cases, not a single drug addict was maltreated. If the Nazis wished to eliminate drug addicts, or cared to develop a coherent policy

---

1013 Erika Hickel, "Das kaiserliche Gesundheitsamt (Imperial Health Office) and the Chemical Industry in Germany During the Second Empire: Partners or Adversaries?" in *Drugs and Narcotics in History*, ed. Roy Porter and Mikuláš Teich (Cambridge: Cambridge University Press, 1995), 97-113.

1014 Edward M. Brecher, *Licit and Illicit Drugs: The Consumers Union Report on Narcotics, Stimulants, Depressants, Inhalants, Hallucinogens, and Marijuana – Including Caffeine, Nicotine, and Alcohol* (Boston: Little, Brown, 1972), 413-414 n.8.

against drug addicts, the opportunity was there for the taking, and they certainly knew how to commit the deed.

In addition, there were also two political factors in the drug policy of the Third Reich that should not be ignored: addicts stemmed from a higher class in society. Physicians were the most susceptible professional group to drug addiction. Instead of antagonizing this group, the German government – whether imperial, republican or dictatorial – tried to include physicians and pharmacists in their program to control drugs. The German authorities agreed that the war produced addiction – in other words, that the prized veterans of World War I were susceptible to addiction. And none of the political parties in the Weimar Republic, least of all the National Socialist Party, wished to antagonize this group of men.

But the most important factor was that drug addiction, unlike mental deficiency and alcoholism, was non-hereditary. Being non-hereditary, it presented no danger to the master race. Drug addiction might have been the scourge of youth in America, but in Nazi Germany it was a disease that could be cured, patients' relapses notwithstanding – and in the awful calculations of the Third Reich, those who were not considered a threat to the race were deemed worthy of life.

Bibliography

Abbreviations:

BArch.	German Federal Archive, Berlin
GSa. PKb.	Secret State Archives, Prussian Cultural Heritage Institute, Berlin
HUJI	Hebrew University/National Library Medical Archive, Jerusalem
Larch.	State Archive, Berlin
Brand. Lharch.	Brandenburg Main State Archive, Potsdam
Pol. Arch. AA.	Political Archive, Ministry of Foreign Affairs, Berlin
NARA	National Archives, College Park
NARA (DC)	National Archives, Washington DC
StA.	State Archive, Munich
USHMM	United States Holocaust Memorial Museum Archive, Washington DC

Archival Sources:

Archives Division of the Wisconsin Historical Society, series 1616.

BArch. R 43 II/736

BArch. RD 19/29

BArch. RD 19/30

Barch. SSO Lolling, Enno, 19.07.1888.

BArch. SSO Thomas, Werner, 12.03.1895.

Brand. Lharch. Re12 B, Nr. 107.

GSa. PKb. I.HA Re76 VIII B Nr. 1246

GSa. PKb. I.HA Re77 Tit. 235 No. 1 vol. 13

HUJI-ML, IZAK 76D 8694

Larch. 5-50z 723

Library of Congress, CLC RM 41.

NARA RG 170 Acc# 170-73-1

NARA RG 170 Acc# 170-174-0005

NARA RG 170, Acc# 170-74-4

NARA (DC) RG 36 Customs Case Files 1909-1938

Pol. Arch. AA R 43.291

Pol. Arch. AA R 43.327

Pol. Arch. AA R 43.328

Pol. Arch AA R 43.43.289

Pol. Arch. AA. R 96839

StA., Pol. Dir. 7582

StA., Staanwa. No. 17584

StA., Staanwa. No. 17670

USHMM, RG 14.070M

Published Primary Sources:

Abraham, Karl, *Selected Papers of Karl Abraham*, edited by Ernst Jones (London: Hogarth Press, 1942).

Adams, E. W., "What is Addiction?" *British Journal of Inebriety*, vol. 31 (1935).

"Alcoholism," *Medical News*, vol. 59/4 (1891).

Allen, Martha M., Alcohol-A Dangerous and Unnecessary Medicine, How and Why: What medical Writers Say (New York, 1900).

Anslinger, Harry J. and Courtney R. Cooper, "Marijuana: Assassin of Youth," in *American Magazine*, vol. 124/1 (July, 1937).

Aschaffenburg, Gustav, *Das Verbrechen und seine Bekämpfung* (Heidelberg, 1903).

Atwater, W. O., John S. Billings, H. Bowditch, R. H. Chittenden, and W. H. Welch (Sub-Committee of the Committee of Fifty to Investigate the Liquor Problem), *Physiological Aspects of the Liquor Problem*, vol. 2 (Boston, 1903).

"Aus den Vereinen: Academie des Sciences zu Paris," Centralblatt für Nervenheilkunde, Psychiatrie und gerichtliche Psychopathologie, vol. 8/6 (1885).

Averill, W. A., "The Teetotaler in the Empire of Beer," in *The Independent*, vol. 68/3211 (16 June 1910), 1344-1345.

Ayass (ed.), Wolfgang, 'Gemeinschaftsfremde': Quellen zur Verfolgung von 'Asozialen', 1933-1945 (Koblenz: Bundesarchiv, 1998).

Baer, Abraham Adolph, "Gesetzliche Maßregeln zur Bekämpfung der Trunksucht" *Preußische Jahrbücher*, vol. 46 (1880).

--------- Der Verbrecher in Anthropologischer Beziehung (Leipzig, 1893).

Bailey, Pearce, "The Heroin Habit," *New Republic*, vol. 6/77 (1916).

Balestier (ed.), Charles W., *James G. Blaine, a Sketch of his Life* (New York, 1884).

Ball, B., "The History of Mental Medicine" *The Lancet*, vol. 115/2941 (1880).

"Balkan Products, Ltd.," *Time Magazine* (3 April 1933).

"Banks say No to Marijuana Money; Legal or Not," *New York Times* (11 January 2014)

Beard, George M., Stimulants and Narcotics: Medically, Philosophically, and Morally Considered (New York, 1871).

"Bekämpfung des mißbrauchs von Betäubungsmitteln," *Ministerialblatt des Reichs- und Preußischen Ministeriums des Innern* (12 Novemner 1941).

Benjamin, Walter, *On Hashish*, edited by Howard Eiland, (Cambridge MA, Harvard University Press, 2006).

---------"Haschisch in Marseilles," *Frankfurter Zeitung* (4 December 1932).

---------"Myslowitz-Braunschweig-Marseilles," *Uhu*, vol. 7/2 (1930).

von Bibra, Ernst, Die narkotischen Genußmittel und der Mensch (Nuremberg, 1855).

Bishop, Ernest S., *The Narcotic Drug Problem* (New York, 1981 [1920]).

Bleuler, Eugen, Der geborene Verbrecher: Eine kritische Studie (Munich, 1896).

--------- *Lehrbuch der Psychiatrie* (Berlin, 1916).

Bloomberg, Wilfred, "Treatment of Chronic Alcoholism with Amphetamine (Benzedrine) Sulfate" in *New England Journal of Medicine*, vol. 220/4, (26 January 1939).

Böll, Heinrich, *Heinrich Böll: Briefe aus dem Krieg 1939 – 1945*, vol. 1 edited by Jochen Schubert (Cologne: Kiepenheuer & Witsch, 2001).

von Brühl-Cramer, C., Ueber die Trunksucht und eine rationelle Heilmethode derselben (Berlin, 1819).

Bürger-Prinz, Hans, *Ein Psychiater berichtet* (Hamburg: Hoffmann & Campe, 1971).

Calkins, Alonzo, Opium and the Opium Appetite: With Notices of Alcoholic Beverages, Cannabis Indica, Tobacco and Coca, and Tea and Coffee, in their Hygienic Aspects and Pathologic Relations (Philadelphia, 1871).

Casper, Johann Ludwig, A Handbook of the Practice of Forensic Medicine, based upon Personal Experience, George William Balfour (tr.), (London, 1865 [1856]).

Cecil, Russel L. and Foster Kennedy (eds.), *A Textbook of Medicine by American Authors*, 3rd edition, (Philadelphia, 1938).

Cherrington, Ernest Hurst, *America and the World Liquor Problem* (Westerville OH, 1922).

"A Chinese Trick," *New York Times* (20 July 1864).

Clarus, Johann Christian August, "Die Zurechnungsfähigkeit des Mörders Johann Christian Woyzeck, nach Grundsätzen der Staatsarzneikunde aktenmäßig erwiesen" (Leipzig, 16 September 1821 and 1 August 1824) in C. M. Marc, War der am 27ten August 1824 zu Leipzig hingerichtete Mörder Johann Christian Woyzeck zurechnungsfähig? (Bamberg, 1825).

--------- Beiträge zur Erkenntniß und Beurtheilung zweifelhafter Seelenzustände, (Leipzig, 1828).

"Charged against Cocaine" *New York Times* (23 August 1886).

Cobbe, William Rosser, Doctor Judas: A Portrayal of the Opium Habit (Chicago, 1895).

"Cocaine's Destructive Work" *New York Times* (24 January 1887).

"Cocaine Forbidden in the U.S. Mails," *New York Times* (17 July 1908).

"The Cocaine Habit," Journal of the American Medical Association, vol. 36/5 (1901).

"Cocaine Sniffing," *New York Tribune* (21 June 1903).

Committee of Fifty, The Liquor Problem: A Summary of Investigations Conducted, 1893-1903 (New York, 1970 [1905]).

Coxe, John R., *The American Dispensatory* (Philadelphia, 1818).

"Crazed by Drugs" *New York Times* (8 March 1887).

Crothers, Thomas D., Morphinism and Narcomanias from other Drugs, their Etiology, Treatment and Medicolegal Relations (Philadelphia, 1902).

--------- The Disease of Inebriety from Alcohol, Opium and Other Narcotic Drugs, its Etiology, Pathology, Treatment and Medico-Legal Relations (New York, 1893).

--------- Inebriety: A Clinical Treatise on the Etiology, Symptomology, Neurosis, Psychosis and Treatment and the Medico-Legal Relations (Cincinnati, 1911).

--------- "Some New Studies of the Opium Disease," *The Journal of the American Medical Association*, vol. 18/8 (1892).

Dai, Bingham, *Opium Addiction in Chicago* (Montclair NJ: Patterson Smith, 1970 [1937]).

Dalcke, Albert, Strafrecht und Strafprozeß: Eine Sammlung der wichtigsten das Strafrecht und das Strafverfahren betreffenden Gesetze (Berlin, 1929 [1879]).

Dansauer, Friedrich and Adolf Rieth (eds.), *Über Morphinismus bei Kriegs-beschädigten*, (Berlin, 1931).

"The Denouement," *Los Angeles Times* (28 June 1882).

Diagnostic and Statistical Manual of Mental Disorders, 2nd ed. (Washington DC, 1968).

Diefendorf (ed.), A. Ross, Clinical Psychiatry: A Text-book for Students and Physicians, abstracted and adapted from the seventh German edition of Kraepelin's 'Lehrbuch der Psychiatrie' (New York, 1915 [1907]).

Diez, "Bemerkungen über Zurechnungsfähigkeit und Todesstrafe, in Beziehung auf den neuen Strafgesetzentwurf für Baden" in J. Schneider, J. H. Schürmayer and F. Hergt (eds.), Annalen der Staatsarzneikunde, vol. 3/2, (Tübingen, 1838).

"Dipsomania a Disease," *Chicago Daily Tribune* (11 October 1891).

Doré, Gustave and Blanchard Jerrold, *London, a Pilgrimage* (New York: B. Blom, 1970 [1872]).

Dittmar, F., "Pervitinsucht und acute Pervitinintoxikation," *Deutsche Medizinische Wochenschrift*, vol. 68/11 (1942).

"Drug Held Cure for Alcoholism," *New York Times*, (28 December 1938).

Druit, Robert, "Drunkenness as Modified by Race; with an analysis of the Report on Drunkenness in Various Parts of the World, issued by the Massachusetts State Board of Health," *Medical Times and Gazette*, vol. 1 (1871).

Earle, Charles W., "The Opium Habit," *Chicago Medical Review*, vol. 2 (1880).

Erlenmeyer, Albrecht, *Die Morphiumsucht und ihre Behandlung* (Berlin, 1887 [1883]).

---------"Ueber die Wirkung des Cocaïn bei der Morphiumentziehung," *Centralblatt für Nervenheilkunde, Psychiatrie und gerichtliche Psychopathologie*, vol. 8/13 (1885)

---------"Über Cocainsucht. Vorläufige Mitteilung," *Deutsche Medizinalzeitung*, vol. 7/44 (1886).

--------- On the Treatment of the Morphine Habit (Detroit, 1889).

Fallada, Hans, *Drei Jahre kein Mensch* edited by Günter Caspar (Berlin: Aufbau-Verlag, 1997).

"Federal Dry Tasks Big Pending Repeal," *New York Times*, (23 February 1933).

von Feuerbach, Anselm, "Johann Pürner oder Beispiel einer Tötung in höchster Trunkenheit" (1828?) in R. A. Stemmle (ed.) *Anselm Ritter von Feuerbach: Merkwürdige Verbrechen in aktenmäßiger Darstellung*, (Munich: Bruckmann, 1963).

Feuerstein, Gerhart, Rauschgiftbekämpfung-ein wichtiges Interessengebiet der Gemeindverwaltung (Berlin, 1936).

--------- (ed.), *Suchtgiftbekämpfung* (Berlin, 1944).

Floret, Theobald, "Klinische Versuche über die Wirkung und Anwendung des Heroins" in *Therapeutische Monatshefte,* vol. 12/9 (1898).

--------- "Weiteres über Heroin" in *Therapeutische Monatshefte*, vol. 13/6 (1899).

Forel, August, "Abstinenz oder Mäßigkeit?" *Grenzfragen des Nerven- und Seelenlebens*, vol. 74 (1910).

Formey, Johann Ludwig, Versuch einer medicinischen Topographie von Berlin (Berlin, 1796).

Freud, Siegmund, "Über Coca," *Centralblatt für die gesammte Therapie*, vol. 2/7 (1884).

---------"Beiträge über die Anwendung des Cocaïn: Bemerkungen über Cocaïnsucht und Cocaïnfurcht mit Beziehung auf einen Vortrag W. A. Hammonds," *Wiener Medizinische Wochenschrift*, vol. 37/28 (1887).

--------- *Civilization and its Discontents* (New York, 1961 [1930]).

--------- The Standard Edition of the Complete Psychological Works of Sigmund Freud, vol. 1, (London: Hogarth Press, 1953).

--------- *Cocaine Papers*, edited by Robert Byck (New York: Stonehill, 1974).

"From the Isthmus," *New-York Daily Times* (27 April 1854).

Gehewe, W., "Reisebericht durch Irrenanstalten Deutschlands und der Schweiz in den Jahren 1869 und 1870" *Allgemeine Zeitschrift für Psychiatrie und psychisch-gerichtliche Medicin* vol. 28/1 (Berlin, 1872).

Glauser, Friedrich, "Morphium-eine Beichte (1932)" in *Morphium, Erzählungen* (Zurich: Arche, 1988).

Glueck, Bernard, *Lehrbuch der Psychiatrie* (Berlin, 1916).

--------- "Psychogenesis in the Psychoses of Prisoners," *Criminal Science Monographs*, no. 2 (1916).

Gompers, Samuel, "Meat vs. Rice: Some Reasons for Chinese Exclusion: American Manhood against Asiatic Coolieism" (Washington DC, 1902) at U.S. Senate, 57th Congress, 1st sess., doc. 137.

Gordon, Alfred, "The Relation of Legislative Acts to the Problem of Drug Addiction," *Journal of the American Institute of Criminal Law and Criminology*, vol. 8/2 (1917).

"Gov. Bigler and the Chinamen," *New-York Daily Times* (21 June 1852).

Gray, M. Geneva and Merrill Moore, "The Incidence and Significance of Alcoholism in the History of Criminals" in *The American Journal of Psychiatry*, vol. 98/3 (November 1941).

Happel, T. J., "Morphinism in its Relations to the Sexual Functions and Appetite, and its Effect on the Offspring of the users of the Drug," *The Medical and Surgical Reporter*, vol. 67 (1892).

Hamlin, Cyrus, "The Anti-Opium Resolution in Parliament" *Our Day*, vol. 8/45 (September, 1891).

Heinroth, Johann Christian August, *System der psychisch-gerichlichen Medicine* (Leipzig, 1825).

Henke, Adolph, Lehrbuch der gerichtlichen Medicin (Berlin, 1841).

--------- Abhandlungen aus dem Gebiete der gerichtlichen Medizin vol. 4/4, (Bamberg, 1840).

Hergt, F., "Bericht über die Leistungen in der gerchitlichen Medicin" in Canstatt and Eisenmann (eds.), *Jahresbericht ueber die Fortschritte der gesammten Medicin in allen Laendern im Jahre 1845*, vol. 7 (Erlangen, 1846).

Himmelsbach, C. K. and L. F. Small, "Clinical Studies of Drug Addiction" *Public Health Report*, (1937).

Holmes, Oliver Wendell, "Currents and Counter-currents in Medical Science," in *The American Journal of the Medical Science*, vol. 40/80 (1860), 462-474.

Homan, J. A., Prohibition-The Enemy of Temperance: An Exposition of the Liquor Problem in the Light of Scripture, Physiology, Legislation and Political Economy. Defending the Strictly Moderate Drinker and Advocating the License System as a Restrictive Measure (Cincinnati, 1910).

"How Germany is trying to solve her Temperance Problem" in *Current Literature*, vol. 50/6 (1911), 636-637.

Hufeland, Christoph Wilhelm, Art of Prolonging Life (London, 1859) [Die Kunst, das menschliche Leben zu verlängern, (1796)]

--------- Ueber die Vergiftung durch Branntwein (Berlin, 1802).

--------- Journal der Practischen Arzneykunde und Wunderarzneykunst, vol. 59/1 (1829).

--------- Enchiridion Medicum oder Anleitung zur medizinischen Praxis (Berlin, 1842 [1836]).

Hunter, William C., *The 'Fan Kwae' at Canton* (Taipei: Ch'eng-wen Pub. Co, 1965 [1882]).

Huss, Magnus, Chronische Alkoholskrankheit, oder Alcoholismus chronicus; ein Beitrag zur Kenntniss der Vergiftungs-Krankheiten, nach eigener und anderer Erfahrung (Stockholm and Leipzig, 1852 [1849]).

"Importation and Use of Opium," *Hearing before the Committee on Ways and Means of the House of Representatives*, 61st Congress, 3rd Session, (14 December 1910 and 11 January 1911).

"Is it True?" *Medical News*, vol. 41/1 (1 July 1882).

Jefferson, Thomas, *Letters, 1743-1826* (New York, 1984).

Jelliffe, Smith Ely, "Drug Addictions: Preliminary Report of the Committee in Section on Nervous and Mental Diseases," *Journal of the American Medical Association*, 46/9 (1906).

Johnson, Samuel, *The Lives of the English Poets* (London, 1825 [1779-1781]).

Kane, H. H., Opium-Smoking in America and China: A Study of Its Prevalence, and Effects, Immediate and Remote, on Individual and the Nation (New York, 1882).

--------- Drugs that Enslave: The Opium, Morphine, Chloral and Hashisch Habits (Philadelphia, 1881).

Kant, Immanuel, *The Metaphysics of Morals* (Cambridge: Cambridge University Press, 1996 [1797]).

Kärber, G., "Unterstellung von Dolantin, Pervitin und Benzedrin unter das Opiumgesetz," *Deutsches Ärzteblatt*, vol. 71/27 (5 July 1941).

Keeley, Leslie E., The Morphine Eater; or, From Bondage to Freedom (Dwight IL, 1881).

--------- The Non-Heredity of Inebriety (Chicago, 1896).

Knight, Robert, "The Psychodynamic of Chronic Alcoholism," *Journal of Nervous and Mental Diseases*, vol. 86/5 (1937).

von Krafft-Ebing, Richard, Grundzüge der Criminalpsychologie auf Grundlage des Strafgesetzbuchs des deutschen Reichs für Aerzte und Juristen (Erlangen, 1872).

--------- Lehrbuch der Psychiatrie auf klinischer Grundlage für Praktische Ärzte und Studierende (Stuttgart, 1890 [1879]).

--------- Text-Book of Insanity based on Clinical Observation for Practitioners and Students of Medicine (Philadelphia, 1905 [1879]).

Kraepelin, Emil, *Psychiatrie: Ein Lehrbuch für Studierende und Aerzte*, 6th ed., vols. 1-2 (Leipzig, 1899).

Kolb, Lawrence, "Types and Characteristics of Drug Addicts," *Mental Hygiene*, vol. 9/2 (1925).

--------- "Drug Addiction: A Study of Some Medical Cases" *Archives of Neurology and Psychiatry*, vol. 20/1 (1928).

--------- and William F. Ossenfort, "The Treatment of Addicts at the Lexington Hospital," *Southern Medical Journal*, vol. 31 (1938).

--------- "The Narcotic Addict: His Treatment," *Federal Probation*, vol. 111/3 (1939).

--------- "Pleasure and Deterioration from Narcotic Addiction," *Mental Hygiene*, vol. 9/4 (1925).

Kalus, F., I. Kucher, and J. Zutt, "Über Psychosen bei chronischem Pervitinmissbrauch," *Nervenarzt*, vol. 15 (1942).

Kopp, Marie E., "Surgical Treatment as Sex Crime Prevention Measure," *Journal of Criminal Law and Criminology*, vol. 28/5 (1938).

Koren, John (an investigation made for the Committee of Fifty under the direction of Henry W. Farnam), *Economic Aspects of the Liquor Problem* (Boston, 1899).

Kremers, Edward, "Agricultural Alcohol: Studies of its Manufacture in Germany," in *Bulletin of the U.S. Department of Agriculture*, No. 182 (2 February 1915).

Laehr, Heinrich, "Ueber Missbrauch mit Morphium-Injectionen" *Allgemeine Zeitschrift für Psychiatrie und psychisch-gerichtliche Medicin*, vol. 28/3 (Berlin, 1872).

"Legal Marijuana Businesses should have Access to Banks, Holder says," *New York Times* (23 January 2014).

Levinstein, Eduard, Die Morphiumsucht: Eine Monographie nach eigenen Beobachtungen (Berlin, 1877 [1883]).

--------- The Morbid Craving for Morphia (die Morphiumsucht): A Monograph founded on Personal Observations, translated by Charles Harrer (London, 1878).

Lewin, Louis, The Incidental Effects of Drugs: A Pharmacological and Clinical Handbook (New York, 1882 [1881]).

--------- Die Nebenwirkungen der Arzneimittel: Pharmakologisch-klinisches Handbuch (Belin, 1898).

--------- and Wenzel Goldbaum, Opiumgesetz: Nebst Internationalen Opiumabkommen und Ausführungs bestimmungen (Berlin, 1928).

Light, Arthur B. and Edward G. Torrance, "The Conduct of the Addict in Relation to Investigative Study" in Arthur B. Light and Edward G. Torrance (eds.), *Opium Addiction* (Chicago, 1930).

von Liszt, Franz, *Lehrbuch des deutschen Strafrechts* (Berlin, 1908).

--------- Lehrbuch des deutschen Strafrechts (Berlin, 1888)

--------- Das Völkerrecht systematisch dargestellt (Berlin, 1902).

--------- and Ernst Delaquis (eds.), *Strafgesetzbuch für das Deutsche Reich* (Berlin, 1914).

MacDonald, Arthur, "Criminal Statistics in Germany, France and England," *Journal of the American Institute of Criminal Law and Criminology*, vol. 1/2 (1910).

Marshall, Edward, "Uncle Sam is the Worst Drug Fiend in the World," *New York Times* (12 March 1911).

Mason, Lewis D., "The Etiology of Dipsomania and Heredity of 'Alcoholic Inebriety'" *Quarterly Journal of Inebriety* (1888), in *The American Journal of Psychology*, vol. 2/3 (1889).

Mattison, J. B., "The Responsibility of the Profession in the Production of Opium Inebriety," *Medical and Surgical Reporter*, vol. 38 (1878).

--------- "Morphinism in Medical Men," *Journal of the American Medical Association*, vol. 186/5 (1894).

--------- "Triple Narcotic Addiction: Opium, Alcohol, Cocaine," *Times and Register*, vol. 21/22 (1890).

--------- "The Dangers of Cocaine," *Medical News*, vol. 50/16 (1887).

--------- "A Case of Opium-Smoking," *Philadelphia Medical Times*, vol. 16/6 (1885).

--------- The Treatment of Opium Addiction (New York, 1885).

--------- The Mattison Method in Morphinism: A Modern and Humane Treatment of the Morphin Disease (New York, 1902).

Merz, Charles, *The Dry Decade* (Seattle, 1969 [1930]).

Mill, John Stuart, *On Liberty* (London, 1985 [1859]).

Moore, Merrill, "Alcoholism: Some 'Causes' and Treatment" in *The Military Surgeon*, vol. 90/5 (May, 1942).

Morse, E. W., "What are the most effective methods of cure of the Opium Habit?" in *Our Day*, vol. 9/55 (July, 1892).

Nash, Wallis, *Two Years in Oregon* (New York, 1882).

Niemann, Albert, "Ueber eine neue organische Base in den Cocablättern: Mittheilung aus der Inaugural-Dissertation," *Archiv der Pharmacie*, vol. 153/2 (1860).

"Niemeyer Pill," in Journal of the American Medical Association, vol. 56/3 (1911).

von Niemeyer, Felix, Lehrbuch der speciellen Pathologie und Therapie: mit besonderer Rücksicht an Physiologie und pathologische Anatomie, vol. 2 (Berlin, 1865).

Nuernberg Military Tribunal "Green" Series, "The Medical Case; Military Tribunals No. I, Case 1" in *Trials of War Criminals Before the Nuernberg Military Tribunals under Control Council Law No. 10*, vol. 1.

Obersteiner, Heinrich, "Ueber Intoxicationspsychosen," *Wiener medizinische Presse*, vol. 24/4 (1886).

Oehler, Friedrich Eduard, "Erstes Gutachten" in Friedrich Julius Siebenhaar and Rudolph Julius Albert Martini (eds.), *Magazin für die Staatsarzneikunde,* vol. 3 (Leipzig, 1844).

"Oinomania; or the Mental Pathology of Intemperance" *The Journal of Psychological Medicine and Mental Pathology*, vol. 8, (1 April 1855).

Oliver, F. E., "The Use and Abuse of Opium," *Massachusetts State Board of Health, Third Annual Report*, (Boston, 1872).

"Our Government may Sell Opium to Filipinos," *New York Times* (22 September 1904).

Parish, Joseph, Alcoholic Inebriety from a Medical Standpoint (Philadelphia, 1883).

Payne, C.R., "Psychology of Alcoholism" *Psychoanalytic Review*, vol. 3/1 (1914).

Pescor, Michael J., "A Statistical Analysis of the Clinical Records of Hospitalized Drug Addicts" *Public Health Reports* (Washington, 1938).

Pettey, George E., The Narcotic Drug Diseases and Allies Ailments: Pathology, Pathogenesis, and Treatment (Philadelphia, 1913).

Ploetz, Alfred, Die Tüchtigkeit unserer Rasse und der Schutz der Schwachen: Ein Verusch über Rassenhygiene und ihr Verhältniss zu den humanen Idealen, besonders zum Socialismus, vol. 1 (Berlin, 1895 [1893]).

"A Physician's Sad Plight; Driven mad by the use of Cocaine to Allay Pain" *New York Times* (16 January 1887).

Pohlisch, Kurt, "Die Verbreitungs des chronischen Opiatmissbrauchs in Deutschland," *Monatsschrift für Psychiatrie und Neurologie*, vol. 79/1 (1931).

Proceedings of the American Medico-Psychological Association at the Seventy-Third Annual Meeting (Baltimore, 1917).

"Prohibition and Inebriety," *Journal of Mental Science* (*British Journal of Psychiatry*), vol. 35/149 (1889).

Radó, Sándor, "The Psychoanalysis of Pharmacothymia (Drug Addiction)," *Psychoanalytic Quarterly*, vol. 11 (1933).

von Richthofen, Ferdinand, *Ferdinand von Richthofen's Tagebücher aus China*, vol. 1, edited by Ernst Tiessen (Berlin, 1907).

"Richtlinien für die Anmeldung von Betäubungsmitteln in der ärztlichen Praxis," in *Deutsches Reichsärzteblatt* (February, 1939).

Ritter, R., "Die Aufgaben der Kriminalbiologie und der kriminalbiologischen Bevölkerungsforschung," *Kriminalistik*, vol. 15/4 (April 1941).

Reich, Eduard, Die Ursachen der Krankheiten der physischen und der moralischen (Leipzig, 1867).

Rösch, Carl, Der Missbrauch geistiger Getränke in pathologischer, therapeutischer, medizinisch-polizeilicher und gerichtlicher Hinsicht (Tübingen, 1839 [1838]).

"Roosevelt asks Narcotic War Aid," *New York Times*, (22 March 1935).

Rush, Benjamin, *Sermons to the Rich and Studious, on Temperance and Exercise* (London, 1772).

--------- An Inquiry into the Effects of the Spirituous Liquors upon the Human Body, and their Influence upon the Happiness of Society (Edinburgh, 1791 [1784]).

--------- *Essays, Literary, Moral & Philosophical* (Philadelphia, 1798 [1796]).

Sacher, Diez, "Über Suchte mit rezeptfreien Schlafmitteln," *Archiv für Psychiatrie und Nervenkrankheiten*, vol. 112/4 (1940).

Samter, J., "Ein Morphiophagie" in Deutsche Klink. Zeitung für Beobachtungen aus Deutschen Kliniken und Krankenhäusern, vol. 16/16 (16 April 1864).

Savage, George H., "Drunkenness in Relation to Criminal Responsibility," *Journal of Mental Science* (*British Journal of Psychiatry*), vol. 32/137 (1886).

Schlager, Ludwig, "Die Bedeutung und die Aufgaben der Irrengesetzgebung im Rechtsstaate" in *Die gerichtliche Psychopathologie* (Tübingen, 1882).

Seige, Max, "Erfolge der Flechsig'schen Brom-Opium-Kur," *Monatsschrift für Psychiatrie und Neurologie*, vol. 22/1 (1907).

--------- "Klinische Erfahrungen mit Neoronal," *Deutsche medizinische Wochenschrift*, vol. 38 (1912), 1828-1830.

"The Soldiers' Home at Dayton, Ohio," *National Repository*, vol. 3 (1878).

Speer, E. "Das Pervetinproblem" *Deutsches Ärzteblatt*, vol. 71 (1941).

Steegmann, "Zur Lehre von der gerichtsärztlichen Beurtheilung der Trunkenheit und der Trunkfälligkeit" *Zeitschrift für die Staatsarzneikunde* vol. 15/4 (1835).

Stromer, Heinrich, Ein getrewe, vleissige und ehrliche Verwarnung widder des hesliche Laster der Trunkenheit (Wittenberg, 1532 [1531]).

Sutton, Thomas, Tracts on Delirium Tremens, on Peritonitis, and on some other internal inflammatory affections, and on Gout (London, 1813).

Tausk, Viktor, "On the Psychology of Alcoholic Occupational Delirium," (31 May 1915) in *Minutes of the Vienna Psychoanalytical Society, 1912-1918*, vol. 4 (New York, 1962).

Trotter, Thomas, An Essay: Medical, Philosophical, and Chemical-On Drunkenness and its Effects on the Human Body (London, 1988 [1804]).

Turner, J. Edward, "An Appeal," Ceremonies, Etc., New York State Inebriate Asylum, Binghamton, New York (New York, 1859).

"Used Morphine and Cocaine" *New York Times* (24 March 1888).

Wall, Patrick M., "The Annals of Manhattan Crime," *New York Magazine*, vol. 21/45 (1988).

Walton, R., Marijuana: America's New Drug Problem (Philadelphia, 1938).

Warner, Harry S., Social Welfare and the Liquor Problems: Studies in the Sources of the Problem and How They Relate to its Solution (Chicago, 1916 [1908]).

Weismann, August, *The Germ-Plasm: A Theory of Heredity* (New York, 1893 [1892]).

Weiss, Soma, "Alcoholism" in Russel L. Cecil and Foster Kennedy (eds.), *A Textbook of Medicine by American Authors*, 3rd ed., (Philadelphia, 1938).

Williams, Edward H., *Alcohol, Hygiene and Legislation* (New York, 1915).

Williams, Fred V., The Hop-Heads: Personal Experiences Among the Users of 'Dope' in the San Francisco Underworld (San Francisco, 1920).

Willoughby, Westel W., Opium as an International Problem: The Geneva Conferences (Baltimore, 1925).

"Without Opium, Chinamen Die," *Los Angeles Times* (17 August 1909).

Wissler, Albert, *Die Opiumfrage* (Berlin, 1931).

"Work of an Awful Habit; the Sad Story of Dr. Charles H. Bradley" *New York Times* (30 November 1887).

Wright, Hamilton, "The International Opium Commission" *The American Journal of International Law* vol. 3/3 (1909).

--------- "Report on the International Opium Commission and on the Opium Problem as seen within the United States and its Possessions" in *Opium Problem: Message from the President of the United States*, U.S. Senate Doc. 377, 61st Congress, 2nd session, (21 February 1910).

Youmans, Edward L., *Alcohol and the Constitution of Man* (New York, 1853).

Zeiz, August Hermann, "Teufel Alkohol. Ein Mann kämpft vergeblich gegen seine Laster," *Berliner Tageblatt*, (7 October 1932).

Zuckmayer, Carl, *Als Wär's ein Stück von Mir* (Frankfurt: Fischer, 1967).

Secondary Sources:

Abrams, Meyer Howard, The Milk of Paradise: The Effect of Opium Visions on the Works of De Quincey, Crabbe, Francis Thompson and Coleridge (Cambridge, MA: Harvard University Press, 1934).

Acker, Caroline Jean, Creating the American Junkie: Addiction Research in the Classic Era of Narcotic Control (Baltimore: Johns Hopkins University Press, 2002).

Ahmad, Diana, *The Opium Debate and Chinese Exclusion Laws in the Nineteenth-Century American West* (Reno: University of Nevada Press, 2007).

Amenda, Lars, "'Welthafen' Hamburg-Kultur- und technikgeschichtliche Perspektiven," in Gudrun Wolfschmidt (ed.), *Hamburgs Geschichte einmal anders: Entwicklung der Naturwissenschaften, Medizin und Technik*, vol. 2 (Norderstedt: Books on Demand, 2009).

--------- Fremde-Hafen-Stadt: Chinesische Migration und ihre Wahrnehmung in Hamburg, 1897-1972 (Hamburg: Dölling und Galitz Verlag, 2006).

Andrus, Burton C., *The Infamous of Nuremberg* (London: Frewin, 1969).

Arikha, Noga, Passions and Tempers: A History of Humours (New York: Ecco, 2007).

Auerhahn, K., "The Split Labor Market and the Origins of Antidrug Legislation in the United States" *Law & Social Inquiry*, vol. 24/2 (1999).

Aurin, Marcus, "Chasing the Dragon: The Cultural Metamorphosis of Opium in the United States, 1825-1935," *Medical Anthropology Quarterly*, vol. 14/3 (2000).

Baumohl, Jim, "Inebriate Institutions in North America, 1840-1920," *British Journal of Addiction*, vol. 85 (1990), 1187-1204.

Bartmann, Wilhelm, Zwischen Tradition und Fortschritt: Aus der Geschichte der Pharmabereiche von Bayer, Hoechst und Schering von 1935 - 1975 (Stuttgart: Franz Steiner Verlag, 2003).

Benn, Maurice B., *The Drama of Revolt: A Critical Study of Georg Büchner* (Cambridge: Cambridge University Press, 1976).

Bennett, J. V., *I Chose Prison* (New York: Knopf, 1970).

Berridge, Virginia, Opium and the People: Opiate Use in Nineteenth-Century England (London: Free Association Books, 1999).

--------- "Morbid Cravings: The Emergence of Addiction," *British Journal of Addiction*, vol. 80 (1985), 233-243.

Bonnie, Richard J. and Charles H. Whitebread II, "The Forbidden Fruit and the Tree of Knowledge: An Inquiry into the Legal History of American Marijuana Prohibition" *Virginia Law Review*, vol. 56/6 (1970).

Boon, Marcus, *The Road of Excess: A History of Writers on Drugs* (Cambridge: Harvard University Press, 2002).

Booth, Martin, *Opium: A History* (New York: St. Martin's Press, 1998).

Brecher, Edward M., Licit and Illicit Drugs: The Consumers Union Report on Narcotics, Stimulants, Depressants, Inhalants, Hallucinogens, and Marijuana – including Caffeine, Nicotine, and Alcohol (Boston: Little, Brown, 1972).

Briesen, Detlef, Drogenkonsum und Drogenpolitik in Deutschland und den USA: Ein historischer Vergleich (Frankfurt a.M: Campus, 2005).

Burnham, John C., Bad Habits: Drinking, Smoking, Taking Drugs, Gambling, Sexual Misbehavior, and Swearing in American History (New York: New York University Press, 1993).

Burns, Eric, *Spirits of America: A Social History of Alcohol* (Philadelphia: Temple University Press, 2004).

Bynum, William F., "Monomania" *The Lancet*, vol. 362/9393 (2003), 1425.

--------- "Alcoholism and Degeneration in 19th century European Medicine and Psychiatry," *British Journal of Addiction*, vol. 79 (1984), 61.

--------- "Chronic Alcoholism in the First Half of the 19th Century" *Bulletin of the History of Medicine*, vol. 42/2 (1968), 161.

Campbell, Nancy D., Discovering Addiction: the Science and Politics of Substance Abuse Research (Ann Arbor: University of Michigan Press, 2007).

--------- J. Olsen and Luke Walden, The Narcotic Farm: The Rise and Fall of America's First Prison of Drug Addicts (New York: Abrams, 2008).

Cheng, Pei-kai, Michael Lestz and Jonathan Spence (eds.), *The Search for Modern China: A Documentary Collection* (New York: Norton, 1999).

Cocks, Geoffrey, *Psychotherapy in the Third Reich: The Göring Institute* (New Brunswick NJ: Transaction Publishers, 1997).

Conrad, Peter and Joseph W. Schneider, *Deviance and Medicalization: From Badness to Sickness* (Philadelphia: Temple University Press, 1992).

Courtwright, David T., *Dark Paradise: A History of Opium Addiction in America* (Cambridge MA: Harvard University Press, 2001).

--------- "Charles Terry, the Opium Problem, and American Narcotic Policy," *Journal of Drug Issues*, vol. 16/3 (1986), 421-434.

--------- Herman Joseph and Don Des Jarlais (eds.), *Addicts who Survived: An Oral History of Narcotic Use in America, 1923-1965* (Knoxville: University of Tennessee Press, 1989).

--------- "The Rise and Fall and Rise of Cocaine in the United States," in Jordan Goodman, Paul E. Lovejoy and Andrew Sherratt (eds.), *Consuming Habits: Drugs in History and Anthropology* (London: Routledge, 1995).

--------- *Forces of Habit: Drugs and the Making of the Modern World* (Cambridge MA: Harvard University Press, 2001).

Crepon, Tom, *Leben und Tode des Hans Fallada* (Leipzig: Mitteldeutscher Verlag, 1992).

Crowley (ed.), John W., *Drunkard's Progress: Narratives of Addiction, Despair, and Recovery* (Baltimore: Johns Hopkins University Press, 1999).

Davenport-Hines, Richard, *The Pursuit of Oblivion* (London: Phoenix Press, 2002).

Davidson, James, Courtesans and Fishcakes: The Consuming Passions of Classical Athens (New York: St. Martin's Press, 1998).

Decker, Gunnar, *Gottfried Benn: Genie und Barbar* (Berlin: Aufbau-Verlag, 2008).

Djang, Feng Djen, The Diplomatic Relations between China and Germany Since 1898 (Shanghai, 1936).

Downs, Jacques M., "The Commercial Origins of American Attitudes Toward China, 1784-1944" in Jonathan Goldstein, Jerry Israel & Hilary Conroy (eds.), *America Views China: American Images of China then and now* (Bethlehem PA: Leigh University Press, 1991).

Dreser, "Pharmakologische über einige Morphinderivate [sic]" in *Therapeutische Monatshefte*, vol. 12/9 (1898).

Driscoll, Lawrence V., Reconsidering Drugs: Mapping Victorian and Modern Drug Discourses (New York: Palgrave, 2000).

Duffy, John, "Medical Practices in the Ante Bellum South" in *The Journal of Southern History*, vol. 25/1 (1959).

Duke, Steven B. and Albert C. Gross, *America's Longest War: Rethinking our Tragic Crusade Against Drugs* (New York: Putnam's Sons, 1993).

van Duyne, Petrus C. and Michael Levi, Drugs and Money: Managing the Drug Trade and Crime-Money in Europe (London, 2005).

Eberstein, Bernd, *Hamburg-China Geschichte einer Partnerschaft* (Hamburg: Christians, 1988).

Eddy, Nathan B., The National Research Council Involvement in the Opiate Problem, 1928-1971 (Washington DC: National Academy of Sciences, 1973),

Engstrom, Eric J., "Forensic Psychiatry in Imperial Germany" *Tabur*, vol. 2. (2009), 25-40. [Hebrew]

Ferentzy, Peter, "From Sin to Disease: Differences and Similarities between Past and Current Conceptions of Chronic Drunkenness," *Contemporary Drug problems*, vol. 28/3 (2001), 363-390.

Fischer, Lothar, *Anita Berber: Göttin der Nacht* (Berlin: Edition Ebersbach, 2006).

Foner, Philip S., History of the Labor Movement in the United States: From Colonial Times to the Foundation of the American Federation of Labor, vol. 1, (New York: International Publishers, 1975).

Foster, Anne L., "Models for Governing: Opium and Colonial Policies in Southeast Asia, 1898-1910," in Julian Go and Anne L. Foster (eds.), *The American Colonial State in the Philippines: Global Perspectives* (Durham: Duke University Press, 2003), 92-117.

--------- "Prohibition as Superiority: Policing opium in South-East Asia, 1898-1925," *International History Review*, vol. 22/2 (2000).

Frevert, Ute, "Professional Medicine and the Working Classes in Imperial Germany," *Journal of Contemporary History*, vol. 20/4 (1985), 637-658.

Friedlander, Henry, *The Origins of the Nazi Genocide: From Euthanasia to Final Solution* (Chapel Hill: North Carolina University Press, 1995).

Friedman, Lawrence M., *A History of American Law* (New York: Simon and Schuster, 1985).

--------- *American Law in the 20th Century* (New Haven: Yale University Press, 2002).

Friedrich, Otto, *Before the Deluge: A Portrait of Berlin in the 1920's* (New York: Fromm International, 1972).

Friman, H. Richard., *NarcoDiplomacy: Exporting the U.S. War on Drugs* (Ithaca: Cornell University Press, 1996).

Galliher, John F., David Keys and Michael Elsner, "Lindesmith v. Anslinger: An early government victory in the failed war on drugs," in *Journal of Criminal Law & Criminology*, vol. 88/2 (1998), 661-682.

Gansel, Carsten and Werner Liersch (eds.), *Hans Fallada und die literarische Moderne* (Göttingen: V&R Uni Press, 2009).

Gasman, Daniel, *The Scientific Origins of National Socialism* (New Brunswick NJ: Transaction Publishers, 2004 [1971]).

Gay, Peter, *Freud: Life for Our Time* (New York: Norton, 1988).

Gellately, Robert, *The Gestapo and German* Society (Oxford: Clarendon Press, 1992).

Gieringer, Dale H., "The Forgotten Origins of Cannabis Prohibition in California," *Contemporary Drug Problems*, vol. 26/2 (1999), 237-288.

Gilbert, Gustave M., *Nuremberg Diary* (New York: Farrar, Straus, 1961 [1947]).

Giles, Geoffrey J., "Drinking and Crime in Modern Germany" in Peter Becker and Richard F. Wetzell (eds.), *Criminals and Their Scientists: The History of Criminology in International Perspective* (Cambridge: Cambridge University Press, 2006).

Gingeras, Ryan, *Heroin, Organized Crime, and the Making of Modern Turkey* (Oxford: Oxford University Press, 2014).

Goldstein, Jan Ellen, Console and Classify: The French Psychiatric Profession in the Nineteenth Century (Chicago: University of Chicago Press, 2001).

Gootneberg, Paul, *Andean Cocaine: The Making of a Global Drug* (Chapel Hill: North Carolina University Press, 2008).

--------- (ed.), *Cocaine: Global Histories* (London: Routledge, 1999).

--------- "Between Coca and Cocaine: A Century or More of U.S.-Peruvian Drug Paradoxes, 1860-1980," *Hispanic American Historical Review*, vol. 83/1 (2003), 121-122.

Grob, Gerald N., *The Deadly Truth: A History of Disease in America* (Cambridge MA: Harvard University Press, 2002).

Gütinger, Erich, Die Geschichte der Chinesen in Deutschland: ein Überblick über die ersten 100 Jahre ab 1822 (Münster: Waxmann, 2004).

Haack, K., S. C. Herpertz and E. Kumbier, "Der 'Fall Sefolge': Ein Beitrag zur Geschichte der forensischen Psychiatrie" *Der Nervenarzt*, vol. 5 (2007).

Haller, John S., *American Medicine in Transition* (Urbana: University of Illinois Press, 1981).

Hamm, Richard F., Shaping the 18th Amendment: Temperance Reform, Legal Culture, and the Polity, 1800-1920 (Chapel Hill: University of North Carolina Press, 1995).

Hanford, James H., "The Progenitors of Golias" in *Speculum, vol. 1/1* (1926).

Hao, Yen-P'ing, "Chinese Teas to America-a Synopsis" in Ernst R. May & John K. Fairbank (eds.) *America's China Trade in Historical Perspective* (Cambridge, MA: Harvard University Press, 1986), 12-31.

Harari, Yuval N., The Ultimate Experience: Battlefield Revelations and the Making of Modern War Culture, 1450-2000 (Basingstoke: Palgrave, 2008).

Hayter, Alethea, *Opium and the Romantic Imagination* (London: Faber, 1968).

Heggen, Alfred, Alkohol und Bürgerliche Gesellschaft im 19. Jahrhundert (Berlin: Colloquium Verlag, 1988).

Helmer, John, *Drugs and Minority Oppression* (New York: Seabury Press, 1975).

Hett, Benjamin Carter, Death in the Tiergarten: Murder and Criminal Justice in the Kaiser's Berlin (Cambridge MA: Harvard University Press, 2004).

Hickel, Erika, "Das kaiserliche Gesundheitsamt (Imperial Health Office) and the Chemical Industry in Germany During the Second Empire: Partners or Adversaries?" in Roy Porter and Mikuláš Teich (eds.), *Drugs and Narcotics in History* (Cambridge: Cambridge University Press, 1995), 97-113.

Hickman, Timothy Alton, The Secret Leprosy of Modern Days: Narcotic Addiction and Cultural Crisis in the United States, 1870-1920 (Amherst: University of Massachusetts Press, 2007).

--------- "'Mania Americana': Narcotic Addiction and Modernity in the United States, 1870-1920," *Journal of American History*, vol. 90/4 (2004), 1269-1295.

Hill, Herbert, "Anti-Oriental Agitation and the rise of Working-Class Racism" in *Society*, vol. 10/2 (1973), 43-54.

Hoffmann, Annika, "Von Morphiumpralinees und Opiumzigaretten: Zur beginnenden Problematisierung des Betäubungsmittelkonsums im Deutschland der 1920er Jahre," in Bernd Dollinger and Henning Schmidt-Semisch (eds.), *Sozialwissenschaftliche Suchtforschung* (Wiesbaden: Springer Verlag, 2007).

--------- Drogenkonsum und –kontrolle: Zur Etablierung eines sozialen Problems im ersten Drittel des 20. Jahrhunderts (Wiesbaden: VS Verlag, 2012).

Höhne, Heinz, *The Order of the Death Heads* (London: Pan, 1969).

Holzer, Tilmann, Die Geburt der Drogenpolitik aus dem Geist der Rassenhygiene: Deutsche Drogenpolitik von 1933-1972 (Norderstedt: Books on Demand, 2007).

Houts, A. C., "Fifty Years of Psychiatric Nomenclature: Reflections on the 1943 War Department Technical Bulletin, Medical 203," *Journal of Clinical Psychology*, vol. 56/7 (2000), 935-967.

Huerkamp, Claudia, "The Making of the Modern Medical profession, 1800-1914: Prussian Doctors in the Nineteenth Century," in Geoffrey Cocks and Konrad H. Jarausch (eds.), *German Professions, 1800-1950* (New York: Oxford University Press, 1990), 66-84.

Hughes, Erika, "Art and Illegality on the Weimar Stage: The Dances of Celly de Rheydt, Anita Berber and Valeska Gert" *Journal of European Studies*, vol. 39/3 (2009), 320 -335.

Jäger, Lorenz, "Ceci n'est pas une pipe à opium: Wie Kommissar Maigret: Walter Benjamin Experimente," *Frankfurter Allgemeine Zeitung* (6 October 1998).

Jay, Mike, *Emperor of Dreams* (London: Daedalus, 2000).

Jelavich, Peter, *Berlin Cabaret* (Cambridge MA: Harvard University Press, 1993).

Jing, Chunxiao, Mit Barbaren gegen Barbaren: die chinesiche Selbststärkungsbewegung und das deutsche Rüstungsgeschäft in späten 19. Jahrhundert (Berlin: LIT, 2002).

Johnson, Paul, *A History of the American People* (New York: Harper Collins, 1997).

Jones, Ernest, *The Life and Work of Sigmund Freud*, vol. 1, (New York: Basic Books 1953).

Jonnes, Jill, Hep-Cats, Narcs, and Pipe Dreams: A History of America's Romance with Illegal Drugs (New York: Scribner, 1996).

Jungblut, Hans Joachim, "Drogenrecht und Drogenpolitik. Internationale Vorgaben und nationale Spielräume," in Bernd Dollinger and Henning Schmidt-Semisch (eds.), *Sozialwissenschaftliche Suchtforschung* (Wiesbaden: VS, Verlag für Sozialwissenschaften, 2007).

Jünger, Ernst, *Annäherungen: Drogen und Rausch* (Stuttgart: Klett, 1970).

Kandall, Stephen R., *Substance and Shadow: Women and Addiction in the United States* (Cambridge MA: Harvard University Press, 1999).

Kelley, Douglas M., *22 Cells in Nuremberg* (New York: Greenberg, 1947).

Kemper, Wolf-Reinhard, Kokain in der Musik: Bestandsaufnahme und Analyse aus kriminologischer Sicht (Munich: LIT, 2001).

Kershaw, Ian , *Hitler, 1936-45: Nemesis* (London: Longman, 2000).

Kielhorn, Friedrich-Wilhelm, "The History of Alcoholism: Brühl-Cramer's Concepts and Observations" *Addiction*, vol. 91/1 (1996), 121-128.

Kinder, Douglas C., "Shutting the Evil: Nativism and Narcotics Control in the United States" in William O. Walker III (ed.), *Drug Control Policy: Essays in Historical and Comparative Perspective* (University Park: Pennsylvania State University Press, 1992), 117-142.

Kobler, John, Ardent Spirits: The Rise and Fall of Prohibition (New York: Putnam, 1973).

Kozma, Liat, "Egyptian Cannabis Prohibition 1880-1939: From Local Ban to the League of Nations," *Middle Eastern Studies*, vol. 41/3 (2011), 443-460.

Kreutel, Margit, *Die Opiumsucht* (Stuttgart: Deutscher Apotheker Verlag, 1988).

Kuhn, Thomas S., *The Structure of Scientific Revolutions* (Chicago: University of Chicago Press, 1962).

Kunitz, Stephen J., "Professionalism and Social Control in the Progressive Era: The Case of the Flexner Report," *Social Problems*, vol. 22/1 (1974), 16-27.

Kyvig, David E., *Repealing National Prohibition* (Chicago: University of Chicago Press, 1979).

Liang, Hsi-huey, *The Berlin Police Force in the Weimar Republic* (Berkeley: University of California Press, 1970).

Lindesmith, Alfred R., *Addiction and Opiates* (Chicago: Aldine Publishing Company, 1968 [1947]).

Leutner, Mechthild and Klaus Mühlhahn (eds.), Deutsch-chinesische Beziehungen im 19. Jahrhundert: Mission und Wirtschaft in interkultureller Perspektive (Münster: LIT, 2001).

Levine, Harry G., "The Discovery of Addiction: Changing Conceptions of Habitual Drunkenness in America," *Journal of Studies on Alcohol*, 39:1 (1978), 143-174.

--------- "The Committee of Fifty and the Origins of Alcohol Control" in *the Journal of Drug Issues*, vol. 13 (1983), 95-116.

Loose, Rik, The Subject of Addiction: Psychoanalysis and the Administration of Enjoyment (London: Karnac Books, 2002).

--------- "The Addicted Subject Caught between the Ego and the Drive: The Post-Freudian Reduction and Simplification of a Complex Clinical Problem," *Psychoanalytische Perspectieven*, vol. 41/24 (2000), 56-81.

Maehle, Andreas-Holger, Drugs on Trial: Experimental Pharmacology and Therapeutic Innovation in the Eighteenth Century (Amsterdam: Rodopi, 1999).

--------- Doctors, Honour and the Law: Medical Ethics in Imperial Germany (New York: Palgrave Macmillan, 2009).

Manvell, Roger and Heinrich Fraenkel, *Herman Göring* (London: New English Library, 1962).

Marrus, Michael, "Social Drinking in the *Belle Epoque*," in *Journal of Social History*, vol. 7/4 (1974), 115-141.

Marx, Otto M., "Nineteenth-Century Medical Psychology: Theoretical Problems in the Work of Griesinger, Meynert, and Wernicke," *Isis*, vol. 61/3 (1970).

McAllister, William B., Drug Diplomacy in the Twentieth Century: An International History (London: Routledge, 2000).

McClellan, Robert, The Heathen Chinee: A Study of American Attitudes toward China, 1890 - 1905 (Columbus OH: Ohio State University Press, 1971).

McIllwain, Jeffrey S., Organizing Crime in Chinatown: Race and Racketeering in New York City, 1890-1910 (Jefferson NC: McFarland & Co. 2004).

McTavish, Janice Rae, *Pain and Profits: The History of the Headache and its Remedies in America* (New Brunswick, NJ: Rutgers University Press, 2004).

McWilliams, John C., The Protectors: Harry J. Anslinger and the Federal Bureau of Narcotics, 1930-1962 (Newark: University of Delaware Press, 1990).

McWilliams, Peter, Ain't Nobody's Business if you do: The Absurdity of Consensual Crimes in a Free Society (Los Angeles: Books on Demand, 1993).

Menninger, Karl A., *Man Against Him Self* (New York: Harcourt, Brace, 1938).

Merlin, Mark David, *On the Trail of the Ancient Opium Poppy* (London: Associated University Press, 1984).

Meier, Kenneth J., The Politics of Sin: Drugs, Alcohol, and Public Policy (New York: M. E. Sharpe, 1994).

Meyer, Kathryn and Terry Parssinen, Webs of Smoke: Smugglers, Warlords, Spies and the History of the International Drug Trade (Lanham: Rowman & Littlefield, 1998).

Mills, James, Cannabis Britannica: Empire, Trade, and Prohibition 1800-1928 (Oxford: Oxford University Press, 2003).

Morgan, H. Wayne, *Drugs in America: A Social History, 1800-1980* (Syracuse: Syracuse University Press, 1981).

--------- (ed.), *Yesterday's Addicts: American Society and Drug Abuse, 1865-1920* (Norman: University of Oklahoma Press, 1974).

Morone, James A., *Hellfire Nation: The Politics of Sin in American History* (New Haven: Yale University Press, 2003).

Morse, Hosea Ballou, *The Trade and Administration of the Chinese Empire* (Taipei: Ch'eng-wen Publishing, 1966 [1907]).

Musser, Joseph F., "The Perils of Relying on Thomas Kuhn," *Eighteenth-Century Studies*, 18:2 (1985), 215-226.

Musto, David F., *The American Disease* (Oxford: Oxford University Press, 1999).

--------- (ed.), *One Hundred Years of Heroin* (Westport CN: Auburn House, 2002).

--------- (ed.), *Drugs in America: A Documentary History* (New York: New York University Press, 2002),

Neave, Airey, Nuremberg: A Personal Record of the Trial of the Major Nazi War Criminals in 1945-6 (London: Hodder and Stoughton, 1978).

Nehmzow, Ralf, "Mitten in Hamburg-eine Zeitreise nach Chinatown," *Hamburger Abendblatt* (28 July 2008).

Noakes, Jeremy, "Nazism and Eugenics: The Background to the Nazi Sterilization Law of 14 July 1933" in R. J. Bullen et al. (eds.), *Ideas into Politics* (London: Croom Helm, 1984), 75-94.

North, Julian, "The Opium-Eater as a Criminal in Victorian Writing" J. B. Bullen (ed.), *Writing and Victorianism* (London: Longman, 1997).

Ohler, Norman, *Der totale Rausch: Drogen im Dritten Reich* (Cologne: Kiepenheuer & Witsch: 2015).

Overmier, Judith A., "John Brown's *Elemena Medicinae*: An Introductory Bibliographical Essay," *Bulletin Medical Library Association*, vol. 70/3 (1982), 310-317.

Parssinen, Terry, *Secret Passions, Secret Remedies: Narcotic Drugs in British Society, 1820-1930* (Philadelphia: Institute for the Study of Human Issues, 1983).

Pendergrast, Mark, *For God, Country and Coca-Cola: The Unauthorized History of the Great American Soft Drink and the Company that Makes it* (New York: Basic Books, 1993).

Peyer, Hans Conrad, *Roche: Geschichte eines Unternehmens* (Basel: Edition Roche, 1996).

Pickens, Donald K., "The Sterilization Movement: The Search for Purity in Mind and State," *Phylon*, vol. 28/1 (1967).

Pieper (ed.), Werner, *Nazis on Speed*, vols. 1-2 (Munich: Grüne Kraft, 2002).

Porter, Roy, "The Drinking Man's Disease: The 'Pre-History' of Alcoholism in Georgian Britain," *British Journal of Addiction*, 80:4 (1985), 385-396.

Proctor, Robert, *Racial Hygiene: Medicine under the Nazis* (Cambridge MA: Harvard University Press, 1988).

Rasmussen, Nicolas, *On Speed: The Many Lives of Amphetamine* (New York: New York University Press, 2008).

Recio, Gabriela, "Drugs and Alcohol: US Prohibition and the Origins of the Drug Trade in Mexico, 1910-1930," *Journal of Latin American Studies*, vol. 34/1 (2002), 21-42

Risse, Guenter B., "Medicine in the Age of Enlightenment," in Andrew Wear (ed.), *Medicine in Society: Historical Essays* (Cambridge: Cambridge University Press, 1998).

Ritter, Hans Jakob and Volker Roelcke, "Psychiatric Genetics in Munich and Basel between 1925 and 1945: Programs-Practices-Cooperative Arrangements," *Osiris*, vol. 20 (2005).

Roazen, Paul, Encountering Freud: The Politics and Histories of Psychoanalysis (New Brunswick NJ: Transaction Publishers, 1990).

--------- *Freud and His Followers* (New York: Knopf, 1979).

Roberts, James S., Drink, Temperance and the Working Class in Nineteenth-Century Germany (Boston: Allen & Unwin, 1984),

--------- "Long-Term Trends in the Consumption of Alcoholic Beverages" in Julian L. Simon (ed.), *The State of Humanity* (Oxford: Oxford University Press, 1995).

Robinson, Benjamin, "'Ist Knastschieben denn schön?' Hans Fallada und die Krise des Willens in der Weimarer Republik" in Moritz Föllmer and Rüdiger Graf (ed.), *Die Krise der Weimarer Republik: Zur Kritik eines Deutungsmusters* (Frankfurt a.m: Campus, 2005).

Room, Robin, "Addiction Concepts and International Control," *The Social History of Alcohol and Drugs*, vol. 20/1 (2006).

Rorabaugh, William J., *The Alcoholic Republic: An American Tradition* (New York: Oxford University Press, 1979).

Rosenberg, Charles E., *No Other Gods: On Science and American Social Thought* (Baltimore: Johns Hopkins University Press, 1976).

Rosenzweig, Michel, Les drogues dans l'histoire entre remède et poison: Archéologie d'un savoir oublié (Brussels: De Boeck & Belin, 1998).

Rumbarger, John J., Profits, Power, and Prohibition: Alcohol Reform and the Industrializing of America, 1800-1930 (Albany: State University of New York Press, 1989).

Scheer, Rainer, "Die nach Paragraph 42 RStGB verurteilten Menschen in Hadamar," in Dorothe Roer and Dieter Henkel (eds.), *Psychiatrie im Faschismus: Die Anstalt Hadamar, 1933-1945* (Bonn: Psychiatrie-Verlag, 1986).

Scheerer, Sebastian, *Sucht*, (Hamburg: Rowohlt, 1995).

--------- Die Genese der Betäubungsmittelgesetze in der Bundesrepublik Deutschland und in den Niederlanden (Göttingen: Otto Schwartz, 1982).

Schivelbusch, Wolfgang, Tastes of Paradise: a social history of spices, stimulants, and intoxicants (New York: Vintage Books, 1993).

Schlimme, Jann, "Towards a Psychiatric Anthropology of Addiction" in Thomas Schramme and Johannes Thome (eds.), *Philosophy and Psychiatry* (Berlin: De Gruyter, 2004).

Sebastian, Anton, *A Dictionary of the History of Medicine*, (New York: Parthenon Publishing Group, 1999).

Sigerist, Henry E., "From Bismarck to Beveridge: Developments and Trends in Social Security Legislation," *Journal of Public Health Policy*, vol. 20/4 (1999 [1943]), 484-496.

Shah, Nayan, Contagious Divides: Epidemics and Race in San Francisco's Chinatown (Berkeley: University of California Press, 2001).

Shahidullah, Shahid M., *Crime Policy in America: Laws, Institutions, and Programs* (Lanham: University Press of America, 2008).

Shryock, R. H., *Medical Licensing in America, 1650-1965* (Baltimore: Johns Hopkins University Press, 1967).

Sinclair, Andrew, *Prohibition: The Era of Excess* (Boston: Little, Brown, 1962).

Snelders, Stephen, Charles Kaplan, and Toine Pieters, "On Cannabis, Chloral Hydrate, and Career Cycles of Psychotropic Drugs in Medicine," *Bulletin of the History of Medicine*, vol. 80/1 (2006), 95-114.

Solomon (eds.), David, *The Coca Leaf and Cocaine Papers* (New York: Harcourt Brace Jovanovich, 1975).

Sournia, Jean-Charles, *A History of Alcoholism* (Oxford: Oxford University Press, 1990).

Speaker, Susan L., "'The Struggle of Mankind Against its Deadliest Foe' Themes of Counter-Subversion in Anti-Narcotic Campaigns, 1920-1940" in *Journal of Social History*, vol. 34/3 (2001), 591-610.

Spillane, Joseph F., Cocaine: From Medical Marvel to Modern Menace in the United States, 1884-1920 (Baltimore: Johns Hopkins University Press, 2000).

Spode, Hasso, Die Macht der Trunkenheit: Kultur- und Sozialgeschichte des Alkohols in Deutschland (Opladen: Leske & Budrich, 1993).

--------- "The First Step Toward Sobriety: The 'Boozing Devil' in 16th Century Germany" *Contemporary Drug Problems*, vol. 2/2 (1994), 453-483.

Stelle, Charles C., "American Trade in Opium to China, Prior to 1820" *The Pacific Historical Review*, vol. 9/4 (1940), 425-444.

Stephens, Robert, *Germans on Drugs: The Complications of Modernization in Hamburg* (Ann Arbor: University of Michigan Press, 2007).

Szasz, Thomas, *Ceremonial Chemistry* (Garden City NJ: Doubleday, 1974).

Taylor, Arnold H., American Diplomacy and the Narcotics Traffic, 1900-1939: A Study in International Humanitarian Reform (Durham, NC: Duke University Press, 1969).

--------- "American Confrontation with Opium Traffic in the Philippines," *Pacific Historical Review*, vol. 36/3 (1967).

Taylor, Blaine, "Hermann Goering and Josef Goebbels: Their Medical Casefiles (Part 1)," *Maryland State Medical Journal*, vol. 25/11 (1976), 35-47.

Teich, Mikuláš, "The Industrialization of Brewing in Germany (1800-1914)" in Erik Aerts et al., (eds.), *Production, Marketing and Consumption of Alcoholic Beverages since the Late Middle Ages*, (Leuven: Leuven University Press, 1990).

Terry, Charles E. and Mildred Pellens, *The Opium Problem* (New York, 1928).

Timberlake, James H., *Prohibition and the Progressive Movement, 1900-1925* (Cambridge MA: Harvard University Press, 1963).

Tlusty, Beverly Ann, *Bacchus and Civic Order: The Culture of Drink in Early Modern Germany* (Charlottesville: University of Virginia Press, 2001).

--------- "Defining 'Drunk' in Early Modern Germany" *Contemporary Drug Problems* vol. 2/2, (1994), 435-436.

Torp, Claudius, *Konsum und Politik in der Weimarer Republik* (Göttingen: Vandenhoeck & Ruprecht, 2011).

Tracy, Sarah W., *Alcoholism in America: From Reconstruction to Prohibition* (Baltimore: Johns Hopkins University Press, 2005).

--------- and Caroline Jean Acker (eds.), Altering American Consciousness: The History of Alcohol and Drug Use in the United States, 1800-2000 (Amherst: University of Massachusetts Press, 2004).

Trebach, Arnold S., *The Heroin Solution* (New Haven: Yale University Press, 1982).

Tsouyopoulos, Nelly, "The Influence of John Brown's Ideas in Germany," *Medical History*, no. 8 (1988), 70.

Tuchman, Arleen M., Science, Medicine and the State in Germany: The Case of Baden, 1815-1871 (Oxford: Oxford University Press, 1993).

Tyrrell, Ian, Woman's World, Woman's Empire: The Woman's Christian Temperance Union in International Perspective, 1880-1930 (Chapel Hill: North Carolina University Press, 1991).

Valverde, Mariana, *Diseases of the Will: Alcohol and the Dilemmas of Freedom* (Cambridge: Cambridge University Press, 1998).

Waddell, Helen, *The Wandering Scholars* (Garden City NJ: Doubleday, 1955 [1926]).

Wakabayashi, Bob Tadashi, "Opium, Expulsion, Sovereignty. China's Lessons for Bakumatsu Japan" *Monumenta Nipponica*, vol. 47/1 (1992).

Warner, Jessica, "Before there was 'Alcoholism': Lessons from the Medieval Experience with Alcohol," *Contemporary Drug Problems*, vol. 19/3 (1992), 409-428.

Wassenberg, Karl, "Die kulturelle Genese der Sucht" in Aldo Legnaro and Arnold Schmieder (eds.), *Suchtwirtschaft* (Münster: LIT, 1999).

Weber, Matthias M., "Ernst Rüdin, 1874-1952: A German Psychiatrist and Geneticist" *American Journal of Medical Genetics. Part B, Neuropsychiatric Genetics*, vol. 67/4 (1996), 323-331.

Weikart, Richard, "Darwinism and Death: Devaluing Human Life in Germany, 1859-1920," *Journal of the History of Ideas*, vol. 63/2 (2002).

--------- "Progress through Racial Extermination: Social Darwinism, Eugenics, and Pacifism in Germany, 1860-1918," *German Studies Review*, vol. 26/2 (2003).

Weiss, Sheila F. , "The Race Hygiene Movement in Germany," *Osiris*, vol. 3 (1987).

Wetzell, Richard F., "Psychiatry and Criminal Justice in Modern Germany, 1880-1933" *Journal of European Studies*, vol. 39/3 (2009), 270-289.

--------- Inventing the Criminal: A History of German Criminology, 1880-1945 (Chapel Hill: North Carolina University Press, 2000).

Wheeler-Bennett, J. W., "Thirty Years of American-Filipino Relations, 1899-1929" *Journal of the Royal Institute of International Affairs*, vol. 8/5 (1929), 503-521.

Whicher (tr.), George F., *The Goliard Poets: Medieval Latin Songs and Satires* (Norfolk CN: New Directions, 1949).

Wiesemann, Claudia, *Die heimliche Krankheit: Eine Geschichte des Suchtbegriffs* (Stuttgart: Frommann-Holzboog, 2000).

Wilhelm, Friedrich, *Die Polizei im NS-Staat* (Paderborn: Verlag Ferdinand Schöningh, 1997).

Wilkins, Mira, "The Impacts of American Multinational Enterprise on American-Chinese Economic Relations, 1786-1949" in Ernst R. May & John K. Fairbank (eds.), *America's China Trade in Historical Perspective: The Chinese and American Performance* (Cambridge MA: Harvard University Press, 1986).

Wilkinson, Rupert, *The Pursuit of American Character* (New York: Harper & Row, 1988).

Williams, Jenny, More Lives than One: A Biography of Hans Fallada (London: Libris, 1998).

Zacharasiewicz, Waldemar, *Images of Germany in American Literature* (Iowa City: University of Iowa Press, 2007).

Zinn, Alexander (Head of the State Press Station), "Hamburgische Werbeprobleme," (1929) *Hamburger Wirtschafts-Chronik*, vol. 6 (2006).

Zheng, Yangwen, *The Social Life of Opium in China* (Cambridge: Cambridge University Press, 2005).

Unpublished Dissertations:

Coonfield, Gordon, "Mapping Addiction" (Ph.D. dissertation, Michigan Technological University, 2003).

Engstrom, Eric J., "Emil Kraepelin: Leben und Werk des Psychiaters im Spannungsfeld zwischen positivistischer Wissenschaft und Irrationalität," (Mgr. thesis, Ludwig-Maximilians-Universität Munich, 1990).

Gabriel, Joseph Michael, "Gods and Monsters: Drugs, Addiction, and the Origins of Narcotic Control in the Nineteenth-Century Urban North" (Ph.D. Dissertation, Rutgers University, 2006).

Gray, Elizabeth Kelly, "American Attitudes Toward British Imperialism, 1815-1860" (Ph.D. Dissertation, College of William and Mary, 2002).

He, Sibing, "Russell and Company, 1818-1891: America's Trade and Diplomacy in Nineteenth-Century China" (Ph.D. Dissertation, University of Miami, 1997).

Jing, Liu, "Wahrnehmung des Fremden: China in deutschen und Deutschland in chinesischen Reiseberichten vom Opiumkrieg bis zum Ersten Weltkrieg," (Ph.D. dissertation, Albert-Ludwigs-Universität zu Freiburg, 2001).

Morrison, Christopher Allen, "A World of Empires: United States Rule in the Philippines, 1898-1913," (Ph.D. dissertation, Georgetown University, 2009).

Rinella, Michael A., "Plato, Ecstasy and Identity," (Ph.D. Dissertation, State University New York-Albany, 1997).

Risse, Guenter B., "The History of John Brown's Medical System in Germany during the Years 1790-1806," (Doctoral dissertation, University of Chicago, 1971).

Roizen, Ron, "The American Discovery of Alcoholism, 1933-1939," (PhD. dissertation, University of California-Berkeley, 1991).

Index